A Case-Based Review of

INFECTIOUS DISEASE

A Case-Based Review of
INFECTIOUS DISEASE

EDIN PUJAGIC

Elsevier
1600 John F. Kennedy Blvd.
Ste 1800
Philadelphia, PA 19103-2899

A CASE-BASED REVIEW OF INFECTIOUS DISEASE

ISBN: 978-0-323-87231-7

Content Strategist: Charlotta Kryhl
Content Development Specialist: Rishi Arora
Publishing Services Manager: Shereen Jameel
Project Manager: Maria Shalini
Design Direction: Bridget Hoette

Printed in India
Last digit is the print number: 9 8 7 6 5 4 3 2 1

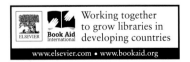

Working together to grow libraries in developing countries

www.elsevier.com • www.bookaid.org

To my family, friends, co-workers, mentors and patients who have supported me during my journey through the world of medicine and helped make this book a possibility!

Contents

Contents

Contents

Contents

Contents

Contents

Contents

A 25-year-old otherwise healthy male presents to the emergency department with low-grade fevers, joint pains, and a skin rash. His symptoms have been ongoing for almost 1 week now and have not responded to conservative therapy. He describes pain in multiple joints that seems to be "getting better in one joint and then moving on to involve another joint." Currently, he has pain and swelling in his left wrist and right ankle. He has had multiple new male sexual partners in the past several months, and he does not use condoms consistently. He drinks alcohol on the weekends and admits to using intravenous (IV) drugs in the past. His temperature is 100.6° F. Vital signs are within normal limits otherwise. Examination reveals a left wrist that is mildly swollen, erythematous, and tender. When asked to grasp his left thumb and adduct his wrist, he has significant pain over his left wrist and thumb. His right ankle is also notably swollen and tender. He has several pustular skin lesions on his extremities that have a red base to them. White blood cell count is 12,000 cells/uL. His renal function and liver function tests are within normal limits. Blood cultures are drawn.

What is the next best step in the management of this patient?

A. Consult Orthopedic Surgery to obtain arthrocentesis.
B. Start ceftriaxone.
C. Obtain HIV screening test.
D. Obtain syphilis screening test.
E. Obtain serum uric acid level.

This patient most likely has disseminated gonococcal infection (DGI). The best next step would be to consult Orthopedics for arthrocentesis (**option A**). Any patient who presents with an inflamed joint (i.e., red, warm, tender, swollen, etc.) should undergo synovial fluid analysis to rule out septic arthritis. Ideally, this should be done before starting antibiotics (**option B**) in order to optimize the yield of cultures.

DGI is a rare complication of infection with *Neisseria gonorrhoeae*, which is a gram-negative diplococcus. The classic presentation is the "arthritis-dermatitis syndrome," which consists of skin lesions (typically small, often acral, "pustular lesions on an erythematous base"), polyarthralgia/arthritis (typically asymmetric), and tenosynovitis. The other way this infection manifests is an oligoarticular or localized purulent arthritis. These infections are typically preceded by asymptomatic infection at other mucosal sites (i.e., pharyngeal, urethral, or cervical). Risk factors for DGI include terminal complement deficiencies, pregnancy, and menses.

The diagnosis can be challenging, so having a high index of suspicion is key. Diagnosis is contingent upon identifying the organism from a nonmucosal site such as blood, synovial fluid, or skin. Cultures of the synovial fluid and skin are commonly negative, and blood cultures are positive in less than 50% of cases. If isolated, the isolates should have antimicrobial susceptibility testing done. In addition, nucleic acid amplification testing (NAAT) for gonorrhea (and chlamydia) at all potentially exposed/involved sites (urine, cervix, pharyngeal, rectal) should be done as well, as this may provide supportive evidence for infection in the event of negative cultures. Interestingly, NAAT of the synovial fluid may be more sensitive than culture. Patients with DGI should also be screened for HIV and syphilis (**options C and D**), but the arthrocentesis takes precedence here.

In general, these patients should be hospitalized, and infectious disease consultation should be considered. Typical initial antibiotic treatment includes ceftriaxone 1 gram IV daily and doxycycline 100 mg PO twice daily × 7 days (to treat for potential concurrent chlamydia infection, especially if unable to rule it out). After 24–48 hours of clinical improvement, the patient can be switched to intramuscular ceftriaxone (at least 500 mg IM daily) to complete at least 7 days of treatment. The purulent arthritis form is often more difficult to manage and may require debridement and a longer course of antibiotic therapy (i.e., 7–14 days). Notable complications of this infection include perihepatitis (Fitz–Hugh–Curtis syndrome), cardiac infection (pericarditis, myocarditis, endocarditis), osteomyelitis, or meningitis.

The patient should be instructed to abstain from sexual activity for 7 days after treatment and until all sex partners are treated. In addition, any sex partner in the preceding 60 days should be evaluated and treated. Retesting for reinfection should be done in 3 months (post-treatment).

Lastly, it is worth noting that crystalline arthropathies (gout, pseudogout) can present as a polyarthritis (**option E**), but ruling out septic arthritis is still paramount because these two clinical entities may coexist.

KEY LEARNING POINT

Any patient presenting with an inflamed joint (e.g., red, warm, tender, swollen) should have an arthrocentesis done (ideally before administration of antibiotics) to exclude septic arthritis.

REFERENCES AND FURTHER READING

- Bennet JE, Dolin R, Blaser MJ, eds. *Mandell, Douglas, and Bennett's Principles and Practice of Infectious Diseases*. 9th ed. Elsevier; 2020.
- Workowski KA, Bachmann LH, Chan PA, et al. Sexually transmitted infections treatment guidelines, 2021. *MMWR Recomm Rep.* 2021;70(4):1–187. https://doi.org/10.15585/mmwr.rr7004a1.

A 25-year-old bisexual male is referred to the infectious disease clinic for an 8-day history of fevers. You review his chart prior to the visit. His temperature has ranged from 99° F to 101° F. Associated symptoms have included sore throat, fatigue, myalgias, enlarged cervical lymph nodes, and a diffuse maculopapular skin rash. Testing for Epstein–Barr virus (EBV) via heterophile antibody test and EBV-specific antibody testing was negative. Testing for cytomegalovirus (CMV) via serum PCR and serology was negative as well. HIV antigen/antibody screen (fourth-generation assay) was negative, as was influenza testing and rapid strep screen. He has not received any antibiotics for this illness.

Which of the following tests would be the most appropriate to do when you see him?

A. Repeat EBV testing.
B. HIV viral load.
C. Repeat CMV testing.
D. *Toxoplasma* serology.
E. No further testing is indicated.

The most appropriate test to do next would be the HIV viral load (quantitative PCR, **option B**). This patient presents with a mononucleosis-like illness. The typical differential for this syndrome is acute EBV infection ("infectious mononucleosis," the most common etiology), other herpes virus infections such as acute CMV and human herpesvirus–6 infection, acute retroviral syndrome (acute HIV infection), other common viral illnesses such as influenza and protracted upper respiratory tract infections, pharyngitis (typically streptococcal), and acute toxoplasmosis. In addition, there are various noninfectious etiologies (such as lymphoma) that can present in a similar fashion. These entities can be difficult to distinguish clinically, but diagnostic testing for all of these is often not necessary. The rationale for this approach is that the results are often unlikely to change your management, especially in an otherwise immune competent and healthy patient.

Acute retroviral syndrome (ARS), on the other hand, should always be considered. This is because acute HIV infection is a critical time for a clinician to make the diagnosis of HIV. This mono-like syndrome develops typically 2 to 4 weeks after becoming infected with HIV. These patients will often have very high levels of viremia, which makes it easier to transmit the infection to others. Consequently, acute HIV infection is an opportune time to start antiretroviral therapy to reduce transmission and to reduce morbidity and mortality associated with HIV. Nearly everyone should be screened for HIV at least once in their lifetime, so it is hardly ever the wrong answer to order an HIV screening test. The caveat here is that the traditional screening test (here, the fourth-generation HIV antibody/p24 antigen assay) may not become positive for at least 2 weeks. The HIV RNA quantitative PCR ("viral load") is able to detect the infection sooner (typically by ~10 days postinfection). Therefore, if you suspect ARS, the best test is actually the HIV viral load, as shown in this case.

Repeating EBV testing (**option A**) can be considered because the initial testing may have been falsely negative because it was done too early. If positive, then the result may be useful for counseling purposes (e.g., splenic rupture risk), but evaluation for ARS is more appropriate and important. Retesting for CMV and testing for toxoplasmosis (**options C and D**) would be unlikely to change your management in this seemingly immune competent adult.

KEY LEARNING POINT

In a patient with a concern for recent HIV infection (i.e., acute retroviral syndrome), HIV antigen/antibody screening test may be falsely negative. The best test to diagnose acute HIV infection is the HIV RNA quantitative PCR ("viral load").

REFERENCES AND FURTHER READING

- Bennet JE, Dolin R, Blaser MJ, eds. *Mandell, Douglas, and Bennett's Principles and Practice of Infectious Diseases.* 9th ed. Elsevier; 2020.
- Centers for Disease Control and Prevention and Association of Public Health Laboratories. Laboratory testing for the diagnosis of HIV infection: updated recommendations. http://dx.doi.org/10.15620/cdc.23447. Published June 27, 2014. Accessed October 22, 2020.

You are seeing a 60-year-old male who is admitted to the hospital. He has a history of poorly-controlled type 2 diabetes mellitus requiring insulin therapy and chronic kidney disease stage 3B. His creatinine at baseline is around 2 mg/dL (creatinine clearance 35 mL/min). He was discharged from the hospital approximately 3 weeks ago on daptomycin for the treatment of methicillin-resistant *Staphylococcus aureus* (MRSA) bacteremia related to a cellulitis of the right foot with an associated abscess. Imaging at that time did not show any bone involvement, and he underwent incision and drainage (I&D) of the abscess. Purulent material was expressed, and cultures grew MRSA that was susceptible to daptomycin. Blood cultures cleared rapidly on the third day of hospitalization. A transesophageal echocardiogram showed no evidence of valvular vegetation. Daptomycin was chosen over vancomycin in light of his chronic kidney disease. The plan was to treat him for 4 weeks. He was discharged to a skilled nursing facility.

He is now readmitted with a 3-day history of fever, cough, and shortness of breath. He has a new oxygen requirement of 3 L/min. Examination is otherwise significant for a temperature of 100.6° F and bilateral crackles in the lungs. He has trace peripheral edema. His right foot I&D site is healing well. White blood cell count is 12,000 cells/uL, with a differential showing 60% neutrophils, 25% lymphocytes, 7% monocytes, and 8% eosinophils, liver function testing is normal, and creatinine is at baseline. Chest x-ray shows bilateral pulmonary opacities interpreted by the radiologist as "bilateral pneumonia versus pulmonary edema." Blood cultures, sputum cultures, respiratory viral panel, and legionella urine antigen have been ordered. The primary hospital physician added cefepime and consulted infectious disease for antibiotic recommendations.

What is the next best step in the management of this patient?

A. Recommend bronchoscopy.
B. Recommend IV furosemide for diuresis.
C. Start prednisone.
D. Obtain a noncontrast CT of the chest.
E. Stop daptomycin and start vancomycin instead.

The best next step here would be to stop the daptomycin and start vancomycin instead (**option E**). This patient's presentation is most consistent with daptomycin-induced eosinophilic pneumonia (DEP). This is a rare complication of daptomycin therapy. The exact cause is unclear, but it has been hypothesized that daptomycin sequestration in the alveoli (caused by binding to pulmonary surfactant) allows daptomycin to cause injury to the lung tissue via immune-mediated mechanisms (Interleukin-5 and eosinophils may play a central role). The diagnosis can be challenging, and criteria have been developed to help with this. These criteria include daptomycin exposure, fever, shortness of breath with new respiratory failure, new infiltrates on chest imaging, bronchoalveolar lavage (BAL) with greater than 25% eosinophils, and clinical improvement following discontinuation of daptomycin. An additional feature may be peripheral eosinophilia. It is important to consider other conditions that can present similarly: infections, inflammatory conditions (aspiration pneumonitis, acute respiratory distress syndrome), and pulmonary edema. The cornerstones of management for DEP include discontinuing the daptomycin and, if no improvement is seen, starting steroids once infection has been sufficiently ruled out.

For this case, the simplest and easiest next step would be to stop the daptomycin and start vancomycin instead to continue management of the patient's MRSA bacteremia. Vancomycin is unlikely to cause significant kidney injury because he likely has a short course of therapy left. If he does not improve after the antibiotic change, and infection is sufficiently ruled out, a trial of steroids (**option C**) may be warranted. This patient's presentation is more consistent with eosinophilic pneumonia than heart failure, and given his lack of edema peripherally plus ongoing concern for potential infection, diuresis (**option B**) likely would not be beneficial. Bronchoscopy (**option A**) is recommended in most cases of DEP to aid in diagnosis (eosinophils >25% on BAL) and to rule out other differential diagnoses, but the offending agent should be stopped first. A chest CT (**option D**) can be considered as well, especially if the patient is not improving clinically because it may show complicated infectious processes (e.g., effusion, empyema) or noninfectious processes (e.g., interstitial lung disease) better.

KEY LEARNING POINT

Daptomycin-induced eosinophilic pneumonia is a rare complication of daptomycin therapy that is managed by discontinuing the offending agent (daptomycin). If there is no improvement, then a trial of steroids may be warranted (once infection has sufficiently been ruled out).

REFERENCES AND FURTHER READING

- Higashi Y, Nakamura S, Tsuji Y, et al. Daptomycin-induced eosinophilic pneumonia and a review of the published literature. *Intern Med*. 2018;57(2):253–258. https://doi.org/10.2169/internalmedicine.9010-17.
- Kumar S, Acosta-Sanchez I, Rajagopalan N. Daptomycin-induced acute eosinophilic pneumonia. *Cureus*. 2018;10(6):e2899. https://doi.org/10.7759/cureus.2899.

4

CASE

A 35-year-old female is admitted to the hospital with a fever of 102° F at home. Associated symptoms include chills and diarrhea. She has a history of non-Hodgkin's lymphoma, for which she is currently receiving chemotherapy. Her last cycle of chemotherapy was 10 days ago. She receives the chemotherapy via a port in her right chest. She is not on any other medications. On examination, she has a temperature of 101° F, heart rate 100 beats per minute, blood pressure 110/80 mmHg, respiratory rate of 18, and oxygen saturation 96% on room air. She appears ill and cold. Her right chest port shows no outward signs of infection. Heart exam reveals regular tachycardia with no murmurs. Lungs are clear, and abdomen is mildly tender diffusely, but there are no peritoneal signs. The remainder of her examination is within normal limits. White blood cell count is 100 cells/uL with 0 neutrophils. Hemoglobin is 7.5 g/dL, and platelets are 80,000 cells/uL. Renal function and liver function are within normal limits. Septic work-up including blood cultures from the port and periphery are drawn. The patient is placed on vancomycin and piperacillin/tazobactam. Infectious disease is consulted the next day. The patient says she feels much better today. Her blood cultures have been negative to date. White blood cell count is largely unchanged. *Clostridium difficile* stool testing was negative as well.

What is the next best step in the management of this patient?

A. Stop vancomycin only.
B. Stop piperacillin/tazobactam only.
C. Stop vancomycin and piperacillin/tazobactam.
D. Add fluconazole.
E. Start granulocyte colony-stimulating factor (G-CSF).

The best next step here is to stop the vancomycin (**option A**), because there is no indication for vancomycin in this patient with febrile neutropenia (FN). FN (also referred to as neutropenic fever) is defined as having a fever (temperature 100.4° F on two separate occasions at least 1 hour apart OR a one-time temperature of ≥101° F) AND neutropenia (absolute neutrophil count <500 cells/uL or <1000 cells/uL and anticipated to decline to <500 cells/uL in 48 hours) (Fig. 4.1). This is a syndrome seen almost exclusively in the oncologic population. These patients get infected with their own microbes, usually as a translocation event from the gastrointestinal tract (enteric pathogens) or skin (staphylococcal and streptococcal species) as a result of chemotherapy-induced skin/mucosal breakdown. In addition, they may not manifest the usual signs of infection (e.g., radiographic infiltrate) due to lack of neutrophils, so having a high index of suspicion is necessary. Evaluation (at the minimum) should include a thorough history and physical examination, CBC with differential, metabolic panel including renal function and liver function testing, urinalysis with microscopy, and two sets of blood cultures including from a line if present and no other clear source of infection.

Patients should be risk stratified, and this can be done using a scoring system like the Multinational Association for Supportive Care in Cancer (MASCC) system. Based on this scoring system, patients can be stratified as low-risk (score ≥21) or high-risk (score <21). Low-risk, reliable patients can be managed as outpatients with a regimen consisting of a fluoroquinolone (usually ciprofloxacin) plus amoxicillin/clavulanate (or clindamycin if penicillin-allergic). High-risk patients should be admitted and started on antipseudomonal therapy with cefepime, carbapenems (not ertapenem because this will not cover pseudomonas), or piperacillin/tazobactam. Vancomycin should be added if clinically suspecting a catheter/line infection, skin/soft tissue infection, pneumonia, or if there is hemodynamic instability or a history of methicillin-resistant *Staphylococcus aureus* (MRSA). Initiation of empiric antifungal therapy (**option D**) should be done in those with persistent fever (for at least 4–7 days) and anticipated duration of neutropenia of greater than 7 days. Growth factors (like G-CSF and granulocyte-macrophage colony-stimulating factor, **option E**) are more useful for primary prophylaxis in high-risk patients or as secondary prophylaxis in those with history of FN. Growth factors have been shown to decrease duration of FN and the time to neutrophil recovery but have not been shown to decrease mortality.

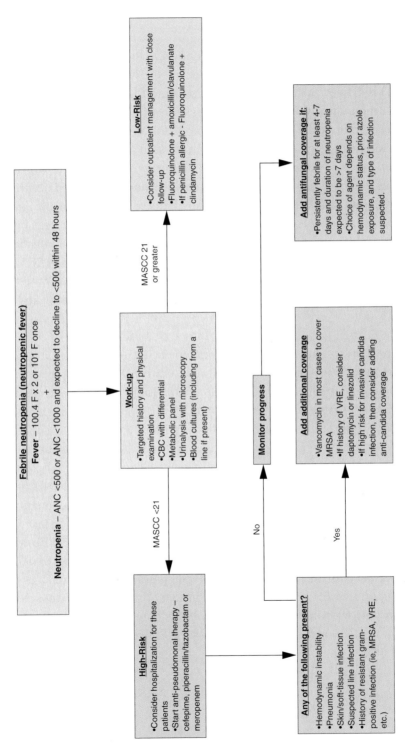

Figure 4.1 – Approach to management of febrile neutropenia

Febrile neutropenia (neutropenic fever)
Fever – 100.4 F x 2 or 101 F once
+
Neutropenia – ANC <500 or ANC <1000 and expected to decline to <500 within 48 hours

Work-up
•Targeted history and physical examination
•CBC with differential
•Metabolic panel
•Urinalysis with microscopy
•Blood cultures (including from a line if present)

MASCC <21

MASCC 21 or greater

High-Risk
•Consider hospitalization for these patients
•Start anti-pseudomonal therapy – cefepime, piperacillin/tazobactam or meropenem

Low-Risk
•Consider outpatient management with close follow-up
•Fluoroquinolone + amoxicillin/clavulanate
•If penicillin allergic - Fluoroquinolone + clindamycin

Any of the following present?
•Hemodynamic instability
•Pneumonia
•Skin/soft-tissue infection
•Suspected line infection
•History of resistant gram-positive infection (ie, MRSA, VRE, etc.)

Yes

No

Add additional coverage
•Vancomycin in most cases to cover MRSA
•If history of VRE, consider daptomycin or linezolid
•If high risk for invasive candida infection, then consider adding anti-candida coverage

Monitor progress

Add antifungal coverage if:
•Persistently febrile for at least 4-7 days and duration of neutropenia expected to be >7 days
•Choice of agent depends on hemodynamic status, prior azole exposure, and type of infection suspected.

KEY LEARNING POINT

In a patient with febrile neutropenia, indications to add vancomycin include history of MRSA, hemodynamic instability, suspected pneumonia, suspected skin/soft-tissue infection, or suspected line infection.

REFERENCES AND FURTHER READING

- AJMC Evidence-Based Oncology. Guidelines in the Management of Febrile Neutropenia for Clinical Practice. In *Perspectives in Febrile Neutropenia*; 2017. https://cdn.sanity.io/files/0vv8moc6/ajmc/aebd70e7888488b98f50d3ad26db7fc425539880.pdf.

You are seeing a 50-year-old man who was admitted several weeks ago with acute necrotizing pancreatitis related to alcohol abuse. His hospital course has been complicated by development of multiple intra-abdominal fluid collections. He has had some of these collections drained, but some have not been accessible percutaneously. There are no plans for surgical intervention at this time. He has been on vancomycin and ertapenem since before his first drain was placed. Cultures from his drainage procedures have shown the following (Table 5.1):

Table 5.1 – Summary of microbiologic results

Culture	Drain 1	Drain 2	Drain 3
Gram stain	• GPC pairs/chains (many) • GNR (many) • Budding yeast (few)	• GPC pairs/chains (many) • GNR (many) • GPR (few)	• GPC pairs/chains (many) • GNR (few) • Budding yeast (few)
Cultures	• *Enterococcus faecium* • *Candida krusei*	• *E. faecium*	• *E. faecium* • *C. krusei*

GPC, Gram-positive cocci; *GPR*, gram-positive rods; *GNR*, gram-negative rods.

Susceptibility testing is pending on the organisms that have grown so far. He has ongoing abdominal pain and fevers despite current antibiotic therapy.

Which of the following antimicrobial regimens would the most appropriate for this patient?

A. Continue current antibiotic therapy and optimize source control.
B. Change to linezolid, meropenem, and fluconazole.
C. Change to daptomycin, ertapenem, and fluconazole.
D. Change to daptomycin, ertapenem, and caspofungin.
E. Change to linezolid, meropenem, and caspofungin.

The most appropriate therapy here would be daptomycin, ertapenem, and caspofungin (**option D**). This patient has a complicated intra-abdominal infection with inadequate source control, as suggested by the ongoing fevers and abdominal pain, lack of appropriate antimicrobial coverage, and undrained foci of infection. Source control is very important to the management of this case, but it appears we have reached our limit there. Therefore, we need to optimize his antimicrobial regimen to provide coverage for the usual enteric pathogens (gram-negative rods and anaerobes), *Enterococcus faecium* (which is often vancomycin-resistant enterococcus [VRE]), and *Candida krusei* (which is intrinsically resistant to fluconazole). Looking at the gram stains, the gram-positive cocci pairs/chains are likely the enterococcus, while the budding yeast are likely the *Candida* species. Both of these grew because neither was being adequately covered in the original regimen. He also has various organisms on gram stain (gram-positive rods, gram-negative rods [GNRs]) that may not have grown on culture due to either being anaerobic organisms (which are often difficult to isolate) or dead organisms due to receipt of antibiotics prior to obtaining the gram stain and culture sample. It is tough to know what these could be, given that he was on ertapenem at the time the culture was obtained. This suggests that they could have been resistant GNRs (e.g., extended-spectrum beta-lactamase producers), but likely not *Pseudomonas* because we would expect *Pseudomonas* to grow while on ertapenem (a drug that does not cover *Pseudomonas*). Therefore, we are stuck with ertapenem in this case. Changing to meropenem would really only add unnecessary pseudomonal coverage, so we would avoid doing this. Changing the vancomycin to daptomycin will provide coverage for the *E. faecium* (often VRE), and adding caspofungin will provide adequate coverage for *C. krusei*. Linezolid will also treat *E. faecium*, but because this patient is likely to need a prolonged course of therapy, we would prefer to avoid using linezolid, as it carries significant toxicities when used long term (use >2 weeks is associated with neuropathy, including optic neuropathy and cytopenia).

KEY LEARNING POINT

Enterococcus faecium *is often vancomycin-resistant enterococcus. Until susceptibility is known, empiric therapy should consist of either daptomycin or linezolid, depending on the specific clinical scenario. Long-term use of linezolid (i.e., >2 weeks) is associated with optic and peripheral neuropathy and bone marrow suppression (cytopenia).* *Candida krusei* *is intrinsically resistant to fluconazole but is usually susceptible to echinocandins such as caspofungin.*

REFERENCE AND FURTHER READING

• Solomkin JS, Mazuski JE, Bradley JS, et al. Diagnosis and management of complicated intra-abdominal infection in adults and children: guidelines by the Surgical Infection Society and the Infectious Diseases Society of America. *Clin Infect Dis.* 2010;50(2):133–164. https://doi.org/10.1086/649554.

A 60-year-old male is referred to your infectious disease clinic for recurrent ear infections. For the past few months, he has experienced recurring left ear infections manifesting as pain and drainage. He has been managed by his primary doctor and various urgent care clinics. He has received various antibiotic courses, both systemic and topical, without any relief. He notes that he gets relief while on the antibiotics, but his symptoms return soon after stopping the antibiotics. He has not had any fevers or chills. His medications include metformin and insulin for type 2 diabetes mellitus and amoxicillin/clavulanic acid for the ear infection. Vital signs are within normal limits. Right ear exam shows a normal ear canal and tympanic membrane. Left ear exam reveals tenderness with manipulation of the tragus, edema and redness of external ear canal with yellowish exudate, and poor visualization of the eardrum. The remainder of the exam is normal. Review of prior labs shows glucose ranging from 200 to 300 mg/dL and CRP 10 mg/L (normal <1.0 mg/L). A culture of the ear drainage is obtained.

Which of the following describes the most likely microbiologic cause of this patient's illness?

A. Gram-negative bacillus, lactose-fermenting.
B. Gram-negative bacillus, lactose nonfermenting, oxidase-positive.
C. Gram-negative bacillus, lactose nonfermenting, oxidase-negative.
D. Septate hyphae with acute angle branching.
E. Gram-positive cocci in clusters, coagulase-positive.

This patient's presentation is concerning for malignant otitis externa (MOE). This is an aggressive form of otitis externa seen in immune-compromised patients (classically poorly controlled diabetics). The typical presentation is illustrated in this case, and the diagnosis is often delayed. The most common cause is *Pseudomonas aeruginosa*, which is an aerobic gram-negative rod (bacillus) that is lactose nonfermenting and oxidase-positive (**option B**). Fungal organisms (especially *Aspergillus* [**option D**] and *Candida* species) are the next most common. Occasionally, other gram-negatives and staphylococci can be seen (**options A, B, and E**). A key examination finding is granulation tissue extending to the osteocartilaginous junction of the external auditory canal. Diagnosis and evaluation should include culture (ideally ear tissue culture, but ear drainage may also be cultured), and imaging (usually CT or MRI) to look for complicated disease. In addition, a tissue biopsy should be considered to rule out malignancy (squamous cell carcinoma typically), especially if failing to improve with the usual therapy.

Empiric treatment should involve pseudomonal coverage with drugs such as cefepime, piperacillin/tazobactam, a carbapenem (not ertapenem), or in uncomplicated, stable outpatients, a fluoroquinolone (ciprofloxacin or levofloxacin). Culture results should ultimately guide antibiotic choice. Duration is not well-defined but typically involves at least 4 to 6 weeks of therapy. Ultimately, the duration will be determined by clinical response.

Complications of this infection include cranial nerve involvement (especially facial n. [often first involved], glossopharyngeal n., vagus n., accessory n., and hypoglossal n.), osteomyelitis of the skull base and/or temporal bone, and intracranial extension (meningitis, venous sinus thrombosis). Addressing the underlying immune deficiency is paramount (i.e., better diabetic control in this case). Refractory cases may require surgical intervention. Hyperbaric oxygen likely has no benefit.

KEY LEARNING POINT

The most common cause of MOE is **Pseudomonas aeruginosa,** *an aerobic gram-negative rod (bacillus) that is lactose nonfermenting and oxidase-positive.*

REFERENCES AND FURTHER READING

- Al Aaraj MS, Kelley C. Malignant otitis externa. In: StatPearls [Internet]. Treasure Island (FL): StatPearls Publishing; 2020. https://www.ncbi.nlm.nih.gov/books/NBK556138. Updated August 10, 2020.
- Handzel O, Halperin D. Necrotizing (malignant) external otitis. *Am Fam Physician.* 2003;68(2):309–312.

A 30-year-old male presents to the emergency room after being bit on his right hand by a dog. This event occurred earlier today while at work. The bite is located over his right metacarpophalangeal (MCP) joint. He notes that he has a history of anaphylaxis in response to penicillin that occurred when he was a child. He has not taken any penicillin-type antibiotics since then. He does not take any medications. He drinks alcohol regularly, most nights and on the weekends. Physical examination shows normal vital signs. His right MCP has a shallow, lightly bleeding skin puncture. There is mild tenderness but no redness, warmth, or erythema in the area. He can make a fist with his right hand without any problem. His rabies vaccination is up-to-date, as per requirement for his job. He had a tetanus, diphtheria, and acellular pertussis vaccine 3 years ago. The emergency room team is working on getting the wound cleansed, and they will not be placing any sutures.

Which of the following regimens would be the best choice for antimicrobial prophylaxis in this patient?

A. Amoxicillin/clavulanic acid.
B. Cefdinir plus metronidazole.
C. Moxifloxacin.
D. Ciprofloxacin plus metronidazole.
E. Trimethoprim/sulfamethoxazole plus doxycycline.

Table 7.1 – Management of Animal Bites

Indications for Prophylaxis	First-Line Therapy	Alternative Therapy
Immune compromise. Swelling/edema of the affected area. Moderate-severe injury, especially to sensitive areas (face, hands, genitalia). Injuries that may have penetrated the periosteum or joint capsule. If wound undergoes primary closure.	Amoxicillin/clavulanic acid (Augmentin).	Mild penicillin allergy (i.e., hives): Oral third-generation cephalosporin + metronidazole. Severe penicillin allergy (i.e., anaphylaxis): Moxifloxacin monotherapy. (Doxycycline or TMP/SMX) + anaerobic coverage (clindamycin or metronidazole).

TMP/SMX, Trimethoprim/sulfamethoxazole.

The best choice for antimicrobial prophylaxis in this patient with a dog bite is moxifloxacin (**option C**). Amoxicillin/clavulanic acid (**option A**) is the usual first-line agent, but it should not be given to this patient with history of severe penicillin allergy. Given his alcohol use history, metronidazole-based options would not be ideal either (**options B and D**). **Option E** (trimethoprim/sulfamethoxazole plus doxycycline) would not have adequate coverage for streptococci or anaerobes.

The indications for antimicrobial prophylaxis in bite wounds are listed in the table above (Table 7.1). The typical duration for prophylaxis is 3 to 5 days. The antimicrobial coverage is designed to cover bacteria found on the skin (of the bite recipient), the oral flora (of the biter), and anaerobes. Some classic organisms in animal bites include *Pasteurella multocida* (typically cats) and *Capnocytophaga canimorsus* (more commonly dogs). Human bites are typically associated with *Eikenella corrodens*. The usual prophylaxis regimens are listed above. In addition, one should always consider (and update, if necessary) tetanus vaccination status and rabies prophylaxis. If the bite was from a human, then evaluate and provide prophylaxis for other pathogens such as HIV, hepatitis B virus, or hepatitis C virus (no prophylaxis exists for hepatitis C). In general, the wounds should be cleansed/irrigated thoroughly and allowed to heal by secondary intention (i.e., avoid primary wound closure if possible).

KEY LEARNING POINT

Coverage for animal (and human) bites include coverage for skin flora of the bitten person (mainly staphylococci and streptococci), oral flora of the biter (usual mouth bugs including **Eikenella,** **Capnocytophaga,** *and* **Pasteurella***), and anaerobes. First-line regimen is amoxicillin/clavulanic acid (Augmentin). Alternatives include moxifloxacin monotherapy OR* *anaerobic coverage (metronidazole or clindamycin) plus (oral third-generation cephalosporin or doxycycline or trimethoprim/sulfamethoxazole).*

REFERENCES AND FURTHER READING

- Goldstein E, et al. Bites. In: Bennet JE, Dolin R, Blaser MJ, eds. *Mandell, Douglas, and Bennett's Principles and Practice of Infectious Diseases.* 9th ed. Elsevier; 2020:3765–3770.
- Stevens DL, Bisno AL, Chambers HF, et al. Practice guidelines for the diagnosis and management of skin and soft tissue infections: 2014 update by the Infectious Diseases Society of America. *Clinical Infectious Diseases.* 2014;59(2):e10–e52. https://doi.org/10.1093/cid/ciu296.

A 35-year-old male was admitted to the hospital 4 days ago with low-grade fevers, nonproductive cough, and shortness of breath. These symptoms have been progressive over the past several weeks. He also complains of odynophagia. He has a known history of HIV infection, but he declined antiretroviral therapy. His last CD4 count about 1 year ago was 220 (15%) cells/mm^3. He has a sulfa allergy; he notes sulfa caused a fever and rash when he was younger. He has not been sexually active since his diagnosis. He does not drink or use illicit drugs. Vitals are notable for temperature 101° F, heart rate 110 beats per minute, blood pressure 110/75 mmHg, respiratory rate 24, and oxygen saturation 90% on 3 L/min oxygen via nasal canula. He appears malnourished and chronically ill. Oral mucosa is coated with white lesions. He has increased work of breathing and crackles bilaterally on lung exam. The remainder of the exam is unremarkable. Labs reveal white blood cell count 4,000 cells/uL, hemoglobin 10 g/dL, platelets 80,000 cells/uL, and normal renal and liver function. Initial arterial blood gas showed pH 7.30, pCO$_2$ of 30 mmHg, and pO$_2$ of 50 mmHg. Glucose-6-phosphage dehydrogenase (G6PD) level was previously normal. Chest x-ray shows bilateral, diffuse interstitial opacities. A bronchoscopy is planned.

What is the most appropriate management for this patient?

A. IV trimethoprim/sulfamethoxazole.
B. IV trimethoprim/sulfamethoxazole and prednisone.
C. Clindamycin + primaquine + prednisone.
D. Clindamycin + primaquine.
E. Pentamidine (inhaled).

The best answer to this case is **option C** (clindamycin + primaquine + prednisone). This patient most likely has moderate-severe *Pneumocystis jirovecii* pneumonia (PJP). *P. jirovecii* is a ubiquitous fungus that causes disease in immune-compromised hosts. HIV patients with CD4 counts less than 200 cells/uL (<14%) and those with thrush are at particular risk. PJP typically presents as an indolent infection with fevers, nonproductive cough, chest pain, and shortness of breath (especially with exertion). Other findings include hypoxemia (sometimes only noted with exertion) and diffuse, bilateral, typically ground-glass interstitial infiltrates on chest imaging. Chest x-ray can be normal if obtained early on in the disease process. Spontaneous pneumothorax is suggestive of PJP, but cavitation and pleural effusion are rather uncommon (these findings argue against the diagnosis). A normal CT chest is helpful in ruling out PJP.

Definitive diagnosis requires identifying the organism in induced sputum, bronchoalveolar lavage (BAL), or a tissue sample. Bronchoscopy with BAL is considered the most accurate test. There are various ways to do this, including staining (Grocott-Gomori's methenamine silver stain, direct fluorescent antibody, etc.) or PCR. Lactate dehydrogenase is often elevated (>500), but this finding is nonspecific. 1,3 beta-D-glucan (Fungitell) is often elevated (also nonspecific) but seems to have a high negative predictive value and sensitivity (may rule out PJP reliably in HIV patients). However, in the real world, its use is somewhat controversial in the diagnosis of PJP. It is worth noting that therapy for PJP can be initiated prior to obtaining a sample for diagnosis, because pneumocystis persists in specimens for days to weeks after initiation of therapy.

Management of PJP is contingent upon the severity of the illness, as shown in the table below. Total treatment duration in both cases is 21 days (Table 8.1).

Table 8.1 – Management of PJP

Mild-Moderate PJP	Moderate-Severe PJP
• Criteria—pO_2 ≥70 mmHg and Aa-gradient <35	• Criteria—pO_2 <70 mmHg or Aa-gradient ≥35
• First line—TMP/SMX 2 DS tabs PO TID	• First line—IV TMP/SMX (change to PO after improvement)
• Alternative #1—dapsone + TMP PO	• Alternative #1—IV pentamidine
• Alternative #2—clindamycin PO + primaquine PO	• Alternative #2—clindamycin PO/IV plus primaquine PO
• Alternative #3—atovaquone PO	• Steroids (prednisone or IV methylprednisolone)—start ideally within 72 hours of PJP therapy

Aa, Alveolar-arterial; *PJP, Pneumocystis jirovecii* pneumonia; *SMX,* sulfamethoxazole; *TMP,* trimethoprim.

Trimethoprim/sulfamethoxazole (TMP/SMX) is considered first line because it is more effective than the other regimens used in PJP, so it should be used whenever possible. TMP/SMX is associated with many adverse effects in these patients, but most of these reactions can be managed with supportive medications (assuming the reactions are not immediately life-threatening). If using primaquine or dapsone, then patient should have a normal G6PD level. Aerosolized pentamidine should generally be avoided for PJP treatment, because it has limited efficacy and increases the risk of relapse. Antiretroviral therapy (ART) should be initiated within 2 weeks of the PJP diagnosis if the patient is not already on ART.

Patients often get clinically "worse" in the first several days of therapy, likely due to an inflammatory response to dying pneumocystis organisms. This is more pronounced in those that did not receive concurrent steroids up front. Therefore, providers should wait approximately 1 week before changing therapy (due to suspected clinical failure). In addition, other infectious etiologies should be ruled out as well, and this may include repeating bronchoscopy with BAL.

KEY LEARNING POINT

In advanced HIV patients with moderate-severe PJP, the first-line and most effective agent is TMP/SMX. Alternative agents include IV pentamidine (lots of toxicities) or clindamycin plus primaquine (must have normal G6PD level). In addition, steroids should be given concurrently, and should ideally be started within 72 hours of PJP therapy.

REFERENCES AND FURTHER READING

- Miller R, et al. *Pneumocystis* species. In: *Mandell, Douglas, and Bennett's Principles and Practice of Infectious Diseases.* 9th ed. Elsevier; 2020:3238–3254.
- Panel on Guidelines for the Prevention and Treatment of Opportunistic Infections in Adults and Adolescents With HIV. Guidelines for the prevention and treatment of opportunistic infections in HIV-infected adults and adolescents: recommendations from the Centers for Disease Control and Prevention, the National Institutes of Health, and the HIV Medicine Association of the Infectious Diseases Society of America. https://clinicalinfo.hiv.gov/en/guidelines/hiv-clinical-guidelines-adult-and-adolescent-opportunistic-infections/whats-new. Accessed October 23, 2020.

A 60-year-old male presents to the emergency room with a 1-week history of fevers, chills, cough, and shortness of breath. His wife also notes he has been confused and has had diarrhea. He is a smoker and carries a diagnosis of chronic obstructive pulmonary disease (COPD). Medications include albuterol as needed and inhaled beclomethasone. He has no medication allergies. He works as a pharmaceutical representative, which requires a lot of traveling (never abroad though). Vital signs are significant for temperature 101° F, heart rate 70 beats per minute, blood pressure 110/70 mmHg, respiratory rate 24, and oxygen saturation 88% on presentation (room air) with improvement to 96% on 4 L/min oxygen by nasal cannula. Examination shows a thin man with pursed-lip breathing. Lung exam shows diffuse crackles. He is able to tell you his name and his wife's name, but not where he is today or the month and year. The remainder of his examination is unremarkable. Lab testing shows white blood cell count 14,000 cells/uL, hemoglobin 12 g/dL, platelets 400,000 cells/uL, sodium 128 mEq/L, creatinine 1.5 mg/dL, and normal liver function testing. Chest x-ray reveals bilateral hazy opacities, but no effusion or frank consolidation.

Which of the following tests is the most appropriate to order next for this patient?

A. Standard sputum culture.

B. Blood cultures.

C. Urinary antigen testing.

D. CT of the chest without contrast.

E. Methicillin-resistant *Staphylococcus aureus* nasal swab for PCR.

This patient's presentation is most consistent with legionnaires' disease. Therefore, the most appropriate test would be the *Legionella* urine antigen (**option C**). There are many different *Legionella* species and subspecies/serogroups, but *Legionella pneumophila* serotype L1 is the most common cause of disease (up to 80%). *Legionella* is a waterborne gram-negative, aerobic, intracellular bacillus that requires a specialized media called buffered charcoal yeast extract (BCYE) to grow. *Legionella* infection can present as either a self-limited flu-like illness (Pontiac fever) or a community- or hospital-acquired pneumonia (legionnaires' disease). *Legionella* infections classically affect the elderly, smokers, patients with chronic lung disease (i.e., COPD), and immune-compromised patients. The pneumonia tends to have a higher incidence of central nervous system findings and gastrointestinal upset (especially diarrhea) compared with other pneumonias. In addition, hyponatremia may be more common and is thought to be caused by syndrome of inappropriate antidiuretic hormone. Relative bradycardia (as seen in this patient) may also be seen. Chest x-ray typically shows a bilateral, "atypical-appearing" pneumonia.

The diagnosis of legionnaires' disease requires a high index of suspicion. The *Legionella* urinary antigen test is a rapid test that only detects the L1 serotype of *L. pneumophila*. Therefore, it misses the other *L. pneumophila* serotypes and the other *Legionella* species. The sensitivity ranges from approximately 70% to 100%, while the specificity is 99% to 100%. Respiratory culture is the gold standard, as it will detect all species and subtypes, but it is slow and requires using BCYE agar (the reason that **option A** is wrong). Other less commonly used tests include direct fluorescent antibody and PCR.

Management of legionnaires' disease involves giving either a respiratory fluoroquinolone (i.e., levofloxacin or moxifloxacin) or a macrolide (i.e., azithromycin) for 7 to 14 days. Typically, this is done intravenously initially, followed by switch to oral therapy once the patient has clinically improved. Compared with macrolides, fluoroquinolones (FQs) were shown to have a trend toward lower mortality and decreased length of hospital stay based on a systematic review and meta-analysis done in 2014. A more recent systematic review and meta-analysis comparing FQs and macrolides found no difference in mortality, clinical cure, time to fever resolution, length of stay, and occurrence of complications. For immune-compromised patients, a 21-day course of levofloxacin is recommended. Other antibiotics with potential efficacy include rifampin and doxycycline, but data for these options are limited. Combination therapies (i.e., FQ + azithromycin) have not been shown to be superior to monotherapy, although these are sometimes given to patients who are critically ill or who have extrapulmonary disease (i.e., endocarditis). Lastly, you should always consider whether the infection is part of an outbreak and investigate accordingly.

Blood cultures (**option B**) and sputum cultures (**option A**) are fairly low-yield in community-acquired pneumonia (CAP). They are only recommended in hospitalized patients with severe CAP, or those with concern for methicillin-resistant *Staphylococcus aureus* (MRSA) or *Pseudomonas aeruginosa* (i.e., IV antibiotics in the preceding 90 days or history of infection with these pathogens). Noncontrast CT chest (**option D**) is unlikely to add much to this case at this time but could be considered if patient fails to improve. The MRSA nasal swab/PCR (**option E**) has a high negative predictive value, which means that treatment for MRSA pneumonia can generally be withheld when the MRSA swab is negative, especially in a patient with low pretest probability of MRSA pneumonia. The positive predictive value is not as high; therefore, when the swab is positive, coverage for MRSA pneumonia is generally initiated, but one should send blood and sputum cultures to allow de-escalation of anti-MRSA therapy if negative.

KEY LEARNING POINT

In patients with CAP, the Legionella *urine antigen test is indicated if there is suspicion for* Legionella *or if the patient meets criteria for severe CAP. The* Legionella *urine antigen test is a rapid test that only detects the L1 serotype of* Legionella pneumophila, *which causes most of the clinical disease. Therefore, it is highly specific but not very sensitive.*

REFERENCES AND FURTHER READING

- Jasper AS, Musuuza JS, Tischendorf JS, et al. Are fluoroquinolones or macrolides better for treating *Legionella* pneumonia? A systematic review and meta-analysis. *Clin Infect Dis.* 2021;72(11):1979–1989. https://doi.org/10.1093/cid/ciaa441.
- Edelstein P, et al. Legionnaires' disease and pontiac fever. In: *Mandell, Douglas, and Bennett's Principles and Practice of Infectious Diseases.* 9th ed. Elsevier; 2020:2807–2817.
- Burdet C, Lepeule R, Duval X, et al. Quinolones versus macrolides in the treatment of legionellosis: a systematic review and meta-analysis. *J Antimicrob Chemother.* 2014;69(9):2354–2360. https://doi.org/10.1093/jac/dku159.
- Metlay JP, Waterer GW, Long AC, et al. Diagnosis and treatment of adults with community-acquired pneumonia. An official clinical practice guideline of the American Thoracic Society and Infectious Diseases Society of America. *Am J Respir Crit Care Med.* 2019;200(7):e45–e67. https://doi.org/10.1164/rccm.201908-1581ST.

A 60-year old female is seen for an "infected boil." She notes she was shaving her legs several days ago and accidently nicked herself over her left anteromedial thigh. Over the ensuing days, she notes the area went from looking like a "pimple" to an "infected boil." She denies any fevers or chills. She has no medication allergies. She has a history of chronic kidney disease—her baseline creatinine clearance is 35 mL/min—essential hypertension, *Clostridioides difficile* colitis, and myelodysplastic syndrome, for which she is transfusion-dependent. Medications include lisinopril and vitamin D supplement. She denies any illicit drug use and only drinks alcohol socially. Vital signs are within normal limits except for temperature of 100.5° F. Examination shows a 3 × 4 cm mass over her left proximal anteromedial thigh with fluctuance. There is obvious tenderness, erythema, and warmth extending out with a diameter of approximately 8 cm. An incision and drainage procedure is planned. Which of the following would be the best empiric antibiotic therapy for this patient, while awaiting culture results?

A. Linezolid.

B. Doxycycline.

C. Trimethoprim/sulfamethoxazole.

D. Clindamycin.

E. Cephalexin.

The best antibiotic option for this patient with a purulent skin and soft-tissue infection (SSTI) would be doxycycline (**option B**). In general, SSTI can be purulent ("pus"-containing) or nonpurulent. Purulent SSTIs are usually caused by *Staphylococcus aureus* and usually require incision and drainage (I&D) with or without antibiotics for appropriate management. Nonpurulent SSTIs are typically due to beta-hemolytic *Streptococcus* species and are typically managed with antibiotics targeting strep species. One should always consider the severity and depth of the infection when encountering a SSTI, so as not to miss deeper infections such as necrotizing SSTI, pyomyositis, septic arthritis, or osteomyelitis. This can usually be determined clinically, but if you suspect deeper infection then the patient may need broader antimicrobial coverage and urgent surgical involvement.

The patient in this case has a purulent SSTI (specifically, a skin abscess). Therefore, we would be concerned about *S. aureus* being the cause. In particular, we would be concerned about *methicillin-resistant S. aureus (MRSA)* until the culture results verify whether or not we are dealing with MRSA or *methicillin-susceptible S. aureus (MSSA)*. Her need for transfusions (healthcare exposure) increases her risk for MRSA infection. Patients with purulent SSTI typically require I&D, and the purulent material should be sent for gram stain and culture. Adjunctive antibiotics are indicated if there is systemic inflammatory response syndrome/ sepsis, large abscess (>2 cm), multiple abscesses, greater than 5 cm surrounding cellulitis, immune compromise, or a failure to respond to I&D alone. Two recent randomized trials and a systematic review showed that adjunctive antibiotics improved cure rate, but the rate of adverse events was increased. Additional considerations include outlining the area of cellulitis (to allow monitoring of progression) and elevating the affected extremity. The typical duration of treatment is 5 to 7 days.

Oral options for MRSA coverage include linezolid, tetracyclines (typically doxycycline), trimethoprim/sulfamethoxazole (TMP/SMX), and clindamycin. Linezolid (**option A**) is associated with cytopenia (especially with prolonged use >2 weeks), so it would not be a great option for a transfusion-dependent patient. TMP/SMX (**option C**) is associated with hyperkalemia, so it would not be a good option for a patient with chronic kidney disease on lisinopril. Clindamycin (**option D**) has a black box warning for the risk of *C. difficile*– associated diarrhea, so it would be prudent to avoid in this patient with a history of *C. difficile* infection. Doxycycline has a very low risk of causing *C. difficile* infection, which makes it a great option. Cephalexin (**option E**) will provide coverage for MSSA but not MRSA (Fig. 10.1).

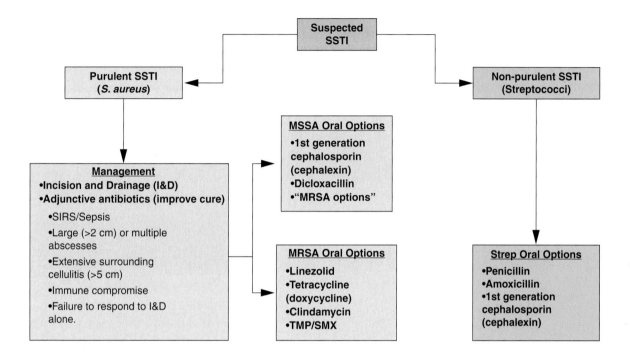

Fig. 10.1 – Management of cellulitis.
Stevens DL, Bisno AL, Chambers HF, et al. Practice guidelines for the diagnosis and management of skin and soft tissue infections: 2014 update by the Infectious Diseases Society of America. Clin Infect Dis. 2014;59(2):e10–e52. https://doi.org/10.1093/cid/ciu296.

KEY LEARNING POINT

Purulent skin and soft-tissue infections are typically caused by Staphylococcus aureus. Management usually requires incision and drainage (I&D), and in many cases antibiotics are indicated, because they improve clinical cure. Coverage for methicillin-resistant S. aureus should be utilized initially, and the antibiotic regimen can be tailored based on the result of the culture from the I&D.

REFERENCES AND FURTHER READING

- Breyre A, Frazee BW. Skin and soft tissue infections in the emergency department. *Emerg Med Clin North Am.* 2018;36(4):723–750. https://doi.org/10.1016/j.emc.2018.06.005.
- Daum RS, Miller LG, Immergluck L, et al. A placebo-controlled trial of antibiotics for smaller skin abscesses. *N Engl J Med.* 2017;376(26):2545–2555.
- Stevens DL, Bisno AL, Chambers HF, et al. Practice guidelines for the diagnosis and management of skin and soft tissue infections: 2014 update by the Infectious Diseases Society of America. *Clin Infect Dis.* 2014;59(2):e10–e52. https://doi.org/10.1093/cid/ciu296.

- Golan Y. Current treatment options for acute skin and skin-structure infections. *Clin Infect Dis.* 2019;68(Suppl 3): S206–S212. https://doi.org/10.1093/cid/ciz004.
- Gottlieb M, DeMott JM, Hallock M, Peksa GD. Systemic antibiotics for the treatment of skin and soft tissue abscesses: a systematic review and meta-analysis. *Ann Emerg Med.* 2019;73(1):8–16. https://doi.org/10.1016/j. annemergmed.2018.02.011.
- Talan DA, Mower WR, Krishnadasan A, et al. Trimethoprim-sulfamethoxazole versus placebo for uncomplicated skin abscess. *N Engl J Med.* 2016;374(9):823–832. https://doi.org/10.1056/NEJMoa1507476.

A 35-year-old female is brought into the emergency room by the paramedics with a several-day history of altered mentation. Apparently, her neighbor had called emergency medical services (EMS) due to concern for her safety because she was acting erratically. Not much is known about her medical history, but EMS brought in her medications. These include tramadol, methadone, and a drug with a partially torn off label. Based on what is left of the label, it appears the drug was indicated for "cellulitis" and was prescribed 5 days ago. There are four tablets left in the bottle. Vital signs show a temperature of 103° F, heart rate 120 beats per minute, blood pressure 160/100 mmHg, respiratory rate 22 with oxygen saturation 92% on room air. Examination shows a confused, disheveled female. She is diaphoretic and confused. She appears tremulous. Heart exam shows a regular tachycardia with no murmurs. Lungs are clear, and abdomen is soft. She does not follow basic commands. Bilateral patellar reflexes are 3+ and equal. The most likely mystery drug in this case works by which of the following mechanisms of action?

A. Inhibition of bacterial cell wall synthesis.

B. Inhibition of bacterial folic acid synthesis.

C. Inhibition of fungal ergosterol synthesis.

D. Inhibition of bacterial protein synthesis.

E. Inhibition of bacterial cell membrane function.

The best answer is **option D** (inhibition of bacterial protein synthesis). This patient's presentation is concerning for serotonin syndrome (SS). SS develops within 6 hours of starting or changing to a medication with serotonergic activity. Various medications have been implicated, including antidepressants, methadone, tramadol, and illicit drugs (i.e., MDMA) to name a few. Usually, these patients are on multiple serotonergic agents. SS is characterized by altered mentation, autonomic nervous system disturbances, and neuromuscular abnormalities that range from mild to life-threatening. Examination classically shows hyperreflexia and clonus. Management is typically supportive, but discontinuing the offending agent is very important.

The most likely etiology of SS in this patient is the concurrent use of tramadol, methadone, and the mystery agent, which is likely linezolid. Linezolid is an antibiotic that is sometimes prescribed for acute bacterial skin and soft-tissue infections. Linezolid provides mainly gram-positive coverage, including streptococcal species, staphylococcal species (including methicillin-resistant *Staphylococcus aureus*), and enterococcal species (including *vancomycin-resistant enterococcus*). The mechanism of action is inhibition of protein synthesis at the 50 S ribosomal subunit. Linezolid also acts as a weak monoamine oxidase inhibitor, which is why it has been associated with SS. The prevalence of SS with linezolid is variable, but likely very low, based on available literature. No randomized trials have been published on this topic. In general, we avoid giving linezolid to patients who are on serotonergic agents if we can. If absolutely necessary, then an appropriate risk-benefit discussion should ensue, and the patient should be monitored closely while on linezolid.

Beta-lactam antibiotics inhibit bacterial cell wall synthesis (**option A**). Trimethoprim/sulfamethoxazole inhibits bacterial folate synthesis (**option B**). Azole antifungals act by inhibition of fungal ergosterol synthesis (**option C**). Daptomycin and polymyxin act on bacterial cell membranes (**option E**).

KEY LEARNING POINT

Linezolid is a bacterial protein synthesis inhibitor and weak monoamine oxidase inhibitor that has rarely been associated with serotonin syndrome, especially when given concurrently with other serotonergic drugs.

REFERENCES AND FURTHER READING

- Karkow DC, Kauer JF, Ernst EJ. Incidence of serotonin syndrome with combined use of linezolid and serotonin reuptake inhibitors compared with linezolid monotherapy. *J Clin Psychopharmacol.* 2017;37(5):518–523. https://doi.org/10.1097/JCP.0000000000000751.
- Quinn DK, Stern TA. Linezolid and serotonin syndrome. *Prim Care Companion J Clin Psychiatry.* 2009;11(6):353–356. https://doi.org/10.4088/PCC.09r00853.

A 20-year-old male presents to the emergency room with fevers and a headache. He was last doing well about 3 days prior to presentation, and he was at a friend's lake house doing some tubing and swimming. He notes that the next day he woke up with a dull headache, which progressively got worse over the next couple days. He notes associated fevers up to 102° F, chills, loss of his sense of smell and taste, nausea, and vomiting. The symptoms seemed to be getting worse, so he came into the hospital for evaluation. He is otherwise healthy and takes no medications. He drinks alcohol on the weekends and smokes marijuana occasionally. He denies any other illicit drug use. He denies any recent travel, animal exposures, or tick exposures. He is sexually active and has had three lifetime female partners. He always used condoms with his prior partners. He is currently in a monogamous relationship with a girlfriend, and they do not use condoms regularly during sexual intercourse. He is a college student and was vaccinated for meningococcus with the quadrivalent conjugate vaccine. Vital signs show temperature 102° F, heart rate 120 beats per minute, blood pressure 100/70 mmHg, respiratory rate 20, and oxygen saturation 95% on room air. He appears ill and prefers to have the lights off in the room. His mentation is a bit slowed. Nuchal rigidity is present. He has no focal neurologic deficit on neurologic exam. Skin exam shows no rashes. The remainder of his examination is noncontributory. Noncontrast head CT is within normal limits. HIV screen is negative. Blood cultures are drawn, and he is started on vancomycin, ceftriaxone, and dexamethasone. Lumbar puncture shows the following:

Opening pressure: 40 cmH$_2$O (normal range: 7–18 cmH$_2$O)

Cell count/differential: 1200 cells/uL, 95% neutrophils

Glucose: 35 mg/dL (normal range: 40–70 mg/dL)

Protein: 500 mg/dL (normal range: <45 mg/dL)

Gram stain and culture: Pending, no organisms or growth so far

Cryptococcal antigen: Negative

Herpes simplex virus 1 and 2 PCR: Negative

Which of the following exposures/routes of infection is the most likely the cause of this patient's illness?

A. Sexual exposure.

B. Close contact/droplet exposure.

C. Airborne particle exposure.

D. Water exposure.

E. Occult tick exposure.

The best answer to this question is water exposure (**option D**). This patient's presentation is concerning for primary amebic encephalitis (PAM). Acute PAM is usually due to *Naegleria fowleri*, a free-living amoeba typically found in freshwater or improperly chlorinated swimming pools that is rarely contracted via nasal irrigation solutions using tap water. The infection is acquired via accidental introduction of the amoeba via the nose, which then leads to central nervous system (CNS) invasion through the cribriform plate. Acute PAM typically occurs in summer months and in patients with recreational freshwater exposure. Acute PAM presents within approximately 1 week of exposure and resembles a bacterial meningitis clinically. Some cases have been associated with abnormal taste or smell and other nasal symptoms. The disease often progresses rapidly and carries a very high mortality rate. Death (typically from cerebral herniation) typically ensues rapidly (median 5 days) after onset of symptoms. A subacute or chronic form of amebic encephalitis called granulomatous amebic encephalitis (GAE) is caused by two other species of free-living amoeba called *Acanthamoeba* and *Balamuthia mandrillaris*. GAE typically progresses much more slowly than acute PAM.

Diagnosis requires a high index of suspicion. Cerebrospinal fluid (CSF) findings in acute PAM show very high opening pressures (median ~30 cmH_2O), elevated red blood cell counts, neutrophilic pleocytosis, elevated protein, and low glucose. Diagnosis of acute PAM can be made by microscopic examination of the CSF or brain tissue (probably the quickest way), immunohistochemistry, indirect immunofluorescence, polymerase chain reaction, or next-generation sequencing. The samples should not be frozen or refrigerated, as this kills the amoeba.

The management of acute PAM is extrapolated from data from prior survivors of the illness. The key to survival seems to be early diagnosis and management. The Centers for Disease Control and Prevention recommends a combination regimen consisting of conventional amphotericin-B (liposomal is actually less effective), miltefosine, azithromycin, fluconazole, rifampin, and dexamethasone.

Close contract/droplet exposure (**option B**) would be more consistent with *Neisseria meningitidis* infection, which can present in a similar manner, but we typically see a skin rash, and death typically occurs more rapidly. Infections classically transmitted by the airborne route (**option C**) that are associated with CNS manifestations include tuberculosis, measles, and disseminated varicella-zoster virus infections. Infections acquired via sexual exposure (**option A**) that can have CNS manifestations include HIV, disseminated gonorrhea, syphilis, and *herpes simplex virus*. Infections acquired via tick exposure (**option E**) that can be associated with CNS manifestations include Lyme disease and Rocky Mountain spotted fever.

KEY LEARNING POINT

Acute primary amebic encephalitis is caused by **Naegleria fowleri,** *a free-living amoeba that is found in freshwater. This amoeba causes infection in the warm summer months by invading the central nervous system via the cribiform plate. Mortality is very high, but survival is more likely with early diagnosis and treatment.*

REFERENCES AND FURTHER READING

- Koshy A, et al. Free-living amebae. In: *Mandell, Douglas, and Bennett's Principles and Practice of Infectious Diseases.* 9th ed. Elsevier; 2020:3287–3298.
- Centers for Disease Control and Prevention. Parasites—*Naegleria Fowleri* —Primary Amebic Meningoencephalitis (PAM)—Amebic Encephalitis. Information for Public Health & Medical Professionals; September 29, 2020. https://www.cdc.gov/parasites/naegleria/health_professionals.html.

A 35-year-old healthy male presents to the emergency room with fevers and a headache. He recently returned from a trip to the Caribbean 1 week ago. He was there for 1 week, and while there he stayed with a local family and enjoyed the local cuisine. He did not go to a travel clinic before his trip. Toward the end of his trip, he started feeling unwell with nausea and vomiting. A couple days ago, he started having fevers and unrelenting headaches. In addition, he notes a pins-and-needles sensation in his hands and feet. Vitals show a temperature of 102° F, heart rate of 120 beats per minute, blood pressure 110/75 mmHg, respiratory rate 20, and oxygen saturation 94% on room air. Examination shows an ill-appearing patient with nuchal rigidity and slowed mentation. White blood cell count is 14,000 cells/uL with 60% neutrophils, 9% eosinophils, and 20% lymphocytes. Blood cultures are ordered. Rapid malaria testing and blood smears have been sent off. Lumbar puncture shows an opening pressure of 40 cmH$_2$O (normal: 7–18 cmH$_2$0), 200 total nucleated cells/uL with 40% neutrophils, 20% eosinophils, and 40% lymphocytes, glucose 70 mg/dL (normal: 40–70 mg/dL), and protein 200 mg/dL (normal: <45 mg/dL). Which of the following organisms is most likely responsible for this patient's illness?

A. *Angiostrongylus cantonensis.*

B. *Coccidiodes immitis.*

C. *Baylisascaris procyonis.*

D. *Gnathostoma spinigerum.*

E. *Toxocara canis.*

The most likely cause of this patient's illness is *Angiostrongylus cantonensis* (**option A**). Angiostrongylus is a nematode parasite (roundworm) that is endemic to southeast Asia (but also reported in other regions including the Caribbean). Two species cause disease in humans: *A. cantonensis* (most common cause of eosinophilic meningitis) and *Angiostrongylus costaricensis*. Rats are the definitive hosts. Infections in humans are typically acquired accidently by ingestion of snails and slugs (the intermediate host) or foods contaminated by these mollusks or their slime (usually raw vegetables). The typical incubation period is 1 to 3 weeks. Initially, patients develop gastrointestinal symptoms (abdominal pain, vomiting, etc.). Later on in the illness, the parasites penetrate the central nervous system (CNS) and cause an intense inflammatory reaction that can manifest as eosinophilic meningitis, encephalitis, cranial neuropathies, and radiculitis (paresthesia). There have also been reports of ocular infection.

Diagnosis requires a high index of suspicion. Cerebrospinal fluid (CSF) analysis will show very high CSF opening pressure, eosinophilic pleocytosis (defined as >10 eosinophils/uL), elevated protein, and often a normal glucose. Peripheral eosinophilia is fairly common. CSF polymerase chain reaction seems to be the most reliable way to make the diagnosis. Rarely, one will find larvae on CSF examination. If initial testing is negative, then a repeat CSF evaluation should be pursued. CNS imaging is mainly helpful to rule out other causes/ differential diagnoses.

Most infections follow a self-limited course, even without treatment. Management of intracranial pressure is important, and this can be done via anti-inflammatory drugs and serial lumbar punctures. Corticosteroids (high-dose) have been shown to be beneficial in decreasing duration of headache and need for serial lumbar puncture. The use of antihelminthic drugs (e.g., albendazole) is controversial due to risk of worsening inflammation and potentially worsening clinical outcome. A trial comparing steroids alone versus albendazole/steroid combination failed to show any benefit for the combination, but adverse events were higher in the combination group. In general, if using antihelminthic agents, then they should be given in combination with steroids.

The differential diagnosis of eosinophilic meningitis includes other less common infections such as *Gnathostoma spinigerum*, *Baylisascaris procyonis* (raccoon roundworm), cysticercosis (*Taenia solium* [pork tapeworm]), schistosomiasis, *Paragonimus* spp., *Toxocara* spp., *Cryptococcus* spp., and *Coccidiodes*. In addition, one should consider malignancy (especially lymphoma) and various drugs, including nonsteroidal anti-inflammatory drugs (NSAIDs) and certain antibiotics (trimethoprim/sulfamethoxazole, ciprofloxacin), in the differential.

KEY LEARNING POINT

Angiostrongylus cantonensis *is the most common cause of eosinophilic meningitis.*

REFERENCES AND FURTHER READING

- Ansdell V, Wattanagoon Y. *Angiostrongylus cantonensis* in travelers: clinical manifestations, diagnosis, and treatment. *Curr Opin Infect Dis.* 2018;31(5):399–408. https://doi.org/10.1097/QCO.0000000000000481.
- Wang Q-P, Lai D-H, Zhu X-Q, et al. Human angiostrongyliasis. *Lancet Infect Dis.* 2008;8(10):621–630.

A 25-year-old female is referred urgently to your clinic for a suspected urinary tract infection. For the past 2 days, she has experienced urinary frequency, urgency, and dysuria. She has not had any fevers, chills, nausea, vomiting, flank pain, or abdominal pain. She is currently pregnant with her first child and is at 12 weeks' gestation. She does not have any medication allergies. Medications include prenatal vitamin and folic acid. Vital signs are within normal limits. Examination reveals tenderness over the suprapubic region. She does not have any flank tenderness. Urine dipstick shows the presence of nitrites and leukocyte esterase. Urine culture is pending.

Which of the following is the most appropriate management?

A. Await the results of the culture prior to treating.
B. Cephalexin.
C. Trimethoprim/sulfamethoxazole.
D. Ciprofloxacin.
E. Nitrofurantoin.

The most appropriate management would be cephalexin (**option B**). This patient presents with acute cystitis in the first trimester (TM) of pregnancy. Cystitis typically presents with urinary frequency, urinary urgency, dysuria, hematuria, and suprapubic discomfort. There should be no signs or symptoms of upper tract involvement (i.e., pyelonephritis) such as fevers, chills, nausea, vomiting, flank pain, or costovertebral angle tenderness. Urinary tract infections (UTIs) are fairly common in pregnancy due to various pregnancy-induced physiologic changes. The causative organisms are similar to the pathogens that cause UTI in nonpregnant patients. Management of UTI in pregnancy is contingent upon the specific presentation and the TM of the pregnancy. The spectrum of UTI presentations in pregnancy can be classified as follows (with associated management) (Table 14.1):

Table 14.1 –Overview of UTI in Pregnancy

	Asymptomatic Bacteriuria (ASBU)[a]	Cystitis	Pyelonephritis
Symptoms	• Asymptomatic	• Frequency, urgency, dysuria, hematuria, suprapubic pain	• Fevers, chills, nausea, vomiting, flank pain + cystitis symptoms
Urinalysis	• +Leukocyte esterase • +Nitrites	• +Leukocyte esterase • +Nitrites	• +Leukocyte esterase • +Nitrites
Urine culture	• Positive	• Positive (usually)	• Positive (usually)
Management[b]	• Amoxicillin ± clavulanate • Cephalexin • Fosfomycin • Nitrofurantoin: not first TM (unless no better option) or near term • TMP/SMX: not first TM or near term • Duration: 3–7 days	• Antibiotic options similar to ASBU • Duration-7 days	• Hospitalize in most cases. • Beta-lactams typically used due to safety profile: piperacillin/tazobactam, ceftriaxone, cefepime, carbapenem, aztreonam • Duration: 10–14 days

After treatment, urine culture should be repeated in 1 to 2 weeks and then once per month.

SMX, Sulfamethoxazole; TM, trimester; TMP, trimethoprim.

[a]General indications to treat ASBU.

[b]Empiric therapy can be guided by prior urine culture results.

Awaiting results of culture prior to treating (**option A**) may result in worsening infection (i.e., pyelonephritis), so this option should be avoided. Trimethoprim/sulfamethoxazole (**option C**) should not be used in the first TM due to risk of teratogenicity (folate antagonist effect). If there wasn't a better option, then nitrofurantoin (**option E**) would be a feasible option. Lastly, fluoroquinolones (**option D**) are typically contraindicated during pregnancy due to risk of fetal cartilage abnormalities.

KEY LEARNING POINT

In general, the beta-lactam antibiotics are considered first-line agents for management of urinary tract infection in pregnancy.

REFERENCES AND FURTHER READING

- Habak PJ, Griggs RP Jr. *Urinary Tract Infection in Pregnancy*. Treasure Island (FL). StatPearls Publishing; 2020. https://www.ncbi.nlm.nih.gov/books/NBK537047/.
- Matuszkiewicz-Rowińska J, Małyszko J, Wieliczko M. Urinary tract infections in pregnancy: old and new unresolved diagnostic and therapeutic problems. *Arch Med Sci*. 2015;11(1):67–77. https://doi.org/10.5114/aoms.2013.39202.

A 60-year-old male presents to the emergency room with right knee pain that started 1 week ago and has progressively worsened. He also notes swelling in the knee over the past few days. He denies any trauma or injury. He has a medical history significant for type 2 diabetes mellitus and osteoarthritis. Medications include acetaminophen, metformin, insulin, atorvastatin, and aspirin. He has a history of hives due to penicillin that occurred when he was a teenager. Surgical history is notable for bilateral total knee arthroplasties done about 5 years ago. He denies alcohol use or illicit drug use. He has no regular animal exposures. Vital signs show temperature 99° F, heart rate 85 beats per minute, blood pressure 135/80 mmHg, respiratory rate 16, and oxygen saturation 98% on room air. Body mass index is 35 kg/m². Physical examination reveals a right knee that is swollen, warm, and tender with active and passive range of motion. There is no erythema present. The left knee is normal. He has bilateral well-healed surgical scars over both knees. The remainder of the examination is unremarkable. Labs show a white blood cell (WBC) count 12,000 cells/uL (80% neutrophils), creatinine 1 mg/dL (creatinine clearance 70 mL/min), normal liver function testing, and C-reactive protein (CRP) 15 mg/L (normal <1.0 mg/L). X-ray of the right knee shows soft-tissue swelling, but no gas or prosthetic loosening. Blood cultures are drawn. Arthrocentesis is planned. What is the next best step in management?

A. Start vancomycin.
B. Start vancomycin and ceftriaxone.
C. Start vancomycin and aztreonam.
D. Hold off on giving antibiotics until further work-up is completed.
E. Obtain an x-ray of the left knee.

The best next step would be holding off on giving antibiotics until further work-up is completed (**option D**). This patient's presentation is concerning for a prosthetic joint infection (PJI) of the right knee. In general, a PJI is acquired by one of three mechanisms: seeding at time of implantation, hematogenous dissemination/seeding from infection at a different site (i.e., urinary tract infection), or spread from a contiguous source of infection near the prosthesis (i.e., cellulitis). Various pathogens are capable of causing PJI, including bacterial (gram-positive most commonly, but also gram-negative and anaerobic), fungal, and mycobacterial (tuberculosis and nontuberculous mycobacteria).

PJIs can be difficult to diagnose, because so many of the clinical findings can be nonspecific. Like most conditions, the diagnosis requires synthesis of clinical findings (symptoms and signs) and ancillary data (lab studies, imaging findings, and microbiologic data). PJI should generally be suspected in a patient with a painful prosthesis or who has chronic wound drainage (or impaired surgical wound healing) or a sinus tract overlying the prosthesis. In addition, you may occasionally (usually with acute infections) see the classic signs of inflammation such as fevers, chills, or involved joint erythema, warmth, pain/tenderness, swelling, and impaired function. In general, the evaluation should include basic labs such as complete blood count with differential, metabolic panel including renal function and liver function testing, inflammatory markers (CRP and erythrocyte sedimentation rate [ESR]), blood cultures (if systemically ill), plain radiograph (x-ray) of the affected joint, and arthrocentesis.

The joint fluid should be sent for cell count with differential, crystal analysis, and gram stain/culture for at least aerobic and anaerobic organisms. The synovial fluid cell count has to be interpreted with respect to the type of prosthesis and timing since prosthetic placement. Based on one prospective study in patients with prosthetic knees (which excluded patients with inflammatory joint disease), a synovial fluid WBC count greater than 1,700 cells/uL, or a differential of greater than 65% neutrophils was shown to be highly sensitive and specific for the diagnosis of PJI. For prosthetic hip infections, the cut-off is a bit higher based on one study that showed the optimal cut-off to be greater than 4,200 cells/uL and greater than 80% neutrophils. Interestingly, the number could be reduced to greater than 3,000 cells/uL when interpreted in combination with ESR and CRP. The cut-offs are even higher in early-onset PJI. Some centers utilize novel synovial fluid markers such as the alpha-defensin. Alpha-defensin is a neutrophil-derived antimicrobial peptide that is released in the synovial fluid in response to pathogens. This marker is highly sensitive and specific and is unaffected by prior antibiotic administration. If the patient is taken to surgery (debridement, revision arthroplasty, etc.), then at least three (but sometimes up to six) tissue samples should be submitted for histopathologic examination (can be very helpful for diagnosis of definitive PJI) and at least aerobic and anaerobic gram stain/culture. If there is suspicion for fungal or mycobacterial infection, then tissue cultures for fungal and acid-fast organisms should be sent as well. Furthermore, if the prosthesis is removed, it can also be sent for microbiologic evaluation (sonication of the prosthesis has been shown to increase yield). Identifying the same organism(s) in multiple tissue cultures is highly indicative of PJI. Finally, the intraoperative findings may be diagnostically helpful as well (i.e., purulence, "dishwater" fluid, etc.), so these should be sought out as well.

Interestingly, it is recommended that antibiotics can be withheld in medically stable patients (i.e., not systemically ill or hemodynamically unstable) in order to optimize the chance that the organism responsible for the PJI can be recovered (either from arthrocentesis or perioperatively). If the patient was on antibiotics previously, then these should be withheld for at least 2 weeks in stable patients in order to optimize diagnostic yield. Identification of the organism is very important, because these patients typically get prolonged courses of antibiotic therapy, so keeping this therapy as targeted (narrow) as possible helps limit unnecessary antibiotic exposure and the associated negative consequences (i.e., toxicities, etc.).

Management can be rather complex. There are various surgical options, such as debridement, antibiotics, and implant retention ("DAIR," typically involves polyethylene liner exchange), one-stage exchange, two-stage exchange, and even permanent resection arthroplasty and amputation in refractory cases. The choice of the procedure is ultimately decided by the orthopedic surgeon, and various factors are weighed in the decision (Table 15.1). As far as antimicrobial therapy goes, the empiric coverage will depend on various factors including clinical stability, prior organisms/cultures, risk for resistant pathogens, comorbid conditions (renal or hepatic dysfunction), medication allergies, and suspected mechanism of the infection. In general, vancomycin will provide coverage for the majority of the gram-positive pathogens (the most likely etiology) including staphylococci, streptococci, enterococci, and indolent organisms like *Cutibacterium* (formerly *Propionibacterium*) *acnes* and *Corynebacteria*. A third-generation cephalosporin such as ceftriaxone will typically cover the common gram-negative pathogens. If there is concern for resistant pathogens (*Pseudomonas spp.*, vancomycin-resistant enterococci, extended-spectrum beta-lactamase producers, or Amp-C beta-lactamase producers) or the patient is significantly ill, then expanded coverage should be provided accordingly. In patients with beta-lactam intolerances (i.e., allergies), a fluoroquinolone (FQ) can provide appropriate gram-negative coverage, as FQs have good bone/joint penetration.

Table 15.1 – Approach to Definitive Management of Prosthetic Joint Infections

Procedure	Indications for Procedure	Subsequent Management
Debridement, Antibiotics, and Implant Retention (DAIR)[a]	• Symptoms <3 weeks or early-onset PJI (within 30 days of implantation) • Prosthesis well-fixed – no loosening, etc. • Absence of sinus tract (more suggestive of chronic PJI) • Organism susceptible to at least one oral antimicrobial	• Staphylococci—targeted antimicrobials (IV typically) × 6 weeks, then step-down to oral therapy with rifampin if susceptible (for biofilm penetration) + highly bioavailable agent with good bone penetration × 6 months (knee) or 3 months (hip and other joints) • Nonstaphylococci—similar to staphylococci, except no role for rifampin
One-Stage Exchange (Not commonly done in the United States)[a]	• PJI of hip with good soft-tissue coverage • Pathogen known and susceptible to at least one bioavailable agent • Able to use antibiotic bone cement and no need for bone grafting	• Similar approach overall to DAIR, but with the following exception: • Staphylococci—step down to oral therapy with rifampin for only 3 months total (regardless of joint)
Two-Stage Exchange	• Poor soft-tissue coverage or difficult-to-treat organism (but antimicrobial options available) • Can tolerate multiple surgeries, and surgeon thinks reimplantation will be possible based on anatomy and will give good functional outcome	• Targeted antimicrobials (IV typically) × 4–6 weeks (typically 6 weeks), then • Antimicrobial-free period (typically at least a couple weeks) followed by repeat arthrocentesis at the end of this period to "document clearance" prior to reimplantation
Amputation	• Preferred over PRA or AD if necrotizing skin/soft-tissue infection, severe bone loss precluding PRA/AD, poor soft-tissue coverage, no antimicrobial available to treat the PJI, improved functional outcome (c/w PRA or AD), or prior failed PRA/AD	• If adequate source control (i.e., clean soft tissue and bone margins of resection), then typically can stop antimicrobials completely
Permanent Resection Arthroplasty (PRA) or Arthrodesis (AD)	• Not meeting criteria for amputation and can tolerate/is willing to undergo a procedure • Failed prior two-stage exchange + risk of recurrent infection with another two-stage exchange is unacceptably high • Patient nonambulatory	• Targeted antimicrobials × 4–6 weeks

[a]For DAIR and one-stage exchange, consider long-term oral suppressive therapy after completion of initial treatment course (especially if unable to use rifampin therapy concurrently for staphylococci, or with certain organisms—not typically done for gram-negative organisms).

Eventually, the therapy should be deescalated to target the causative organism(s). The duration of therapy will depend on the organism, the clinical course/response, and the type of surgical intervention performed, as outlined in Table 15.1.

Option A (start vancomycin) and option B (start vancomycin and ceftriaxone) would both be feasible options, but the appropriate work-up should be obtained first in this stable patient. Option C (start vancomycin and aztreonam) could be an option, but aztreonam should only be used for gram-negative coverage in a patient with a penicillin allergy who cannot tolerate other beta-lactams (i.e., higher-generation cephalosporins or carbapenems) or FQs. Option E (x-ray left knee) is unnecessary, as we have no clinical reason to suspect anything is wrong with the left knee.

KEY LEARNING POINT

In clinically stable patients (e.g., hemodynamically stable and not systemically ill) with suspected prosthetic joint infections, antimicrobials may be withheld until appropriate work-up can be obtained in order to optimize diagnostic yield.

REFERENCES AND FURTHER READING

- Osman DR, Berbari EF, Berendt AR, et al. Diagnosis and management of prosthetic joint infection: clinical practice guidelines by the Infectious Diseases Society of America. *Clin Infect Dis.* 2013;56(1):e1–e25.
- Schinsky MF, Della Valle CJ, Sporer SM, Paprosky WG. Perioperative testing for joint infection in patients undergoing revision total hip arthroplasty. *J Bone Joint Surg Am.* 2008;90(9):1869–1875. https://doi.org/10.2106/JBJS.G.01255. Erratum in: J Bone Joint Surg Am. 2010;92(3):707.
- Tande AJ, Gomez-Urena EO, Berbari EF, Osmon DR. Management of prosthetic joint infection. *Infect Dis Clin North Am.* 2017;31(2):237–252. https://doi.org/10.1016/j.idc.2017.01.009.
- Trampuz A, Hanssen AD, Osmon DR, Mandrekar J, Steckelberg JM, Patel R. Synovial fluid leukocyte count and differential for the diagnosis of prosthetic knee infection. *Am J Med.* 2004;117(8):556–562. https://doi.org/10.1016/j.amjmed.2004.06.022.
- Trampuz A, Piper KE, Jacobson MJ, et al. Sonication of removed hip and knee prostheses for diagnosis of infection. *N Engl J Med.* 2007;357(7):654–663. https://doi.org/10.1056/NEJMoa061588.

A 60-year-old male is admitted to the hospital with a 2-day history of low-grade fevers, suprapubic pain, and hematuria. He has a history of type 2 diabetes mellitus, benign prostatic hyperplasia with recent placement of a Foley catheter for urinary retention, and chronic kidney disease. Medications include aspirin, metformin, insulin, atorvastatin, tamsulosin, and finasteride. He has no medication allergies. Vital signs show temperature 100.5° F, heart rate 90 beats per minute, blood pressure 120/75 mmHg, respiratory rate 16, and oxygen saturation 98% on room air. Physical examination shows tenderness in the suprapubic region, but no costovertebral angle tenderness. Rectal examination reveals a smoothly enlarged prostate without any frank tenderness or bogginess. The remainder of the examination is unremarkable. Labs show a white blood cell (WBC) count of 11,000 cells/uL, creatinine 1.2 mg/dL (at his baseline), normal electrolyte panel, and liver function testing. Urinalysis shows presence of blood and leukocyte esterase. Urine microscopy shows greater than 50 red blood cells per high-powered field and greater than 100 WBC/hpf. Renal ultrasound was unremarkable. Blood cultures are drawn, and the patient is started on ceftriaxone. Eventually, the urine culture reveals greater than 100,000 CFU/mL of *Candida krusei*.

What is the most appropriate treatment for this patient?

A. Fluconazole.

B. Caspofungin.

C. Amphotericin-B deoxycholate.

D. Amphotericin-B liposomal.

E. Flucytosine.

The best treatment for this patient is amphotericin-B deoxycholate (**option C**). This patient is presenting with a catheter-associated urinary tract infection (UTI) due to *Candida krusei*, specifically cystitis or potentially early pyelonephritis (as evidenced by the fever, which is atypical for cystitis). When *Candida* spp. are discovered in the urine (candiduria), one should always attempt to find out why it is there. Candiduria is common in critically ill patients with indwelling urinary devices, diabetics, and those with prior antibiotic exposure. Most of the time, candiduria represents either contamination of the urinary specimen (i.e., a poorly collected urine sample with excessive squamous epithelial cells) or colonization (asymptomatic candiduria [ASCU]). ASCU should only be treated if the patient is pregnant (drug of choice is typically amphotericin-B here as well), is neutropenic, or has an impending urologic procedure. Treatment of patients with ASCU who do not meet these criteria will only result in development of resistance and potential adverse effects without improving outcome. The other way candiduria occurs is by hematogenous seeding of the urine from a candidemia. This etiology can be evaluated with routine blood cultures, as *Candida* will grow on routine blood cultures (i.e., you do not need fungal blood cultures). Blood cultures should be considered, because candidemia may not always be clinically obvious. *Candida* may cause a spectrum of urinary infections similar to most UTI pathogens (i.e., cystitis, pyelonephritis, etc.), but, unlike the usual bacterial pathogens, *Candida* may rarely form urinary tract fungus balls. This complication can cause urinary tract obstruction and should be suspected in patients (usually immune-compromised) with persistent candiduria of unclear etiology. The approach to the diagnosis of *Candida* urinary infections is similar to that for most other UTIs, and may include urinalysis with microscopy, urine culture, blood cultures, imaging to rule out obstruction (will also detect fungus balls), and pregnancy testing in females of child-bearing age.

Management of *Candida* UTI depends on the subspecies and the presentation. In all cases, one should consider removing or exchanging any indwelling urinary devices (i.e., stents, catheters), and attaining appropriate source control (i.e., relieve obstruction, drain perinephric abscess), if feasible. For susceptible isolates, fluconazole is the drug of choice, as it achieves excellent urinary concentrations and has randomized trial data supporting its efficacy. In general, assuming no prior azole exposure, most *Candida* species are predictably susceptible to fluconazole, except for *Candida auris*, *C. krusei*, and *Candida glabrata*. *C. auris* is a highly resistant species of UTI that is fortunately not very common (updated information can be found on the relevant Centers for Disease Control and Prevention webpage). *C. krusei* is intrinsically resistant to fluconazole and flucytosine (5-FC), so alternative agents need to be used. *C. glabrata* can either be susceptible dose–dependent (SDD) to fluconazole or resistant

Table 16.1 – Management of Candida Urinary Tract Infections

Candida Species	Cystitis	Pyelonephritis	Fungus Ball
Fluconazole-susceptible species	• Fluconazole (3 mg/kg daily—typically 200 mg) × 2 weeks	• Fluconazole (6 mg/kg daily—typically 400 mg) × 2 weeks	• Surgical removal + antifungals, similar to pyelonephritis
Fluconazole-resistant *Candida glabrata*	• Amp-B deoxycholate × 1–7 days, OR 5-FC × 7–10 days	• Amp-B deoxycholate +/− 5-FC × 1–7 days, OR 5-FC × 14 days (weaker recommendation)	
Candida krusei	• Amp-B deoxycholate × 1–7 days	• Amp-B deoxycholate × 1–7 days	

Amp-B, Amphotericin-B; *5-FC*, flucytosine.

to fluconazole. SDD means that the resistance can be overcome by higher doses of fluconazole. The remaining azoles (itraconazole, voriconazole, posaconazole, and isavuconazole) do not penetrate into the urine very well and have insufficient data for their use in *Candida* UTIs. The echinocandins (e.g., caspofungin [**option B**], micafungin, anidulafungin) generally have poor urinary penetration as well, and, despite some case reports of success, they are not recommended for *Candida* UTIs. 5-FC (**option E**) is active against most *Candida* species except *C. krusei*, so it cannot be used for the patient in this case. 5-FC can cause cytopenia, and resistance can develop rapidly when 5-FC is used alone (monotherapy). Amphotericin-B will cover most *Candida* species, except for *Candida lusitaniae*, which is usually resistant to amphotericin. When used for urinary infections, the deoxycholate formulation of amphotericin-B should be used, because the lipid formulations (such as **option D**) do not achieve adequate urinary penetration. Table 16.1 summarizes the treatment of *Candida* urinary infections.

KEY LEARNING POINT

Urinary tract infections due to resistant Candida *species can be treated with amphotericin-B (Amp-B) deoxycholate. The lipid formulations of Amp-B (e.g., liposomal Amp-B) are ineffective.*

REFERENCE AND FURTHER READING

• Pappas PG, Kauffman CA, Andes DR, et al. Clinical practice guideline for the management of candidiasis: 2016 update by the Infectious Diseases Society of America. *Clin Infect Dis.* 2016;62(4):e1–e50. https://doi.org/10.1093/cid/civ933.

A 40-year-old man presents to the emergency room with a 1-week history of fevers (102° F–103° F), malaise, fatigue, night sweats, myalgias, headache, nonproductive cough, and shortness of breath. He has no medication allergies and is otherwise healthy. There is no family history of malignancy. He recently finished training and is now working as a large-animal veterinarian. He denies ever working with birds or rodents. It is not uncommon for him to find ticks on himself, but he does not recall ever seeing one attached or engorged. He has not been exposed to anyone with a similar illness. He lives in rural Iowa and denies any recent travel. He does not use any substances and only rarely consumes alcohol. He does not consume unpasteurized dairy products. He has never been incarcerated or spent prolonged time in a homeless shelter. He is married and in a monogamous relationship with his wife. Vitals reveal temperature 102° F, heart rate 110 beats per minute, blood pressure 110/70 mmHg, respiratory rate 24, and oxygen saturation 94% on 3 to 4 L/min oxygen by nasal cannula. On examination, he appears ill and visibly dyspneic. There is no icterus, nor are there conjunctival abnormalities. Examination of the oral mucosa reveals no oral ulcerations. Heart exam shows regular tachycardia without murmurs. Lung exam reveals diffuse, bilateral crackles. Abdominal exam shows no tenderness, but there is hepatomegaly. There is no skin rash, joint swelling or tenderness, spinal tenderness, or lymphadenopathy. Labs reveal white blood cell (WBC) count 15,000 cells/uL (neutrophils 85%), hemoglobin 12 g/dL, platelets 75,000 cells/uL, creatinine 0.8 mg/dL, ALT 90 U/L, AST 75 U/L, and normal alkaline phosphatase and bilirubin. Chest x-ray shows bilateral interstitial opacities. What is the most likely cause of this patient's illness?

A. *Coxiella burnetii.*

B. *Chlamydophila psittaci.*

C. *Legionella pneumophila.*

D. *Histoplasma capsulatum.*

E. *Leptospira interrogans.*

The most likely cause is *Coxiella burnetii* (**option A**). *Coxiella* is a gram-negative intracellular organism that causes a zoonotic illness known as Query fever, or simply Q fever. This infection can be acquired in a variety of ways, including contact with animal excretions/bodily fluids (especially birth products), being bitten by an infected tick, and inhalation of aerosols contaminated with *Coxiella* (can be transmitted to people miles away from the source). Rarely, it can be acquired via person-to-person transmission, transfusions, and organ transplantation. People in certain occupations are at higher risk, such as veterinarians, farmers, or others who work with livestock. The incubation period is typically a few weeks long. In most cases (up to 60%), the infection is asymptomatic. Symptomatic patients can present with an acute form, which typically manifests as a flu-like illness with pneumonia and hepatitis (abnormal liver function tests in ~80%). Labs may show normal or increased WBC count and platelet abnormalities (thrombocytopenia initially followed by thrombocytosis). Rarely, acute Q fever can manifest as carditis, meningoencephalitis, severe headache, maculopapular skin rash, and cholecystitis. If left untreated, patients can be symptomatic for weeks to months. Both symptomatic and asymptomatic patients can rarely develop a chronic form of the illness at any point after acute infection. This is more common in the immune-compromised (including pregnant patients). Chronic Q fever is usually characterized by endovascular infection in at-risk patients (endocarditis if pre-existing valvular disease, graft infections if pre-existing endovascular graft, infection of pre-existing aneurysm, etc.). Alternative presentations could be chronic hepatitis, chronic pneumonia, or osteoarticular infections. If the chronic form is left untreated, then it is universally fatal. In pregnant patients, acute infection during the first trimester is most problematic, as it can be dangerous to mother and baby. In addition, the infection can recur in subsequent pregnancies. Lastly, some patients can go on to develop a chronic fatigue syndrome called post–Q fever fatigue syndrome that is often managed conservatively (similar to chronic fatigue syndrome).

The diagnosis of Q fever can be challenging. The diagnosis should include synthesis of clinical presentation (symptoms and signs) and ancillary data (laboratory tests, imaging, etc.), similar to other infectious diseases. In general, diagnosis most commonly employs serology (antibodies) and polymerase chain reaction (PCR). Serology can be confusing, as there are two antigenic phases (phase I and phase II), and each has an IgM and an IgG component. Compared with IgG, the IgM antibody is less useful due to low-level titer cross-reactivity (especially with *Bartonella* species) and lower specificity. Culture is usually not done, due to the hazardous nature of the organism.

Acute infection can be definitively diagnosed by showing at least a four-fold rise in phase II IgG antibody titer (typically done via immunofluorescence assay) between acute and convalescent sera (typically separated by at least 3 weeks to allow seroconversion). In general, phase II titer should be greater than phase I titer in acute infection. Furthermore, in resolved infections, the phase I IgG and IgM titers may continue to increase but usually do not exceed phase II titers. A single positive convalescent serum sample (IgG phase II ≥1:128) in a patient who has been ill for greater than 1 week indicates a probable acute infection. Serology in acute infection is typically supplemented by PCR of blood or serum, because this test will become positive very early in infection (and stay positive out to ~2 weeks), but it may also become negative quickly once antibody titer rises or after administration of antibiotics.

Chronic Q fever is diagnosed by showing an elevated phase I IgG antibody titer (1:1024 or greater, and higher than phase II IgG titer) plus an identifiable chronic infection (e.g., endocarditis). The valvular vegetations are notoriously difficult to detect (even with transesophageal echocardiogram), so diagnosing endocarditis may involve application of Duke's criteria. A phase I IgG antibody titer greater than 1:800 or a blood culture positive for *Coxiella* is a very helpful finding. In addition, identifying *Coxiella* in tissue specimens via immunohistochemical staining, PCR, or culture can provide a definitive diagnosis of acute or chronic Q fever.

Management is fairly complicated as well. Even without treatment, most infections resolve on their own in a few weeks. There are indications as to who should be treated (see later) for acute and chronic infections. In general, treatment should not be given for just positive serology (i.e., without compatible presentation). The US Centers for Disease Control and Prevention guidelines contain an algorithm that can be very helpful when managing Q fever. Table 17.1 summarizes the management of Q fever.

Chlamydophila psittaci (**option B**) is an atypical bacterium that causes the disease psittacosis. This infection can present in a similar fashion as Q fever, but typically there will be a history of bird exposure, which this patient does not have. *Legionella pneumophila* (**option C**) presents as either a self-limited flu-like illness (Pontiac fever) or a severe pneumonia, typically associated with central nervous system symptoms, gastrointestinal symptoms, and hyponatremia (Legionnaire's disease) (Table 17.2). In addition, this disease usually affects patients who are elderly, smokers, immune-compromised, or have chronic lung disease. *Histoplasma capsulatum* (**option D**) typically manifests as an acute or chronic pneumonia, but in immune-compromised patients (not the case with this patient) it can disseminate to involve the reticuloendothelial system, leading to bone marrow involvement (often pancytopenia, instead of isolated thrombocytopenia, as in this case), hepatosplenomegaly, and liver enzyme

Table 17.1 – Overview of Q Fever Management

Stage	Indications	First-Line	Alternative(s)
Acute Q fever	• Symptomatic (compatible syndrome) • Asymptomatic but at risk for chronic infection (can consider treatment in these cases) • **Do NOT withhold antibiotics if suspicious but testing negative or pending**	• **Doxycycline** 　• Most effective if given early (within 3 days) 　• Shortens duration of illness and reduces risk of complications • **Duration = 14 days**	• Trimethoprim-sulfamethoxazole (TMP/SMX), macrolides, fluoroquinolones (FQ), rifampin
Chronic Q fever	• Positive serology (phase I IgG ≥1:1024) + compatible presentation • **Treatment should only be given to CONFIRMED cases**	• **Doxycycline + hydroxychloroquine (HCQ)** • **Duration for endovascular infection:** ≥18 (native infections) to 24 (prosthetic infections) months • **Duration for other infections is ill-defined**	• Doxycycline + FQ
Pregnancy and Q fever	• Only treat postpartum if serologic titers remain elevated >12 months after delivery	• **TMP/SMX with folic acid supplementation (during pregnancy)** • **Delivery with airborne precautions** • **Doxycycline + HCQ postpartum**	• Not defined • Avoid doxycycline and FQ (during pregnancy)

Monitoring recommendations

• Key component is always using the same test every time (i.e., same lab and assay), as there is a lot of variability in the available testing.

• After treatment for acute infections:

　• **If low-risk for chronic infection**, then do clinical and serologic monitoring for at least 6 months.

　• **If high-risk for chronic infection (includes pregnancy)**, then do clinical and serologic monitoring at 3, 6, 12, 18, and 24 months.

　• **After monitoring is completed**, then stop or perform less frequently. Patients should know that they are at risk for developing Q fever in the future and should seek medical attention if compatible symptoms or signs develop.

• While on treatment for chronic infection, perform serial clinical and serologic monitoring.

• If poor response during treatment, then consider checking drug levels of HCQ (goal 0.8–1.2 ug/mL) and/or doxycycline (goal ≥5 ug/mL).

• If using HCQ, then will need to ensure normal glucose-6-phosphate dehydrogenase level and will need to monitor for retinopathy (eye exam at baseline and every 6 months thereafter).

disturbances. Lastly, *Leptospira interrogans* (**option E**) causes leptospirosis, which is acquired via contact with infected bodily fluids of certain animals (classically rodents, but various others are implicated, including domestic animals). The presentation is variable, but tip-offs (not seen here) include conjunctival suffusion, renal failure, and liver failure with jaundice.

Table 17.2 – Pneumonia Associations

Situation	Associations
Community-acquired pneumonia	• *Streptococcus pneumoniae, Haemophilus influenzae, Moraxella catarrhalis*, atypical pathogens *(Mycoplasma, Chlamydophila, Legionella)*, viral • Aspiration/lung abscess: oral flora, gram-negative and anaerobic organisms
Hospital-acquired pneumonia (onset >2 days into hospitalization)	• *Staphylococcus aureus* (including methicillin-resistant *S. aureus*) and resistant gram-negative organisms including *Pseudomonas*; rarely *Legionella*.
Immune-compromised host (association will depend on the type and degree of immune suppression)	• Bacterial—*Nocardia*, mycobacteria, *Coxiella, Rhodococcus* • Viral—adenovirus, cytomegalovirus • Fungal—*Cryptococcus, Pneumocystis jirovecii*, endemic mycoses, various molds including *Aspergillus* and *Mucorales* • Parasites—*Strongyloides, Toxoplasma*
Travel-related pneumonia	• Southwest United States—*Coccidiodes, Hantavirus, Yersinia pestis* (plague) • Southeast Asia—*Mycobacterium tuberculosis, Burkholderia pseudomallei* (meliodosis), severe acute respiratory syndrome coronaviruses • Middle East—Middle East respiratory syndrome coronavirus • Hawaii—*Leptospira interrogans*
Exposure to decaying wood or vegetation	• *Blastomyces* spp. (blastomycosis)
Exposure to birds or bats or their droppings	• *Chlamydophila psittaci, Histoplasma capsulatum, Cryptococcus*
Exposure to farm animals and their secretions/excretions	• *Coxiella* (Q fever)
Consumption of undercooked or raw shellfish	• *Paragonimus westermani*
Bioterrorism	• *Francisella tularensis* (tularemia), *Bacillus anthracis* (anthrax), *Yersinia pestis* (pneumonic plague)
Exposure to cruise ship, hotels, or water	• *Legionella pneumophila*
Unvaccinated (or waning vaccination)	• *Bordetella pertussis, H. influenzae, S. pneumoniae*, influenza, varicella, measles

KEY LEARNING POINT

Acute Q fever typically manifests as a flu-like illness with acute hepatitis (liver enzyme elevation) and, at times, thrombocytopenia and a skin rash. The diagnosis of Q fever is summarized in figure 17.1

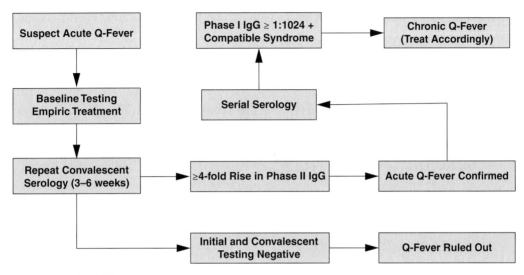

Fig. 17.1- Diagnosis of Q fever

REFERENCES AND FURTHER READING

- Anderson A, Bijlmer H, Fournier PE, et al. Diagnosis and management of Q fever—United States, 2013: recommendations from CDC and the Q Fever Working Group. *MMWR Recomm Rep.* 2013;62(RR-03):1–30. Erratum in: *MMWR Recomm Rep.* 2013;62(35):730.
- Hartzell JD, et al. *Coxiella burnetii* (Q fever). In: *Mandell, Douglas, and Bennett's Principles and Practice of Infectious Diseases.* 9th ed. Elsevier; 2020:2360–2367.
- Hartzell JD, Gleeson T, Scoville S, Massung RF, Wortmann G, Martin GJ. Practice guidelines for the diagnosis and management of patients with Q fever by the Armed Forces Infectious Diseases Society. *Mil Med.* 2012;177(5): 484–494. https://doi.org/10.7205/milmed-d-12-00059.

18 CASE

A 20-year-old male presents to the HIV clinic with a 2-day history of dysuria. He denies any fevers, skin rashes, genital lesions, or joint pains. He has a history of well-controlled chronic HIV infection, for which he is currently taking bictegravir, tenofovir alafenamide fumarate, and emtricitabine. He does not take any other medications and has no medication allergies. He is sexually active, with male partners only. He does not use condoms regularly. Vital signs are within normal limits. Genital exam shows expressible purulent penile discharge, but no inguinal lymphadenopathy or genital ulcerations. Urinalysis shows presence of pyuria. Nucleic acid amplification testing (NAAT) of all involved sites is performed, and a syphilis screening test is obtained. He is eager to leave, because he hates having to come to the doctor. Which of the following is the most appropriate next step in management (based on 2021 US Centers for Disease Control and Prevention [CDC] guidance for sexually transmitted infections)?

A. Ceftriaxone 250 mg intramuscular once.

B. Ceftriaxone 500 mg intramuscular once.

C. Ceftriaxone 250 mg intramuscular once + doxycycline 100 mg PO BID × 7 days.

D. Ceftriaxone 500 mg intramuscular once + doxycycline 100 mg PO BID × 7 days.

E. Await results of testing prior to treatment.

The most appropriate next step would be ceftriaxone 500 mg intramuscular once and doxycycline 100 mg PO BID × 7 days (**option D**). This patient is presenting with urethritis, which is characterized by urethral inflammation that manifests as dysuria and urethral discharge (often mucopurulent). There are several causes of urethritis, including *Chlamydia trachomatis* (most commonly), *Neisseria gonorrhoeae*, *Trichomonas vaginalis*, *Mycoplasma genitalium*, *Ureaplasma* spp., and some viruses including *herpes simplex virus* and *adenovirus*. There are some reports of enteric pathogens causing urethritis in men who have sex with men. Noninfectious etiologies include trauma/irritation and some inflammatory disorders (reactive arthritis, for example).

Diagnostic testing may include point-of-care gram stain, which will show inflammation (at least two white blood cells per field) and potentially gram-negative intracellular diplococci (suggesting *N. gonorrhoeae*). Urinalysis may show pyuria (leukocytes in the urine) as well, which indicates inflammation. Alternatively, and probably more commonly, practitioners can use NAATs for diagnosis. NAAT is highly sensitive and specific for the diagnosis of gonorrhea and chlamydia. NAAT can and should be done on all exposed sites, including first-void urine (or urethral swab), oropharynx, and rectum. A saline wet mount of cervical secretions in women can identify *Trichomonas* infections and should be done in all women presenting with vaginal discharge. Validated testing for *Trichomonas* in males is limited and not widely available.

Management depends on the situation/causative organism, patient allergies, and patient reliability (see Table 18.1 for options). In many cases, it is not wrong to wait for the results prior to treatment (**option E**), but in patients with obvious infection and low likelihood of returning for treatment (such as this patient), empiric treatment should be given. In this case, treatment for gonorrhea and chlamydia should be given (see Table 18.1). This is why **options A and B** are incorrect.

Anytime a patient is diagnosed with a sexually transmitted illness (STI), several other steps should be taken. First, they should be evaluated for other STIs such as HIV and syphilis. In addition, they should abstain from sexual activity for at least 7 days after treatment. Furthermore, the patient's sexual partners in the preceding 60 days (90 days for syphilis) should be referred for evaluation and treatment. The patient should not have sexual contact with these partners for at least 7 days after they are treated. Lastly, for those diagnosed with gonorrhea, chlamydia, or trichomoniasis, repeat testing should be done in 3 months, as the risk of reinfection is considerable.

Table 18.1 – Common Sexually Transmitted Illnesses (STIs)

Presentation	First-Line Treatment	Alternative Treatment
Undifferentiated urethritis or both *Neisseria gonorrhoeae* and *Chlamydia trachomatis* detected		
Undifferentiated urethritis OR both ***N. gonorrhoeae* and *C. trachomatis* detected**	• Ceftriaxone 500 mg IM once + doxycycline 100 mg PO BID × 7 days	• See gonorrhea and chlamydia later
Cervicitis		
Cervicitis	• Doxycycline 100 mg PO BID × 7 days	• Azithromycin 1 g PO once
	• **Consider concurrent treatment for gonococcal infection if the patient is at risk for gonorrhea or lives in a community where the prevalence of gonorrhea is high**	
Chlamydial infections (*C. trachomatis*)		
Adults and adolescents	• Doxycycline 100 mg PO BID × 7 days	• Azithromycin 1 g PO once, or • Levofloxacin 500 mg daily × 7 days
Pregnancy	• Azithromycin 1 g PO once	• Amoxicillin 500 mg PO TID × 7 days
Gonococcal infections (*N. gonorrhoeae*)		
Uncomplicated infection of cervix, urethra, or rectum in adults and adolescents[a]	• Ceftriaxone 500 mg IM once	• If cephalosporin allergic → gentamicin 240 mg IM once + azithromycin 2 g PO once • Alternative if cannot use ceftriaxone → cefixime 800 mg PO once
Uncomplicated infection of the pharynx in adults and adolescents[a]	• Ceftriaxone 500 mg IM once	• N/A
Disseminated gonococcal infection[a]	• Ceftriaxone 1 g IM/IV daily × at least 7 days	• Cefotaxime 1 g IV every 8 hours
Pregnancy[a]	• Ceftriaxone 500 mg IM once	• N/A
Conjunctivitis	• Ceftriaxone 1 g IM once + saline lavage eye	• N/A
Lymphogranuloma venereum	• Doxycycline 100 mg PO BID × 21 days	• Azithromycin 1 g PO once weekly × 3 weeks (if using, consider test of cure after 4 weeks)

[a]If chlamydial infection has not been excluded, treat for chlamydia with doxycycline 100 mg PO BID × 7 days (if pregnant, use azithromycin 1 g PO once)

Trichomoniasis (*Trichomonas vaginalis*)		
Men	• Metronidazole 2 g PO once	• Tinidazole 2 g PO once
Women	• Metronidazole 500 mg PO BID × 7 days	• Tinidazole 2 g PO once

(Continued)

Table 18.1 – Common Sexually Transmitted Illnesses (STIs) *(cont'd)*

Presentation	First-Line Treatment	Alternative Treatment
Mycoplasma genitalium (a rare cause of persistent/recurrent nongonococcal urethritis)		
If macrolide-resistant or resistance not known	• Doxycycline 100 mg PO BID × 7 days then Moxifloxacin 400 mg PO daily × 7 days	• **For settings without resistance testing and when moxifloxacin cannot be used →** doxycycline 100 mg BID × 7 days + • Azithromycin 1 g initially then azithromycin 500 mg once daily × 3 days → consider test of cure 21 days after completion of therapy
If macrolide-susceptible	• Doxycycline 100 mg PO BID × 7 days, then azithromycin 1 g PO once initially then 500 mg PO once daily for 3 additional days (2.5 g total)	
Other syndromes		
Bacterial vaginosis (*Gardnerella vaginalis*)	• Metronidazole 500 mg PO BID × 7 days, or • Metronidazole gel × 5 days, or • Clindamycin cream × 7 days	• Clindamycin 300 mg PO BID × 7 days, or • Clindamycin ovules × 3 days, or • Secnidazole 2 g PO granules once, or • Tinidazole – 2 g PO once daily × 2 days OR 1 g PO once daily × 5 days
Epididymitis	• If suspect STI → Ceftriaxone 500 mg IM once (use 1 g if ≥ 150 kg) + Doxycycline 100 mg PO BID × 10 days • If suspect due to enteric organisms (i.e., men who have sex with men) → Levofloxacin 500 mg PO daily × 10 days • If undifferentiated → Ceftriaxone 500 mg IM once (use 1 g if ≥ 150 kg) + Levofloxacin 500 mg PO daily × 10 days	

Failure to improve after appropriate treatment for urethritis suggests reinfection, potentially poor treatment adherence, unrecognized infection (*Trichomonas*, or *M. genitalium* if doxycycline was used for initial treatment), complication (i.e., prostatitis), and, very rarely, treatment resistance.

Lastly, the most recent iteration of the STI management guidelines from the CDC came with two major changes. First, the dose of ceftriaxone for uncomplicated gonococcal infection was increased from 250 mg to 500 mg due to concerns over rising resistance in gonococci. Second, doxycycline became the first-line therapy for chlamydial infections due to data showing improved microbiologic cure and better efficacy in rectal infections. This explains why choices **A and C** are incorrect. Table 18.1 shows a summary of some common STIs.

KEY LEARNING POINT

In patients with undifferentiated urethritis with low likelihood of follow-up, treatment for both gonorrhea (ceftriaxone 500 mg IM once) and chlamydia (doxycycline 100 mg PO BID × 7 days) should be provided.

REFERENCES AND FURTHER READING

- Workowski KA, Bolan GA, Centers for Disease Control and Prevention. Sexually transmitted diseases treatment guidelines, 2015. *MMWR Recomm Rep.* 2015;64(RR-03):1–137. Correction appears in *MMWR Recomm Rep.* 64(33):924. https://doi.org/10.15585/mmwr.rr7004a1.
- Workowski KA, Bachmann LH, Chan PA, et al. Sexually transmitted infections treatment guidelines, 2021. *MMWR Recomm Rep.* 2021;70(4):1–187. https://doi.org/10.15585/mmwr.rr7004a1.

A 25-year-old female presents to the HIV clinic for routine follow-up. She has no complaints. She was diagnosed with HIV at the age of 20 years, as part of a routine screening. Her CD4 cell count at that time was 820 cells/uL. She was started on antiretroviral therapy and has been adherent since, as evidenced by ongoing virologic suppression. She is currently on bictegravir, tenofovir alafenamide fumarate, and emtricitabine (Biktarvy). She is not taking any other medications. She has been sexually active, with only male partners, since the age of 16 years. She had an initial Pap smear (cervical cytology) at the age of 20 years, which was normal. Repeat Pap smears at ages 21 and 22 years were normal as well. Which of the following is the best recommendation for cervical cancer screening in this patient?

A. Repeat Pap smear today.
B. Repeat Pap smear with HPV testing today.
C. Repeat Pap smear in 2 years.
D. Repeat Pap smear with HPV testing in 2 years.
E. Repeat Pap smear with HPV testing at the age of 30 years.

The correct answer is repeat Pap smear today (**option A**). Cervical cancer screening recommendations for patients with HIV are summarized in Table 19.1. For patients with HIV, cervical cancer screening is continued throughout the patient's lifetime.

KEY LEARNING POINT

In HIV-positive women aged 21 to 29 years, Pap smear should be done annually until at least three consecutive normal results are obtained. After that, Pap smear can be performed every 3 years as long as results are normal.

Table 19.1 – Cervical Cancer Screening in HIV-Positive Patients

Situation	Typical Recommendation	Dealing With Abnormal Results
When to start screening?	• Within 1 year of onset of sexual activity and no later than age 21 years • At time of initial diagnosis	• N/A
Age 21–29 years	• Annual Pap smear until at least three consecutive normal results, then can do every 3 years	• ASCUS, reflex HPV positive → colposcopy • ASCUS, reflex HPV not done → repeat Pap 6–12 months • LSIL, ASC-H, AGC, HSIL → colposcopy

Age 30 years and older	• Option 1 = same as for age 21–29 years
	• Option 2 = cotesting (Pap+HPV):
	• At time of diagnosis or at age 30 years
	• If both normal → repeat in 3 years
		• ASCUS, HPV negative → repeat Pap 6–12 months or repeat cotesting 12 months
		• ASCUS, HPV positive → colposcopy
		• ASCUS, HPV not done → repeat Pap 6–12 months
		• LSIL, ASC-H, AGC, HSIL → colposcopy
		• If HPV positive (but normal Pap):
		  • HPV 16 or 18 → colposcopy
		  • Other HPV → repeat cotesting in 1 year

Terminology		

Cotesting (Pap smear and HPV testing) is not recommended for women under the age of 30 years (**options B and D**). Cotesting can start at the age of 30 years (**option E**), but this patient should still have a Pap smear done at the current visit. *AGC*, Atypical glandular cells; *ASC-H*, atypical squamous cells cannot exclude *HSIL*; *ASCUS*, atypical squamous cells of undetermined significance; *HSIL*, high-grade squamous intraepithelial lesions; *LSIL*, low-grade squamous intraepithelial lesion.

REFERENCE AND FURTHER READING

- CDC. Guidelines for the Prevention and Treatment of Opportunistic Infections in HIV-Infected Adults and Adolescents: Recommendations from the Centers for Disease Control and Prevention, the National Institutes of Health, and the HIV Medicine Association of the Infectious Diseases Society of America. https://clinicalinfo.hiv .gov/en/guidelines/hiv-clinical-guidelines-adult-and-adolescent-opportunistic-infections/whats-new. Accessed October 30, 2020.

A 40-year-old male presents to the emergency room with acute onset of high fevers (up to 104° F), cough, and shortness of breath. He has no major medical problems and does not take any medications. He has no medication allergies. He works as a mail delivery man. He lives in New Mexico and denies any recent travel outside of that area. He smokes half a pack of cigarettes per day but does not drink alcohol or use illicit drugs. He has not been around any animals recently. Vital signs show temperature 103° F, heart rate 125 beats per minute, blood pressure 90/62 mmHg, respiratory rate 28, and oxygen saturation 90% on 6 L/min oxygen by nasal cannula. Examination shows a toxic-appearing male. His mentation is a bit slowed, but he is fully oriented. Heart exam reveals regular tachycardia. Lung exam shows increased work of breathing with decreased breath sounds over the left lower lobe posteriorly. There are no rashes or lymphadenopathy. The remainder of the exam is unremarkable. Labs reveal white blood cell count 20,000 cells/uL (90% neutrophils), hemoglobin 9 g/dL, creatinine 1.5 mg/dL (creatinine clearance 35 mL/min), and normal liver function testing. Chest x-ray is shown in Fig. 20.1.

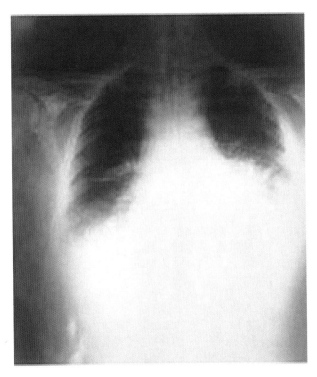

Figure 20.1 – Patient's chest X-ray
Image courtesy of the CDC Public Health Image Library.

Blood cultures are drawn. Diagnostic thoracentesis is performed and shows a bloody effusion, which is sent for analysis. Microbiologic studies of the pleural fluid are most likely to show which of the following?

A. Gram-positive cocci in pairs.

B. Anaerobic gram-positive rods.

C. Gram-negative coccobacilli.

D. Aerobic gram-positive rods.

E. Small spherules.

The correct answer is aerobic gram-positive rods (**option D**). This patient's presentation is concerning for acute inhalational anthrax. Anthrax is a disease caused by *Bacillus anthracis*, an aerobic gram-positive, spore-forming rod that typically forms long chains on gram stain. The disease can be acquired via skin contact (cutaneous anthrax), ingestion (gastrointestinal [GI] anthrax), and inhalation (inhalational anthrax). The cutaneous form is the most common, but the inhalational form carries the highest mortality. Cutaneous anthrax starts soon after exposure as a papular lesion at the site of inoculation that evolves into a vesiculopustular lesion and finally into a painless black eschar with surrounding edema (Fig. 20.2). Patients

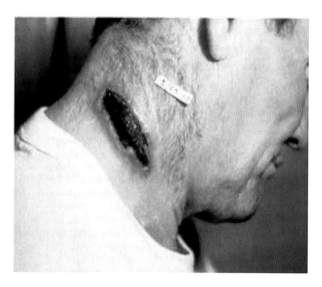

Figure 20.2 – Cutaneous anthrax lesion
Image courtesy of the CDC Public Health Image Library.

may also have fevers and lymphadenopathy. Notably, the injectional form may not have an eschar. GI anthrax presents soon after ingestion of raw or undercooked meat from an infected animal, with severe GI upset including mucosal ulceration, bloody diarrhea, and even ascites. Inhalational anthrax can present soon after exposure (i.e., spore inhalation as in biowarfare, or from infected animal products), but the incubation can be several weeks in some cases. The disease starts out with flu-like symptoms (rhinorrhea is characteristically absent) and often rapidly evolves into severe respiratory failure and septic shock. Complications include hemorrhagic effusions (pleural and pericardial), hemorrhagic mediastinitis, and dissemination with resultant meningitis (central nervous system [CNS] disease is frequently fatal). Importantly, the disease is not considered contagious, so only standard precautions are necessary.

Diagnosis must be confirmed and typically involves blood cultures and cultures of any involved bodily fluid (i.e., pleural fluid in this case). The microbiology lab should be notified of the suspicion, as this organism is considered biohazardous. Chest imaging typically will show widened mediastinum (mediastinitis) or pleural effusions. A lumbar puncture should be considered to rule out meningitis.

The management depends on the form of the disease (Table 20.1). Uncomplicated cutaneous anthrax can be managed with a fluoroquinolone or doxycycline for 7 to 10 days (if acquisition involved possible inhalational component, then patient will need 60 days of treatment as for postexposure prophylaxis—see later). In addition, penicillin can be used if the organism is known to be susceptible. Systemic disease should be managed in the intensive care unit. The choice of regimen depends on whether or not meningitis has been ruled out. If meningitis is ruled out, the treatment consists of a fluoroquinolone plus a protein synthesis inhibitor to suppress toxin production (clindamycin or linezolid). If meningitis is not ruled out, then a similar regimen is recommended, except the protein synthesis inhibitor should be linezolid (no data on CNS penetration for clindamycin), and meropenem should be added. In addition, dexamethasone should be considered as per usual meningitis therapy. These regimens are continued for at least 2 to 3 weeks and until the patient has significantly improved, whichever is longer. After this phase is complete, patients can be transitioned to a single oral agent to prevent relapse from surviving spores (the regimens are the same as for postexposure prophylaxis--see later). Additional considerations should be antitoxin treatments (raxibacumab or anthrax immunoglobulin) and obtaining adequate source control (i.e., drain effusions, which can be loaded with toxin). Postexposure prophylaxis includes a three-dose vaccine series and antimicrobials (either ciprofloxacin or doxycycline) for 60 days.

Table 20.1 – Summary of US Centers for Disease Control and Prevention (CDC) Category A Bioterror Agents

Disease	Clinical Features	Diagnosis/Precautions	Management
Anthrax (*Bacillus anthracis*)[a]	• Forms of illness include cutaneous, gastrointestinal (GI), and inhalational • Dissemination in any form can cause meningitis	• Blood cultures • Culture affected areas • CONTACT PRECAUTIONS in cutaneous anthrax with uncontained drainage (standard precautions in other cases)	• Skin – fluoroquinolone (FQ) or doxycycline×7–10 days • Systemic–FQ +toxin-agent (clindamycin or linezolid) +meropenem (if meningitis), then as for postexposure prophylaxis (ciprofloxacin or doxycycline×60 days)
Plague (*Yersinia pestis*)[a]	• Forms of illness include bubonic (painful buboes), septicemic, pneumonic, meningeal, and cutaneous • Transmitted by rodent fleas, esp. in the west and southwest United States	• Cultures of sputum, blood, or lymph node aspirates • "Safety-pin" appearance on gram stain • Standard precautions in most cases • Pneumonic – add Droplet Precautions until 48 hours after effective antibiotic therapy	• Aminoglycosides (streptomycin or gentamicin) or FQ×10–14 days • Doxycycline is an alternative and may be equivalent to gentamicin for bubonic plague • Postexposure prophylaxis (PEP)–doxycycline or FQ×7 days
Tularemia (*Francisella tularensis*)[a]	• Forms of illness include glandular, ulceroglandular, oculoglandular, oropharyngeal, pneumonic, typhoidal (septicemic) • Transmitted by contact with certain animals (classically rabbits), bites of ticks or deer flies, ingestion of contaminated water or food, or inhalation of contaminated aerosols	• Culture is definitive • Polymerase chain reaction, direct fluorescent antibody, immunohistochemistry staining→presumptive diagnosis • Serology–≥four-fold rise between acute & convalescent sera (tested at least 4 weeks apart) • Standard Precautions	• Streptomycin or gentamicin × 10 days. • Alternative treatments – doxycycline or FQ×14 days • PEP–doxycycline or FQ×14 days
Smallpox (*Variola major*)[a]	• Incubation~2 weeks • Then develop fevers and centrifugal "chickenpox-like" rash (but lesions in same stages of development) • Complications–encephalitis, blindness	• Risk-based testing – follow CDC algorithm • Airborne And Contact Precautions for duration of illness • Infectious until rash scabs over and sloughs	• Vaccination can decrease symptoms if given within 1 week of exposure, but it has complications • Antivirals (tecovirimat, cidofovir, brincidofovir) effective in animal studies and *in vitro*, but not proven in humans
Botulism (*Clostridium botulinum*)	• Forms – GI, wound, inhalational, iatrogenic • Toxin blocks presynaptic acetylcholine release→impaired neurotransmission • **Ds**: diplopia, dysarthria, dysphagia, descending paralysis (symmetric, flaccid)	• Largely a clinical diagnosis • Can identify toxin in serum, gastric secretions, stool, or food • Xenodiagnosis (mouse inoculation) is gold standard • Standard Precautions	• Intensive supportive care • Antitoxin can halt progression but only affects unbound toxin • Antibiotic therapy and surgical debridement for source control in wound botulism.

[a]Notify the microbiology lab and local authorities (public health department, etc.).

Gram-positive cocci in pairs (**option A**) suggest *Streptococcus pneumoniae*, but the presentation is not consistent with this pathogen. *S. pneumoniae* is the most common cause of pneumonia, and certainly can cause a parapneumonic effusion, but the hemorrhagic nature of the effusion argues against this pathogen. Anaerobic gram-positive rods (**option B**) could suggest *Clostridium*, *Actinomyces*, or *Cutibacterium acnes* (Fig. 20.3). Thoracic actinomycosis can cause a syndrome called "empyema necessitans," which typically presents less acutely and does not classically cause a hemorrhagic effusion. Gram-negative coccobacilli (**option C**) could suggest either *Francisella tularensis* (tularemia) or *Yersinia pestis* (pneumonic plague). In this case, there were not any of the typical exposures associated with these infections, such as rabbits or ticks (tularemia) or prairie dogs (plague). Lastly, small spherules (**option E**) suggest coccidioidomycosis. This infection can be acquired in the Southwest United States, which is where this patient lives. The usual presentation is a pneumonia, but dissemination to other organs (CNS, bone/joints, skin, etc.) may occur. Similar to the other diseases mentioned above, a bloody effusion is not consistent.

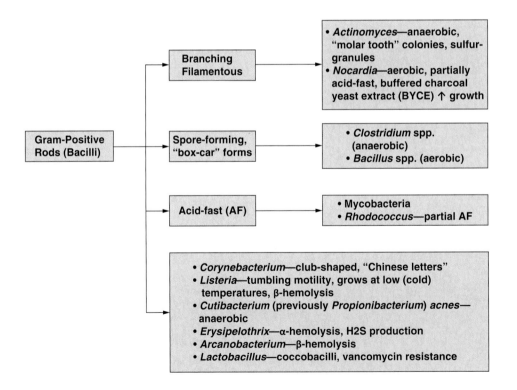

Figure 20.3 – Overview of gram-positive rods (bacilli)

KEY LEARNING POINT

Key features suggesting acute inhalational anthrax include occupational exposure (i.e., postal worker) and hemorrhagic mediastinitis/pleural effusions.

REFERENCES AND FURTHER READING

- Adalja AA, Toner E, Inglesby TV. Clinical management of potential bioterrorism-related conditions. *N Engl J Med.* 2015;372(10):954–962. https://doi.org/10.1056/NEJMra1409755.
- Hynes N, et al. *Bioterrorism: an overview.* In: *Mandell, Douglas, and Bennett's Principles and Practice of Infectious Diseases.* 9th ed : Elsevier; 2020.
- Centers for Disease Control and Prevention. Bioterrorism agents/diseases. https://emergency.cdc.gov/agent/agentlist-category.asp. Accessed October 3, 2020.

A 35-year-old female is referred to the infectious disease clinic with a 1-month history of fevers. Associated symptoms have included night sweats, a 10-pound unintentional weight loss, fatigue, and low back pain. The remainder of the review of systems is unremarkable. She is otherwise healthy. Her only medications are acetaminophen and ibuprofen as needed for her fever and pain. She has no medication allergies. She lives in Iowa and works as a schoolteacher. She enjoys attending wine and cheese tastings. She has not traveled anywhere recently. She denies any illicit drug use. She denies any history of incarceration or prolonged stays at a homeless shelter. She is married and monogamous. Vital signs show temperature 100.6° F, heart rate 95 beats per minute, blood pressure 110/75 mmHg, respiratory rate 18, and oxygen saturation 98% on room air. Physical examination shows an ill-appearing woman. Heart exam reveals a grade II/VI early systolic murmur heard loudest at the apex. Lungs are clear. Abdominal exam reveals hepatosplenomegaly. There is tenderness with palpation over her lower back, particularly over the right sacroiliac region. The rest of the examination is unremarkable. Review of ancillary studies done prior to the current visit shows:

White blood cell count 3,500 cells/uL

HIV antigen/antibody negative

Hemoglobin 9 mg/dL with MCV 80 fL

Blood cultures—no growth for 5 days

Platelet count 90,000 cells/uL

Erythrocyte sedimentation rate 80 mm/h

Creatinine 1.0 mg/dL

C-reactive protein 8 mg/L (normal <1 mg/L)

Alanine aminotransferase 80 U/L

HLA-B27 positive

An x-ray of the low back reveals erosion of the right sacroiliac joint. She has not been given any antimicrobial treatment to date. What is the most likely diagnosis in this patient?

A. Reactive arthritis.

B. Osteoarticular tuberculosis.

C. Brucellosis.

D. Multiple myeloma.

E. Disseminated histoplasmosis.

The most likely diagnosis is brucellosis (**option C**). Brucellosis is a zoonotic illness that can present in various ways ("a great imitator"). There are several species of *Brucella* that can cause disease in humans, including *B. abortus* (cattle), *B. melitensis* (goats, sheep, camels), *B. canis* (dogs), and *B. suis* (pigs). There are other less common species as well. *Brucella* is a gram-negative intracellular coccobacillus that is acquired by ingestion of unpasteurized dairy products (as is likely the cause in this case) or contaminated meat or by contact with certain animals, with transmission via exposure to their secretions or inhalation of aerosols. Consequently, people in certain occupations are at high risk, including veterinarians or others who work with large animals/livestock. The incubation period is approximately 2 to 4 weeks. The presentation is variable and may include constitutional symptoms (fevers, weight loss, night sweats, fatigue, anorexia), arthralgias, myalgias, headaches, lymphadenopathy, hepatosplenomegaly, arthralgia and arthritis, spondylitis and sacroiliitis, osteomyelitis, central nervous system infections (neurobrucellosis), cardiac infections (typically "culture-negative" endocarditis, which could be suggested by the heart murmur in this case), and epididymitis/orchitis. Laboratory studies may show leukopenia with relative lymphocytosis, anemia of chronic disease, and liver function test abnormalities.

Definitive diagnosis is made by identifying *Brucella* in culture. Culture is considered the gold standard, and the microbiology lab should always be notified, because *Brucella* is a biohazard concern, and the lab may need to hold the cultures for a longer period of time to aid diagnosis. Culture can take time to become positive (up to 21 days) and is more likely to be positive in acute cases (much less likely in chronic cases). In addition, culture of the bone marrow is considered more sensitive than blood cultures. Alternatively, definitive diagnosis can be established by showing at least a four-fold rise in *Brucella* antibody titer between acute and convalescent samples (drawn at least 2 weeks apart). IgM predominates in acute infection, and IgG and IgA predominate in chronic and relapsing infections. There are several causes of false-positive serology, including *Francisella tularensis*, *Salmonella* spp., *Escherichia coli O157*, and *Yersinia enterocolitica*. In addition, some species of *Brucella* (*B. canis*, or *B. abortus RB-51*) are not detected by serologic tests, so if there is suspicion for infection with these species, then further testing may be warranted. Presumptive diagnosis can be made by antibody titer 1:160 or higher (via agglutination-based tests) or detection of *Brucella* DNA by PCR.

Management consists of combination therapy for prolonged periods of time. The usual regimen for nonfocal brucellosis is doxycycline plus rifampin or an aminoglycoside (gentamicin or streptomycin) for at least 6 weeks. Doxycycline plus an aminoglycoside is considered the most effective regimen. For more complicated cases, the recommendation is to treat for a longer total duration (several months) and may involve combination therapy (at least three drugs). Trimethoprim-sulfamethoxazole (TMP/SMX) may have some efficacy and is used in combination with rifampin in pregnant patients with brucellosis. In addition, fluoroquinolones (in combination with rifampin) may be a suitable alternative. Relapses may occur in up to 15% of cases, usually within the first 6 months after treatment. Postexposure prophylaxis consists of a 3-week course of doxycycline plus rifampin in most cases. If there is concern for the *B. abortus RB-51*, which is resistant to rifampin, then doxycycline plus TMP/SMX can be used instead. Serial monitoring with serology (not applicable to *B. canis* or *B. abortus RB-51*) should be considered, as per US Centers for Disease Control and Prevention protocol.

Reactive arthritis (**option A**) typically presents a few weeks after a genitourinary (*Chlamydia trachomatis*) or diarrheal illness (*Salmonella, Shigella, Yersinia, Campylobacter*). The classic manifestations include uveitis, aphthous ulceration, asymmetric oligoarthritis, spondylitis or sacroiliitis, and occasionally dermatologic manifestations (circinate balanitis, keratoderma blennorrhagicum). Cytopenia (as seen in this patient) would be unusual, though. Osteoarticular tuberculosis (TB; **option B**) can present very similarly to brucellosis and is one of the most common causes of unilateral sacroiliitis. This patient has no risk factors for TB, which makes this diagnosis less likely. Multiple myeloma (**option D**) can cause pancytopenia and skeletal destruction, but it would be very unusual in a patient of this age. Additional features of myeloma (not seen in this patient) would be hypercalcemia, protein gap (total protein minus albumin greater than 4), and acute kidney injury. Disseminated histoplasmosis (**option E**) can cause constitutional symptoms, pancytopenia, and liver function test abnormalities similar to this case. Disseminated histoplasmosis would be unusual in an immune-competent patient with no known recent exposure (i.e., recent cave exploration).

KEY LEARNING POINT

Brucellosis can manifest in many different ways, which can make the diagnosis challenging. A history of ingestion of unpasteurized dairy or contaminated raw or undercooked meat or exposure to large animals/livestock can be suggestive of the diagnosis.

REFERENCES AND FURTHER READING

- Centers for Disease Control and Prevention. Brucellosis Reference Guide: Exposures, Testing, and Prevention. Available at: https://www.cdc.gov/brucellosis/pdf/brucellosi-reference-guide.pdf. Accessed October 31, 2020.
- Gul H, et al. In: Bennet JE, Dolin R, Blaser MJ, Mandell D, eds. *Bennett's Principles and Practice of Infectious Diseases*. 9th ed. Elsevier; 2020:2753–2758.
- Solís García del Pozo J, Solera J. Systematic review and meta-analysis of randomized clinical trials in the treatment of human brucellosis. *PLoS One*. 2012;7(2). https://doi.org/10.1371/journal.pone.0032090.

A 40-year-old male is admitted to the intensive care unit with shock requiring vasopressor support. He has a history of dental caries and was recently given clindamycin for an odontogenic infection. Toward the end of the course, he started experiencing profuse watery diarrhea, abdominal cramping, and fevers. Upon presentation, vitals showed temperature 102° F, heart rate 120 beats per minute, blood pressure 80/55 mmHg, respiratory rate 20, and oxygen saturation 95% on room air. Examination revealed diffuse abdominal tenderness without rebound. Stool guaiac was negative. Laboratory studies showed white blood cell (WBC) count 20,000 cells/uL, creatinine 2 mg/dL (creatinine clearance 29 mL/min), and lactic acid 5 mmol/L. Abdominal x-ray reveals a nonobstructive gas pattern with concern for ileus. Stool testing for *Clostridioides difficile* has been sent. In addition to surgical consultation, what is the next best step in management?

A. Vancomycin 125 mg PO four times daily.

B. Metronidazole 500 mg IV every 8 hours.

C. Vancomycin 500 mg PO four times daily + rectal vancomycin + metronidazole 500 mg IV q8h.

D. Vancomycin 125 mg PO four times daily + rectal vancomycin + metronidazole 500 mg IV q8h.

E. Fidaxomicin.

The best next step would be vancomycin 500 mg QID + rectal vancomycin + metronidazole 500 mg IV q8h (**option C**). The reason why the other options are incorrect will be evident based on the discussion below.

This patient's presentation is concerning for fulminant *Clostridioides* (formerly *Clostridium*) *difficile* infection. *C. difficile* is a gram-positive spore-forming rod (bacillus) that causes a toxin-mediated diarrheal illness (pseudomembranous colitis). The main risk factors are hospital exposure, antibiotic use (clindamycin has a black box warning), and use of antisecretory drugs

Table 22.1 – Management of *Clostridioides difficile* Infection

Situation	Definition	Management Recommendation
Initial episode—nonsevere	• WBC count <15,000 cells/uL and serum creatinine <1.5 mg/dL	• Preferred—fidaxomicin 200 mg PO BID × 10 days, OR • Alternative—vancomycin 125 mg PO QID × 10 days, OR • Alternative (if above agents cannot be used and nonsevere infection)—metronidazole 500 mg PO every 8 hours × 10–14 days
Initial episode—severe	• WBC count ≥15,000 or serum creatinine ≥1.5 mg/dL	
Fulminant	• Shock/hypotension, ileus, or toxic megacolon	• Vancomycin 500 mg PO QID + metronidazole 500 mg IV every 8 hours + rectal vancomycin (500 mg in 100 mL normal saline every 6 hours via retention enema) if ileus present • Consider surgical consultation (options include subtotal colectomy with rectal preservation or diverting loop ileostomy with colon lavage and antegrade vancomycin flushes)
First recurrence	• Second episode overall	• Preferred—fidaxomicin 200 mg BID×10 days, OR fidaxomicin 200 mg BID×5 days followed by once every other day for 20 days • Alternative 1—prolonged tapered and pulsed oral vancomycin for 6–12 weeks' duration • Alternative 2 (if metronidazole was used for initial episode)—vancomycin 125 mg PO QID × 10 days • Adjunctive therapy—bezlotoxumab 10 mg/kg IV once during administration of standard-of-care *Clostridioides difficile* treatment. Caution with congestive heart failure (CHF)
Second and subsequent recurrences	Third or greater episode overall	• Preferred—fidaxomicin 200 mg BID × 10 days, OR fidaxomicin 200 mg BID × 5 days followed by once every other day for 20 days • Alternative 1—prolonged tapered and pulsed oral vancomycin for 6–12 weeks' duration • Alternative 2—vancomycin 125 mg PO QID × 10 days then rifaximin 400 mg PO TID × 20 days • Fecal microbiota transplant (FMT)—should try medical therapy for at least three total episodes before considering FMT • Adjunctive therapy—bezlotoxumab 10 mg/kg IV once during administration of standard-of-care *C. difficile* treatment. Caution with CHF

such as proton-pump inhibitors (PPIs). *C. difficile* infection can be classified as community-acquired or hospital-acquired, severe (WBC ≥15,000 cells/uL or creatinine ≥1.5 mg/dL) or nonsevere (does not meet severe criteria), or fulminant (presence of shock, ileus, or toxic megacolon). This case is considered fulminant because the patient is in shock and likely has an ileus.

Management of *C. difficile* is contingent upon the severity of illness and whether the infection represents an initial episode or recurrent disease (Table 22.1). In most cases, it is reasonable to start empiric therapy while awaiting results of *C. difficile* testing, especially in fulminant cases. Additional management considerations include discontinuing the offending antibiotic(s) if possible and placing the patient on contact precautions/isolation (even while awaiting the results of testing). Antimotility agents (i.e., loperamide) should generally be avoided. There are some data that show that antisecretory drugs (especially PPIs) increase risk of recurrence, so, if possible, one should discontinue or de-escalate the antisecretory therapy.

KEY LEARNING POINT

Fulminant Clostridioides difficile *is defined by the presence of shock, ileus, or toxic megacolon. Management involves high-dose oral vancomycin, IV metronidazole, and, if ileus is present, rectal vancomycin (retention enema). In addition, consideration should be given to surgical consultation.*

REFERENCES AND FURTHER READING

- McDonald LC, Gerding DN, Johnson S, et al. Clinical Practice Guidelines for *Clostridium difficile* Infection in Adults and Children: 2017 update by the Infectious Diseases Society of America (IDSA) and Society for Healthcare Epidemiology of America (SHEA). *Clin Infect Dis.* 2018;66(7):e1–e48. https://doi.org/10.1093/cid/cix1085.
- Johnson S, Lavergne V, Skinner AM, et al. Clinical Practice Guideline by the Infectious Diseases Society of America (IDSA) and Society for Healthcare Epidemiology of America (SHEA): 2021 Focused Update Guidelines on Management of *Clostridioides difficile* Infection in Adults. *Clin Infect Dis.* 2021;73(5):e1029–e1044. https://doi.org/10.1093/cid/ciab549.

A 30-year-old male is admitted to the hospital with a 3-week history of fevers and confusion. He has a history of poorly-controlled chronic HIV infection. He has not been adherent to his antiretroviral therapy. His medical history is also significant for recurrent pneumonias, herpes zoster, and depression. Medications include sertraline, and acetaminophen as needed. He has no medication allergies. Vital signs show temperature 101° F, heart rate 60 beats per minute, blood pressure 150/90 mmHg, respiratory rate 14, and oxygen saturation 96% on room air. Physical examination shows a confused, malnourished man who has difficulty following simple commands. Fundoscopic examination shows blurred optic disc margins bilaterally. The remainder of the exam is unremarkable. Noncontrast head CT is unremarkable. Work-up reveals:

LABORATORY STUDIES

White blood cell count—3500 cells/uL

Hemoglobin—9 g/dL

Platelets—90,000 cells/uL

Creatinine—1 mg/dL

Albumin—2 g/dL

Liver function testing—normal

CD4 T-lymphocyte count (1 year ago)—110 cells/uL

Toxoplasma IgG—positive

Syphilis screen (treponemal-specific)—negative

Tuberculosis interferon-gamma release assay (TB-IGRA)—negative

Serum cryptococcal antigen—positive

CEREBROSPINAL FLUID ANALYSIS

CSF opening pressure—40 cmH$_2$O (normal level [NL] <18)

CSF white blood cell (WBC) count—100 cells/uL, 80% lymphocytes

CSF protein—200 mg/dL (NL <45)

CSF glucose—40 mg/dL (NL 40–70 mg/dL)

CSF gram stain—many WBCs, no organisms

CSF culture—no growth so far

CSF herpes simplex virus PCR—negative

CSF cryptococcal antigen—pending

Which of the following is the most appropriate next step in the management of this patient?

A. Start liposomal amphotericin-B and flucytosine.
B. Start liposomal amphotericin-B and fluconazole.
C. Repeat lumbar puncture (LP) to remove CSF until pressure declines by at least 50%.
D. Start corticosteroids.
E. Restart antiretroviral therapy.

The most appropriate next step is to repeat an LP to remove CSF until the pressure declines by at least 50% (**option C**). This patient has cryptococcal meningitis. There are two species of *Cryptococcus* that cause disease in humans: *C. neoformans* and *C. gattii* (management is the same for both). *C. gattii* is less common and is found in the Pacific Northwest, United States and Australia. *C. neoformans* is found worldwide in the soil and is classically associated with pigeon droppings. In HIV-infected individuals, the major risk factor is a CD4 count less than 100 cells/uL. Cryptococcal infection initially starts as a pulmonary infection (pneumonia) with subsequent dissemination, which can result in a subacute or chronic meningoencephalitis, cutaneous manifestations (usually umbilicated papular lesions resembling molluscum contagiosum), and other less common manifestations (i.e., genitourinary, etc.). The usual meningitis findings (nuchal rigidity, photophobia, etc.) are not very common, and patients (such as the patient in this case) may present with signs of elevated intracranial pressure (visual disturbances, altered mentation, cranial neuropathies, etc.).

The diagnosis of cryptococcal meningitis should involve an LP. Patients with HIV-associated cryptococcal meningitis typically have very high opening pressures. The CSF profile classically shows a lymphocytic pleocytosis, normal to low glucose, and elevated protein. CSF cryptococcal antigen and culture are positive in most cases. The serum cryptococcal antigen is typically positive in both meningeal and nonmeningeal infections and can be detected well before onset of symptoms. Furthermore, identifying cryptococcus at any site should prompt an LP to rule out central nervous system infection. Lastly, routine blood cultures can detect *Cryptococcus* and are positive in about half of cases.

Management (in the ideal situation) of cryptococcal meningitis in HIV patients can be summarized as follows (Fig. 23.1). The induction phase consists of a combination of amphotericin-B (typically the liposomal formulation, which is better tolerated) and flucytosine (5-FC). The addition of 5-FC is associated with improved survival and more rapid sterilization of the CSF. Alternative induction regimens (**option B**) are considered inferior to this combination. After at least 2 weeks of induction therapy, an LP is repeated. If the repeat CSF culture is negative and the patient has substantially improved, then the therapy can be advanced to the consolidation phase, which consists of at least 8 weeks of higher-dose fluconazole (typically at least 400 mg daily assuming normal renal function). This is followed by the maintenance phase that consists of at least 1 year of lower-dose fluconazole (typically at a dose of 200 mg daily assuming normal renal function). After completion of this phase, the fluconazole can be discontinued if the patient is asymptomatic with a CD4 of at least 100 cell/uL for at least 3 months and a suppressed HIV viral load in response to antiretroviral therapy (ART).

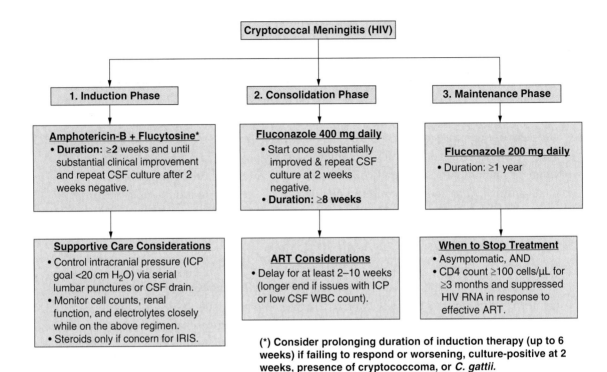

Figure 23.1 – Management of cryptococcal meningitis in HIV-positive patients.
ART, Antiretroviral therapy; *ICP*, intracranial pressure; *IRIS*, immune-reconstitution inflammatory syndrome; *RNA*, ribonucleic acid.

The other vital component to management of cryptococcal meningitis is control of CSF opening pressure (if it is elevated >25 cmH$_2$O). This is typically done via serial (daily) LPs to remove enough CSF to reduce the CSF pressure by at least 50% and to consistently improve symptoms and signs. If refractory or unable to tolerate serial LP, then CSF drainage should be pursued. Corticosteroids (**option D**) have been shown to have increased adverse effects without improving survival. In addition, they have no benefit for reduction of intracranial pressure (ICP). The only potential role for steroids in these patients is for treatment of immune reconstitution inflammatory syndrome (IRIS). Restarting ART (**option E**) is typically delayed by at least 2 weeks and up to 10 weeks in those at higher risk for IRIS (low CSF WBC count, ART-naïve, elevated viral load) or those who had issues with ICP elevation. Restarting ART earlier has been associated with worse outcomes (6-month mortality).

KEY LEARNING POINT

The initial management of cryptococcal meningitis in patients with HIV consists of induction therapy with amphotericin-B and flucytosine. In addition, antiretroviral therapy should be deferred for at least 2 weeks. If cerebrospinal fluid opening pressure is greater than 25 cmH$_2$O, then daily lumbar puncture should be done to relieve the pressure.

REFERENCE AND FURTHER READING

- Panel on Guidelines for the Prevention and Treatment of Opportunistic Infections in Adults and Adolescents with HIV. Guidelines for the Prevention and Treatment of Opportunistic Infections in HIV-infected Adults and Adolescents: Recommendations from the Centers for Disease Control and Prevention, the National Institutes of Health, and the HIV Medicine Association of the Infectious Diseases Society of America. https://clinicalinfo.hiv.gov/sites/default/files/inline-files/adult_oi.pdf. Accessed October 31, 2020.

A 40-year-old female is referred to the infectious disease clinic for a positive *Trypanosoma cruzi* serologic test that was discovered while donating blood. She denies any chest pain, cough, shortness of breath, orthopnea, peripheral edema, exertional difficulty, syncope, dysphagia, abdominal pain, or constipation. She is otherwise healthy and does not take any medications. She has no medication allergies. She was born in Argentina and moved to the United States at the age of 30 years. Vitals signs and physical examination are within normal limits. Labs and electrocardiogram (ECG) are normal. What is the next best step in the management of this patient?

A. Obtain *T. cruzi* serum polymerase chain reaction (PCR).
B. Repeat serology using a different testing format.
C. Obtain a peripheral blood smear.
D. Start nifurtimox.
E. Start benznidazole.

The best answer here is to repeat serology using a different test (**option B**). This patient's presentation is concerning for chronic asymptomatic Chagas disease (the indeterminate form). Chagas disease (American trypanosomiasis) is caused by a protozoan parasite called *T. cruzi*. This parasite is typically transmitted by the bite of the triatomine (reduviid) bug, which is endemic to Central and South America. The bug may also be found in the southern United States. Other modes of transmission include blood transfusions (the United States blood supply is routinely screened), vertical transmission, transplantation, oral ingestion of contaminated foods or drinks, and laboratory accidents.

Acute infection is often asymptomatic. If symptomatic, acute infection presents within a couple of weeks of exposure with fevers, malaise, lymphadenopathy, and hepatosplenomegaly. At the site of inoculation, some patients may develop eyelid swelling (Romana sign, Fig. 24.1)

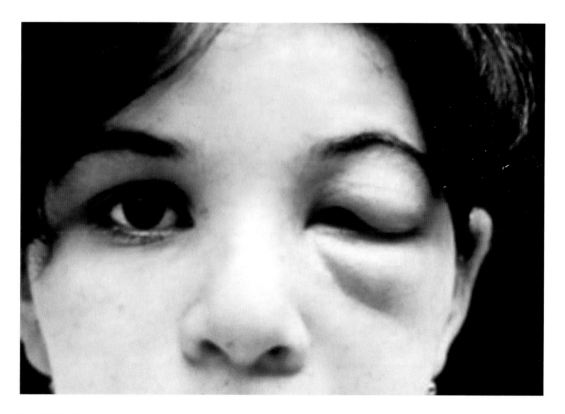

Figure 24.1 – Romana sign.
Photo courtesy of WHO/TDR.

or a skin abscess (chagoma). Additional manifestations of acute infection include myocarditis and meningoencephalitis.

The diagnosis of acute Chagas disease can be established via blood smear (**option C**, Fig. 24.2) or PCR (**option A**). These two tests are also used in the diagnosis of congenital Chagas and reactivation-related Chagas (typically seen in immune-compromised patients). Eventually, after the acute phase resolves, the disease goes on to a chronic asymptomatic form called the indeterminate form of Chagas disease. Most patients will stay in this phase for their entire life, but approximately 20% of patients will progress to the determinate form, which is characterized by cardiomyopathy and/or gastrointestinal (GI) disease. The cardiac manifestations can include congestive heart failure or cardiac rhythm disturbances. The GI manifestations are typically motility disorders (due to destruction of enteric neurons) that result in megaesophagus or megacolon. The diagnosis of the chronic form is typically made with serology (IgG). Based on the World Health Organization recommendation, serologic diagnosis requires positive testing on at least two separate assays that are based on different formats or antigens.

The evaluation should include annual history and physical examination, along with annual ECG. The patient's family members should be referred for evaluation, and patients should not donate blood products. The drug of choice is benznidazole (**option E**), and it is given for

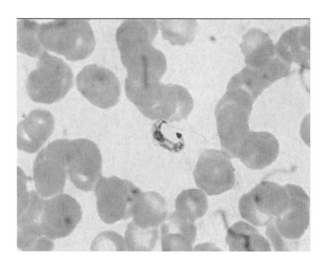

Figure 24.2 – *Trypanosoma cruzi* trypomastigote in blood film.
Nabarro, Laura, et al. Arthropod-Borne Disease. In: *Peter's Atlas of Tropical Medicine and Parasitology*. 7th ed. Elsevier Inc; 2019. Accessed 8/4/21 from https://www.clinicalkey.com/#!/content/book/3-s2.0-B9780702040610000017?scrollTo=%23hl0002390.

60 days. Benznidazole is typically better tolerated than the alternative, which is nifurtimox (**option D**). In addition, nifurtimox has to be given for 90 to 120 days, which makes it less ideal. In general, both drugs can be difficult to tolerate, and adverse effects are not uncommon. Based on the US Centers for Disease Control and Prevention recommendations, the treatment is indicated for patients with acute infection, congenital infection, reactivation-related infection, or chronic infection in patients 18 years of age or younger. Treatment should be considered in those with chronic infection who are 50 years or younger and do not have advanced cardiomyopathy, women of childbearing age, and those with impending immune suppression. Patients older than 50 years can be treated on a case-by-case basis. In general, the treatment is more likely to be effective when it is given as early as possible in the course of the illness. A landmark trial (BENEFIT) showed that benznidazole (compared with placebo) significantly reduced parasitemia but did not affect cardiac clinical deterioration at 5-year follow-up in patients with established Chagas cardiomyopathy. Pregnant patients and those with the determinate form do not benefit from treatment. Some authorities advocate for monitoring annual serology after treatment, because some patients may revert to negative eventually, but this practice is controversial.

KEY LEARNING POINT

In patients with a positive **Trypanosoma cruzi** *serologic test and history consistent with potential Chagas infection, the first step should be to repeat the serology using a different testing platform.*

REFERENCES AND FURTHER READING

- Bern C, Montgomery SP, Herwaldt BL, et al. Evaluation and treatment of Chagas disease in the United States: a systematic review. *JAMA.* 2007;298(18):2171–2181. https://doi.org/10.1001/jama.298.18.2171.
- Bern C. Chagas Disease. *NEJM.* 2015;373(5):456–466. https://doi.org/10.1056/nejmra1410150.
- Meymandi S, Hernandez S, Park S, Sanchez DR, Forsyth C. Treatment of Chagas disease in the United States. *Curr Treat Options Infect Dis.* 2018;10(3):373–388. https://doi.org/10.1007/s40506-018-0170-z.
- Morillo CA, Marin-Neto JA, Avezum A, et al. Randomized trial of benznidazole for chronic Chagas' cardiomyopathy. *N Engl J Med.* 2015;373(14):1295–1306.
- Nabarro L, et al. *Arthropod-borne disease. Peter's Atlas of Tropical Medicine and Parasitology.* 7th ed. Elsevier; 2019.
- Viotti R, Vigliano C, Lococo B, et al. Long-term cardiac outcomes of treating chronic Chagas disease with benznidazole versus no treatment: a nonrandomized trial. *Ann Int Med.* 2006;144(10):724–734.

A 50-year-old male is admitted to the hospital with a 3-day history of worsening cough, sputum production, and shortness of breath. He has a history of chronic obstructive pulmonary disease (COPD) and continues to smoke. He was born in Vietnam and moved to the United States with his family about a decade prior. He does not drink alcohol or use illicit drugs. Vital signs show temperature 100° F, heart rate 100 beats per minute, blood pressure 130/80 mmHg, respiratory rate 24, and oxygen saturation 92% on 4 L/min of oxygen by nasal cannula. Physical examination shows increased work of breathing with pursed-lip breathing, and bilateral expiratory wheezing on lung exam. Labs show white blood cell (WBC) count 12,000 cells/uL (70% neutrophils, 20% lymphocytes, 10% eosinophils). Chest x-ray shows hyperinflation but no infiltrates. He is started on doxycycline, bronchodilators, and high-dose steroids for presumed exacerbation of COPD. The plan is to continue on antibiotics and high-dose steroids for 7 days. He initially improves over the ensuing few days but remains hospitalized due to need for skilled nursing care placement. On the seventh day of hospitalization, he develops fevers, hypotension, altered mental status, and worsening respiratory failure. Labs are repeated and show WBC count 15,000 cells/uL (80% neutrophils, 5% lymphocytes, 0% eosinophils). Repeat chest x-ray shows bilateral airspace opacities. Blood cultures are repeated and are showing polymicrobial growth, including *Klebsiella pneumoniae* and *Enterococcus faecalis*. Sputum cultures are pending. CT scan of the abdomen with contrast shows a nonspecific colitis, but no abdominal abscess or free air. The patient was started on piperacillin/tazobactam and vancomycin and has stabilized. What is the next best step in the management of this patient?

A. De-escalate antibiotic therapy to ertapenem monotherapy.

B. Repeat blood cultures.

C. Obtain targeted serologic testing.

D. Start ivermectin.

E. Start albendazole.

The next best step would be to start ivermectin (**option D**). This patient's presentation is highly concerning for severe strongyloidiasis (disseminated infection or hyperinfection). Strongyloidiasis is typically caused by a nematode known as *Strongyloides stercoralis*. This infection is acquired in tropical or subtropical regions of the world, as well as in the southeast United States (Kentucky, Tennessee, etc.). The parasite larvae enter the host via the skin, usually in those who walk barefoot on contaminated soil, but transmission can also occur sexually (fecal-oral contact), with organ transplantation, or via ingestion of contaminated food or water. The infective larval forms then travel (via the bloodstream) to the alveoli, where they can be coughed up and then swallowed to enter the gastrointestinal (GI) tract. There, they mature, reproduce, and undergo the autoinfection cycle (essentially a repeat of the process discussed up until now). Patients with impaired cell-mediated immunity (i.e., someone who receives high-dose steroids, such as this patient, patients with HTLV-1 infection, etc.) can develop severe strongyloidiasis (either hyperinfection or disseminated infection). Hyperinfection represents an accelerated form of the usual cycle with overwhelming infection in the skin, GI tract, and lungs. Disseminated infection involves infection in other organs that are not traditionally involved in the life cycle of the organism. When these severe infections occur, the migrating worms may carry enteric bacteria with them and classically cause a gram-negative bacteremia and even gram-negative meningitis (a classic tip-off).

The clinical presentation is variable, and most acute and chronic infections are asymptomatic. Acute infection typically manifests as an erythematous pruritic or urticarial rash ("ground itch") at the site of entry that resembles cutaneous larval migrans. This is followed by a pulmonary syndrome that resembles bronchitis or pneumonia called Loeffler syndrome. The classic GI symptoms typically show up last. Eventually, a chronic infection is established and is characterized by GI and pulmonary symptoms similar to acute infection. A pathognomonic rash called larva currens (Fig. 25.1) may occur; this is described as a serpiginous maculopapular or urticarial rash (represents intradermal larval migration) and commonly affects the perianal region or the thighs. Approximately three quarters of patients with chronic infection have a mild eosinophilia. Hyperinfection manifests with overwhelming infection in the gut, skin, and lungs, while disseminated infection is characterized by widespread dissemination to multiple organs (gram-negative bacteremia and meningitis is a classic association). These more severe infections carry a very high mortality, and these patients are considered highly infectious (contact precautions should be used when dealing with these patients). Eosinophilia is actually fairly uncommon in these severe forms, probably due to the use of immune suppression (i.e., steroids), which incites the infection but also kills off eosinophils, as seen in this case.

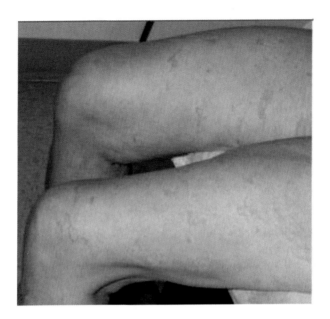

Figure 25.1 – Larva currens
Pichard DC, Hensley JR , Williams E, Apolo AB, Klion AD, DiGiovanna JJ. Rapid development of migratory, linear and serpiginous lesions in association with immunosuppression. *J Am Acad Dermatol*. 2014;70(6):1130-1134.

Stool microscopy and smear (ova and parasites) is considered the gold standard diagnostic test in strongyloidiasis, but up to seven stool samples may be necessary for optimal sensitivity. Duodenal aspirate or biopsy may be more sensitive. Stool culture is time-consuming and not commonly employed. The ELISA IgG serologic test (**option C**) is the most commonly employed serologic test. It cannot distinguish prior infection from current infection, but it can be used to monitor response to therapy (most patients become seronegative within 6 months after treatment). The serologic tests may cross-react (cause false-positives) with other parasitic infections, including *Schistosoma, Ascaris,* and *Filaria*. The serologic test may be falsely negative in patients with severe immune compromise. For severe infections, examination of respiratory and GI specimens may be very high-yield, so the case should be discussed with the microbiology lab if possible.

The management of strongyloidiasis is summarized in Table 25.1. Ivermectin (**option D**) is the drug of choice and is likely the most efficacious. It is reasonable to start ivermectin empirically in patients with suspected severe strongyloidiasis (such as this patient). An alternative drug, albendazole (**option E**), may be used but is likely less efficacious than

Table 25.1 – Management of Strongyloidiasis

Situation	First-Line Treatment	Alternative Treatments
Acute or chronic infection	• Ivermectin 200 ug/kg PO once daily ×1–2 days. Some experts advocate for two doses 2 weeks apart • Contraindications—*Loa Loa* infection (may precipitate encephalopathy, so consider ruling out with blood smear), weight <15 kg, or pregnant/lactating women	• Thiabendazole ×3 days—similar efficacy to ivermectin • Albendazole ×3–7 days (less efficacious than ivermectin) • Mebendazole ×3 days (less efficacious than ivermectin)
Hyperinfection or disseminated infection	• Ivermectin 200 ug/kg PO once daily until resolution of symptoms and negative results on stool and/or sputum smear for at least 2 weeks • Some advocate for dual therapy with ivermectin and albendazole	• If unable to tolerate PO (ileus, obstruction, malabsorption), then consider rectal or subcutaneous (veterinary formulation) administration

Other considerations	• Stop immune suppression if possible
	• Administer antibiotic therapy for concurrent bacterial infections (usually bacteremia or meningitis). This is typically done empirically by some
	• **Monitoring after treatment:**
	  • Serology—Reduction in antibody titers 6–12 months post-treatment may indicate successful treatment. Recommendation is to repeat every 3–6 months for up to 2 years
	  • Repeat complete blood count with differential every 3 months for up to 12 months—reduction in eosinophilia is suggestive of treatment success
	  • Stool microscopy—if initial positive results, then follow-up stool exam should be performed after 2–4 weeks of treatment if symptoms are persistent. If still positive, then retreatment is indicated
	  • Failure to respond should prompt testing for HTLV-1 infection	

Prophylaxis	• Done if anticipated immune suppression and positive serology • Regimen is ivermectin 200 ug/kg PO daily for 2 days and then repeat in 2 weeks	

ivermectin. Thiabendazole is another alternative that likely has similar efficacy as ivermectin but is less well-tolerated. Repeating blood cultures (**option B**) is not routinely necessary in gram-negative bacteremia but can be considered if the patient does not improve or has a line in place that cannot be removed. De-escalation to ertapenem (**option A**) would likely cover the *K. pneumoniae*, but it would not cover *Enterococcus*. Therefore, this would not be a wise choice.

KEY LEARNING POINT

Severe strongyloidiasis infection (disseminated infection or hyperinfection) should be suspected in patients with epidemiologic exposure (i.e., from endemic region) who have received immune suppression. The classic presentation is shock due to gram-negative bacteremia (and often meningitis), and potentially multiorgan system failure. Eosinophilia is not commonly seen, so a high index of suspicion is necessary, as the disease is associated with a very high rate of mortality. Treatment of choice is ivermectin.

REFERENCES AND FURTHER READING

- Boggild AK, Libman M, Greenaway C, McCarthy AE. Committee to Advise on Tropical Medicine and Travel (CATMAT). CATMAT statement on disseminated strongyloidiasis: prevention, assessment and management guidelines. *Can Commun Dis Rep.* 2016;42(1):12–19. https://doi.org/10.14745/ccdr.v42i01a03.
- Buonfrate D, Requena-Mendez A, Angheben A, et al. Severe strongyloidiasis: a systematic review of case reports. *BMC Infect Dis.* 2013;13:78. https://doi.org/10.1186/1471-2334-13-78.
- Centers for Disease Control and Prevention. Strongyloidiasis: Resources for health professionals. Available at: https://www.cdc.gov/parasites/strongyloides/health_professionals/index.html. Accessed November 1, 2020.
- Mejia R, et al. *Intestinal nematodes (roundworms). Mandell, Douglas, and Bennett's Principles and Practice of Infectious Diseases.* 9th ed. Elsevier; 2020:3436–3442.
- Pichard DC, Hensley JR, Williams E, Apolo AB, Klion AD, DiGiovanna JJ. Rapid development of migratory, linear, and serpiginous lesions in association with immunosuppression. *J Am Acad Dermatol.* 2014;70(6):1130–1134. https://doi.org/10.1016/j.jaad.2013.11.036.

A 40-year-old male is brought to the emergency room by paramedics after suffering a tonic-clonic seizure while grocery shopping. Not much is known about the man, as he is confused and can only mumble a few nonsensical things in Spanish. Vitals show temperature 99° F, heart rate 70 beats per minute, blood pressure 150/90 mmHg, respiratory rate 16, and oxygen saturation 98% on 2 L/min oxygen by nasal cannula. Examination shows a confused male of Hispanic descent. There are no focal neurologic findings. Remainder of the examination is unremarkable. Basic laboratory studies are normal. Toxicology screen is negative. Noncontrast head CT shows scattered parenchymal calcifications and obstructive hydrocephalus. There are no foci of hemorrhage evident. Follow-up MRI with contrast shows similar findings, but the radiologist notes that the findings are concerning for neurocysticercosis. Appropriate serologic testing is sent off. Continuous EEG monitoring and antiepileptic drug therapy are initiated. What is the most appropriate next step in management?

A. Albendazole.
B. Praziquantel.
C. Dexamethasone.
D. Neurosurgical consultation.
E. Albendazole plus praziquantel.

The most appropriate next step is to consult the neurosurgical team (**option D**). This patient's presentation is concerning for neurocysticercosis, which is a disease caused by the pork tapeworm called *Taenia solium*. This tapeworm is found worldwide, especially in less developed countries (such as those in Africa, Southeast Asia, Central and South America). The life cycle is somewhat complex. Cysticercosis is only acquired via the fecal-oral route—ingestion of eggs or proglottids (which are shed in the stool) from feces-contaminated food/water or person-to-person transmission. Once ingested, they will hatch in the intestine, invade into the bloodstream, and migrate to various organs or tissues (including the central nervous system [CNS]), where they mature into adult worms called cysticerci. Intestinal taeniasis, on the other hand, is associated with ingestion of adult tapeworms (cysticerci) in undercooked pork and does not cause neurocysticercosis.

The incubation period is typically long, and the presentation depends on various factors, including the characteristics of the cysticerci (i.e., location, size, number, and stage) and the degree of inflammatory response to the degenerating cysts. Intestinal taeniasis manifests as a gastrointestinal illness that may be associated with eosinophilia. Cysticercosis is characterized by cysticerci in various organs, typically striated muscle, as well as in the skin and soft tissue (tender nodules). Neurocysticercosis (NCC) can be parenchymal or extraparenchymal (including the spine and eyes). NCC can present with seizures (by far the most common presentation), cerebral edema, hydrocephalus, chronic meningoencephalitis, ocular involvement, cranial neuropathies, strokes, and even death. Viable cysts often do not cause much inflammation, but degenerating cysts do (due to release of antigens as they degenerate). Calcified lesions are considered nonviable (i.e., dead parasites), but they can still induce seizures. Sometimes, plain x-ray can visualize calcified cysts within skeletal muscle.

The diagnosis of *T. solium* infection should be made in the appropriate host with a consistent clinical presentation, in combination with characteristic imaging findings and positive serology. There are two serologic testing formats: enzyme-linked immunoblot transfer assay (EITB) or commercial enzyme-linked immunoassay. The EITB is the preferred serologic test, as it provides more clinical data and has better sensitivity and specificity, especially with an increased number of lesions. Of note, these serologic tests cannot distinguish between active and inactive disease, and there may be cross-reactivity with other parasitic infections such as *Echinococcus*. Microscopic demonstration of *T. solium* in tissue constitutes a definitive diagnosis. CNS imaging should be considered. CT may be better at showing calcific disease, whereas MRI is better for most other aspects (edema, cyst staging, etc.). Both a brain MRI and a noncontrast head CT are recommended by the Infectious Diseases Society of America

(IDSA)/American Society of Tropical Medicine and Hygiene (ASTMH) guidelines (see references) for appropriate staging. MRI of the spine should be considered as well to look for spinal foci of infection. Cerebrospinal fluid analysis (CSF) classically shows a mononuclear or eosinophilic pleocytosis. Ophthalmologic examination should be considered to rule out ocular infection before providing treatment, because the antiparasitic therapy is associated with an inflammatory response that can cause vision loss.

The treatment of NCC can be a bit nuanced (Fig. 26.1). The mainstay of management is supportive therapy in symptomatic patients, which includes controlling seizures (antiepileptic drugs), relieving hydrocephalus (CSF shunting), and managing cerebral edema. This is why **option D** is the best choice in this case. Antiparasitic therapy (**options A and B**) is hardly ever an urgent matter in these cases. The antiparasitic drug of choice in NCC is typically albendazole ($\geq$2-week course), as it has been shown to be superior to praziquantel for treatment of NCC. Antiparasitic therapy (APT) may worsen symptoms initially because it kills viable cysts, which results in release of more antigen and subsequent inflammatory response (this is why APT is avoided in situations where there is untreated hydrocephalus or diffuse cerebral edema). This inflammatory reaction can be managed with steroids that penetrate into the CNS (usually dexamethasone [**option C**]). In general, steroids should be given whenever APT is given. An important point to remember is to rule out tuberculosis and strongyloidiasis before administering high-dose steroids.

The most recent guidelines from the US Centers for Disease Control and Prevention and IDSA/ASTMH recommend APT in symptomatic patients with multiple, live cysticerci (i.e., not calcified, because APT will not benefit patients with calcified [dead] cysts). Intraventricular cysts should typically be removed surgically, and APT should be avoided due to risk of precipitating obstructive hydrocephalus. Cysticercal encephalitis with diffuse cerebral edema should be managed with steroids, but APT should be avoided due to risk of worsening edema. Ocular infection should be managed with surgical removal. Albendazole monotherapy is sufficient in most cases. Combination therapy (**option E**) can be considered in those with greater than two viable parenchymal cysticerci, or if there is subarachnoid NCC. Subarachnoid NCC typically requires the most aggressive management, with prolonged medical treatment with APT, steroids (methotrexate can be used as a steroid-sparing agent), and surgical intervention. An MRI should be repeated at least every 6 months until resolution of the cystic component. Retreatment should be considered if the lesions persist past 6 months. Intestinal taeniasis can be treated with a one-time dose of praziquantel, but there is a risk of precipitating a seizure if there were underlying NCC lesions that went unnoticed. Other

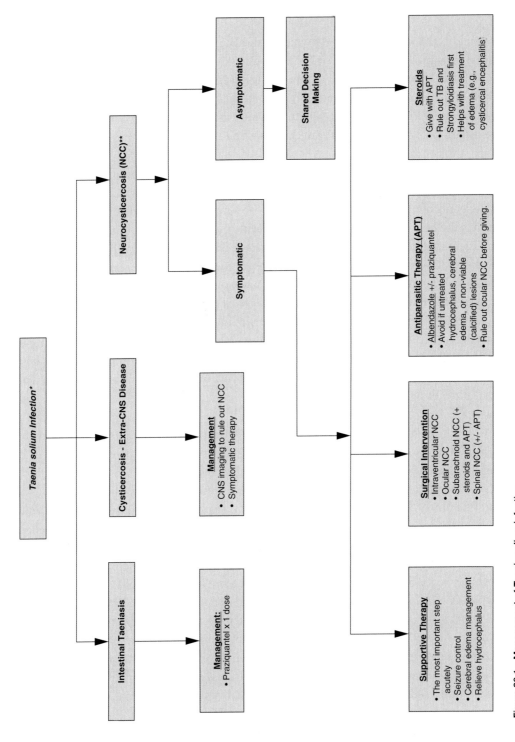

Figure 26.1 – Management of *Taenia solium* infection.

*, Screen household members for infection; **, defer treatment in pregnant patients until after pregnancy; *CNS*, central nervous system; *TB*, tuberculosis.

extraneural disease generally requires only symptomatic therapy, but imaging of the CNS should be pursed to evaluate for NCC. In pregnant patients, treatment should be deferred until after pregnancy. Lastly, household members should also be screened for the infection.

KEY LEARNING POINT

The most important component of managing an acute symptomatic case of neurocysticercosis is supportive care (seizure control, cerebral edema management, hydrocephalus relief, etc.). Antiparasitic therapy (typically either albendazole or praziquantel) and steroids (typically dexamethasone) are hardly ever an emergency.

REFERENCES AND FURTHER READING

- White AC, Coyle CM, Rajshekhar V Jr., et al. Diagnosis and treatment of neurocysticercosis: 2017 Clinical Practice Guidelines by the Infectious Diseases Society of America (IDSA) and the American Society of Tropical Medicine and Hygiene (ASTMH). *Clin Infect Dis.* 2018;66(8):e49–e75. https://doi.org/10.1093/cid/cix1084.
- Centers for Disease Control and Prevention. Parasites—Cysticercosis. Resources for Health Professionals. https://www.cdc.gov/parasites/cysticercosis/health_professionals/index.html. Accessed November 2, 2020.
- Centers for Disease Control and Prevention. DPDx—Laboratory identification of parasites of public health concern—cysticercosis (*Taenia solium*). https://www.cdc.gov/dpdx/cysticercosis/index.html. Accessed November 2, 2020.

A 60-year-old male is admitted to the hospital with shortness of breath and increasing peripheral edema. He has not had any fevers or chills. He has a history of congestive heart failure, chronic kidney disease, and coronary artery disease. Medications include aspirin, atorvastatin, nitroglycerin, metoprolol, lisinopril, and furosemide. Surgical history is notable for placement of an implantable cardioverter-defibrillator (ICD) 2 years ago. Vital signs show temperature 98° F, heart rate 110 beats per minute, blood pressure 95/65 mmHg, respiratory rate 24, and oxygen saturation 95% on 3 L/min nasal cannula. Physical examination reveals a thin male in mild distress. Heart is regular and tachycardic. There is no murmur. Lung exam shows bibasilar crackles. Abdomen is mildly distended, but there is no tenderness. The ICD pocket site looks and feels normal. There is 2 to 3+ peripheral edema extending up to the level of the lower thighs. Labs shows white blood cell count 11,000 cells/uL (75% neutrophils), hemoglobin 16 g/dL, creatinine 1.5 mg/dL (creatinine clearance 35 mL/min), and B-type natriuretic peptide 1000 pg/mL (normal <100 pg/mL). Transthoracic echocardiogram reveals an ejection fraction of 30%, global left-ventricular hypokinesis, and no vegetations on the valves or ICD leads. Blood cultures (two peripheral sets) were drawn on admission and are growing *Staphylococcus epidermidis* in the aerobic bottle of one of the blood culture sets (time to positivity 26 hours). The other blood culture set is negative so far. The patient has not received any antibiotics to date. What is the next best step in management?

A. Start vancomycin.
B. Repeat blood cultures.
C. Obtain a transesophageal echocardiogram (TEE).
D. Obtain antimicrobial sensitivity profile before starting antibiotics.
E. Start cefazolin.

The next best step would be to repeat blood cultures (**option B**). This patient has an acute exacerbation of heart failure, which likely explains the entire clinical presentation. Blood cultures were drawn for an unknown reason and now are growing a coagulase-negative *Staphylococcus* species (*S. epidermidis*) in one out of four blood culture bottles. This low-grade positivity likely represents blood culture contamination, which typically occurs during the process of specimen acquisition and/or processing. Prior to starting antibiotics, blood cultures should be repeated. If repeat blood cultures are negative in the setting of no prior antibiotic therapy, then it is fairly likely that the organism represents blood culture contamination. On the other hand, if an antibiotic is started prior to repeating blood cultures (**options A and E**), and then if the repeat blood cultures are negative, it would be very difficult to decide whether the situation represents a real infection or contamination. Furthermore, if antibiotics were to be started, vancomycin would be a better choice than cefazolin, because many *S. epidermidis* strains are methicillin-resistant. Obtaining a TEE (**option C**) may be useful if there is significant concern for infection of the ICD. *S. epidermidis* can infect prosthetic devices such as ICDs, and if the repeat blood culture is positive there is potentially more cause for concern. Obtaining a TEE at this time may be a bit premature. Lastly, many microbiology laboratories

Table 27.1 – Considerations when interpreting blood culture results

Consideration	Comments
Organism identity	• Common contaminants include coagulase-negative staphylococci, *Bacillus* spp. (but not *B. anthracis*), *Corynebacterium* spp. ("diphtheroids"), *Cutibacterium* (formerly *Propionibacterium*) acnes, *Micrococcus*, and even viridans-group streptococci
Number of positive sets	• Each blood culture set consists of an aerobic bottle and an anaerobic bottle, and in most situations at least two sets are drawn (equivalent to four total bottles: two aerobic and two anaerobic) • More sets positive→higher likelihood of true infection
Number of positive bottles within a set	• Similar concept to the blood set discussion above • More bottles positive→higher likelihood of true infection
Source of culture	• If blood cultures are drawn from a catheter, then positive results can reflect true infection, catheter colonization, or contamination • One should always try to draw a concurrent peripheral blood culture set any time a catheter blood culture is obtained in order to appropriately determine whether a real infection is present
Time to growth	• The faster the organism grows, the more likely it is to represent a true infection
Clinical context	• This is arguably one of the most important considerations • True infection is more likely if the patient was septic at the time of blood culture acquisition and/or if the clinical context is appropriate for infection with the identified organism (i.e., coagulase-negative *Staphylococcus* in a blood culture in a patient with an indwelling device or hardware)

do not routinely perform antimicrobial sensitivity testing (AST) on most *coagulase-negative Staphylococcus species*, unless requested. Obtaining AST prior to starting antibiotics (**option D**) in this case would not be necessary, as there are several worthy options for empiric therapy, but AST may eventually be needed down the line for potential oral treatment options.

In general, almost any organism recovered in blood cultures could potentially cause a true infection. Therefore, one should always analyze each blood culture result in a systematic way. Table 27.1 lists some general considerations that can be applied.

KEY LEARNING POINT

When trying to determine whether a blood culture result represents a true infection or not, always consider the identity of the organism, the number of sets/bottles that are positive, the source of the culture, the time to growth, and, most importantly, the clinical context. In addition, repeating blood cultures before starting antibiotics can be helpful as well.

REFERENCE AND FURTHER READING

- Dargère S, Cormier H, Verdon R. Contaminants in blood cultures: importance, implications, interpretation and prevention. *Clin Microbiol Infect.* 2018;24(9):964–969. https://doi.org/10.1016/j.cmi.2018.03.030.

A 47-year-old male has been hospitalized for approximately 1 month now. He was admitted for conditioning chemotherapy and eventually underwent an allogeneic hematopoietic stem cell transplant 14 days ago for an acute myelogenous leukemia. He has been severely neutropenic (zero neutrophils) for almost 3 weeks now. He is currently on prophylactic antimicrobials including cefepime, voriconazole, and acyclovir. Today, he spiked a temperature of 102° F. He has been hemodynamically stable otherwise. Examination is largely unremarkable. He has a right upper extremity peripherally inserted central catheter (PICC) in place that shows no signs of infection. Labs show white blood cell count 0 cells/uL, hemoglobin 7.2 g/dL, platelet count 12,000 cells/uL, creatinine 1.0 mg/dL (creatinine clearance 70 mL/min), and normal liver function testing. Blood cultures are drawn from the PICC line and the left antecubital vein. The primary care team inquiries about ordering a 1,3-beta-D-glucan (BDG) test for the patient. The BDG test is least likely to be helpful for which of the following fungal infections?

A. *Mucorales* spp.
B. *Aspergillus* spp.
C. *Candida* spp.
D. *Fusarium* spp.
E. *Pneumocystis jirovecii.*

The correct answer is *Mucorales* species (**option A**), as discussed later. The other fungal organisms presented in the case (**options B, C, D, and E**) would likely cause a positive BDG.

1,3-beta-D-glucan (BDG) is found in the cell walls of most fungal organisms except for *Cryptococcus*, *Mucorales*, and *Blastomyces* (which either do not produce BDG or do so in very small amounts that are not detectable). This antigen can be detected even before symptoms of invasive fungal infection (IFI) appear. A positive BDG test is suggestive of IFI, but the result should always be interpreted in context (i.e., clinically correlated with other clinical and microbiologic data). In addition, the utility may be best for patients that are high-risk for IFI (i.e., stem cell transplant recipients, neutropenic patients, etc.). Serially positive BDG tests can be more meaningful that an isolated positive test. The BDG test has a high negative predictive value for *P. jirovecii* infection, so a negative test may be helpful in ruling out pneumocystis infection in patients with a low pretest probability. A single negative BDG test result should not solely be relied on to rule out other IFIs. The sensitivity may be reduced in those receiving prior antifungal therapy. Furthermore, there is some evidence that BDG testing can be used to assess treatment response, as it will decline with appropriate therapy (most of these data comes from invasive *Candida* infections), but this is a controversial practice. Similarly, a rising BDG level may not necessarily indicate treatment failure. There are various causes of false-positive BDG test results, including recent hemodialysis (especially using cellulose membranes), treatment with certain blood products (intravenous immune globulin or albumin), certain antibiotics (classically intravenous amoxicillin/clavulanic acid and piperacillin/tazobactam, but this may be less likely nowadays), infection with some bacteria (i.e., *Pseudomonas*, *Enterococcus*), or exposure to glucan-containing gauze during surgery.

Another commonly used fungal antigen is the serum galactomannan (GAL) test. GAL is a polysaccharide antigen found in the cell walls of certain fungi, and it is most commonly used to diagnose invasive aspergillosis. Other fungal organisms that produce GAL include *Penicillium* spp., *Paecilomyces* spp., *Fusarium* spp., *Blastomyces* spp., and *Histoplasma* spp. The test is most useful for patients with high risk of invasive aspergillosis, such as hematopoietic stem cell transplant recipients. It is not recommended for screening in solid-organ transplant patients or in patients with chronic granulomatous disease. GAL becomes positive before clinical symptoms appear; thus, it can be monitored in high-risk patients to allow preemptive initiation of antifungal therapy. Similar to the BDG test, a single positive test should always be interpreted in context, and a single negative test cannot completely rule out invasive aspergillosis. Serial GAL testing should be considered to help with diagnosis, and at least two consecutive GAL tests should be obtained before officially calling it a positive test. The sensitivity declines with prior use of antifungal therapy with mold activity. GAL levels decline with appropriate therapy, so GAL can be used to monitor therapeutic response. False-positive results can be seen in patients receiving Plasma-Lyte fluid, certain antibiotics (similar to BDG), certain bacteria (i.e., *Bifidobacterium*), and certain food that contain GAL (i.e., pasta) that can translocate the gut during gastrointestinal disruption (i.e., mucositis). The GAL test can also be done on bronchoalveolar lavage (BAL) fluid. Compared with the serum GAL, the BAL GAL is more sensitive but less specific for the diagnosis of invasive aspergillosis.

KEY LEARNING POINT

1,3-beta-D-glucan is a component of the cell walls of many fungal organisms, but not of **Cryptococcus, Mucorales,** *or* **Blastomyces.**

REFERENCES AND FURTHER READING

- Theel E. Detection of (1→3)-β-D-glucan as a marker of invasive fungal disease. *Insights.* news.mayocliniclabs. com/2019/09/09/detection-of-13-%CE%B2-d-glucan-as-a-marker-of-invasive-fungal-disease/. Accessed June 18, 2020.
- Pappas PG, Kauffman CA, Andes DR, et al. Clinical practice guideline for the management of candidiasis: 2016 update by the Infectious Diseases Society of America. *Clin Infect Dis.* 2016;62(4):e1–e50. https://doi.org/10.1093/cid/civ933.
- Ramanan P, Wengenack NL, Theel ES. Laboratory diagnostics for fungal infections: a review of current and future diagnostic assays. *Clin Chest Med.* 2017;38(3):535–554. https://doi.org/10.1016/j.ccm.2017.04.013.
- Patterson TF, Thompson GR III, Denning DW, et al. Practice guidelines for the diagnosis and management of aspergillosis: 2016 update by the Infectious Diseases Society of America. *Clin Infect Dis.* 2016;63(4):e1–e60. https://doi.org/10.1093/cid/ciw326.

A 65-year-old male is admitted to the hospital with fevers, and right-sided facial swelling. He has a history of type 2 diabetes mellitus, peripheral neuropathy, and insomnia. His medications include insulin, metformin, atorvastatin, and amitriptyline. His vaccinations are up to date. Vital signs show temperature 101° F, heart rate 95 beats per minute, blood pressure 115/80 mmHg, respiratory rate 16, and oxygen saturation 98% on room air. Examination shows swelling, warmth, and tenderness over the right parotid region. His dentition is in poor repair, with obvious dental caries. Mucus membranes are dry, and there is no cervical lymphadenopathy. The remainder of the exam is unremarkable. Laboratory testing is significant for white blood cell count 11,000 cells/uL. Blood cultures are drawn. Which of the following pathogens is the most likely cause of this patient's presentation?

A. Mumps virus.

B. *Candida albicans.*

C. *Staphylococcus aureus.*

D. *Mycobacterium tuberculosis.*

E. *Fusobacterium necrophorum.*

The most likely cause is *S. aureus* (**option C**). This patient is presenting with acute suppurative parotitis (ASP), which is also known as acute suppurative sialadenitis. ASP results from any situation in which the natural flow of saliva is impaired. When the flow of saliva is impaired, bacteria (typically *S. aureus*, but also oral flora including gram-negatives and anaerobes [**option E**]) can ascend the parotid (Stenson's) duct and infect the parotid gland. *Streptococcus* spp. and *Hemophilus influenzae* are also fairly common causes. Rarely, the infection can arise from hematogenous dissemination or spread from a contiguous focus of infection (i.e., dental infection). Typical predisposing situations include dehydration/dry mouth (typically elderly or drug-induced, as in this patient), immune suppression, Sjogren's syndrome, ductal stones, malnutrition or debilitation, and postoperative state. This infection can present with fevers, acute onset of painful, often unilateral parotid swelling, warmth and erythema, and purulent discharge from the parotid duct (may require parotid massage to express purulence).

Viral parotitis is more likely to be bilateral and does not usually manifest with purulence. Viral causes include mumps virus (the most common viral cause, **option A**), HIV, enteroviruses, Epstein–Barr virus, influenza, parainfluenza, cytomegalovirus, and lymphocytic choriomeningitis virus. Fungal (**option B**) and mycobacterial (**option D**) etiologies are rare causes of parotitis. Differential diagnosis also includes inflammatory disorders (sarcoidosis, IgG-4–related disease, etc.) and malignancy (primary parotid tumors and lymphoma).

The diagnosis of parotitis should include Gram stain and culture of expressed ductal purulence (caveat being that oral flora may contaminate this process), as well as imaging to rule out stones (sialoliths) and abscess. A reasonable initial imaging test is an ultrasound; if indeterminate, then additional imaging may include CT scan or MRI. Sialography can be used in chronic cases but should be avoided acutely due to risk of ductal rupture and worsening pain. Needle aspiration for Gram stain and culture is considered the most definitive test for identifying the causative organism, and this test is probably most useful if there is an associated fluid collection or abscess.

The management of ASP is multifaceted. Supportive measures that should be employed include hydration, warm compresses, parotid gland massage, avoidance of inciting factors (i.e., anticholinergic medication), and administration of sialagogues to improve salivary flow. If an abscess is present, it should be drained if feasible. Empiric antibiotics should cover *S. aureus* (including methicillin-resistant *S. aureus* [MRSA]) and oral flora. Patients who are immune-compromised or severely ill should receive broader empiric therapy, including coverage for MRSA, *Pseudomonas*, and anaerobic organisms. Eventually the regimen can be tailored to the causative organism(s) plus or minus ongoing coverage for oral flora, regardless of whether oral microbes were recovered or not. Typical treatment duration is 10 to 14 days. Complications include extension into deeper infections such as Ludwig angina, facial nerve dysfunction or paralysis, and fistula formation. Development of any of these complications or failure to improve with conservative management should prompt surgical intervention. Follow-up imaging at the end of therapy can be considered, especially if there is concern for underlying malignancy.

KEY LEARNING POINT

The most common bacterial cause of acute suppurative parotitis is **Staphylococcus aureus.** *The most common viral cause is mumps.*

REFERENCES AND FURTHER READING

- Brook I. Acute bacterial suppurative parotitis: microbiology and management. *J Craniofac Surg.* 2003;14(1):37–40. https://doi.org/10.1097/00001665-200301000-00006.
- Fattahi TT, Lyu PE, Van Sickels JE. Management of acute suppurative parotitis. *J Oral Maxillofac Surg.* 2002;60(4):446–448. https://doi.org/10.1053/joms.2002.31234.
- Wilson KF, Meier JD, Ward PD. Salivary gland disorders. *Am Fam Physician.* 2014;89(11):882–888.

A 50-year-old male is admitted to the hospital with a 2-month history of fevers, weight loss, abdominal pain, diarrhea, and joint pains. He does not like to come to the doctor. He was apparently "dragged in" by his wife because "he was not acting like his usual self." Vital signs show temperature 100.8° F, heart rate 90 beats per minute, blood pressure 105/70 mmHg, respiratory rate 16, and oxygen saturation 96% on room air. Physical examination reveals a thin man with temporal wasting. There is conjunctival pallor. He has palpable cervical lymphadenopathy. Heart exam shows a grade II/VI systolic heart murmur. Lungs are clear. Abdomen is soft and diffusely tender without rebound tenderness. His skin appears tan. He has discomfort with passive range of motion in both knees and his left wrist. He is able to tell you his own name but not his current location or the day of the week. The remainder of the examination is within normal limits. Labs show white blood cell count 12,000 cells/µL, hemoglobin 8 g/dL with mean corpuscular volume 78 fL, platelet count 450,000 cells/µL, creatinine 0.8 mg/dL (creatinine clearance 75 mL/min), albumin 2 g/dL, and C-reactive protein 15 mg/dL (normal <1.0 mg/dL). Tuberculosis skin testing shows 0 mm induration. HIV antigen/antibody screen is negative. Which of the following tests is the most appropriate to do next to establish a definitive diagnosis for this patient's presentation?

A. Transthoracic echocardiogram.
B. Transesophageal echocardiogram.
C. Colonoscopy.
D. Upper endoscopy.
E. Three sets of blood cultures.

The correct answer is upper endoscopy (**option D**). This patient's presentation is most consistent with Whipple disease, which is a rare disease that classically affects middle-aged White men (mean age is mid-50s). This disease is caused by *Tropheryma whipplei*, a gram-positive bacillus that is found commonly in the soil, in sewage workers, and in rural Africa (i.e., Senegal and West Africa). The transmission of this organism is likely oral-oral (saliva) or fecal-oral (feces). This transmission can result in a self-limited acute infection, asymptomatic infection (positive serology but no symptoms) with chronic carriage (saliva, dental plaque, feces), or a chronic infection (classic multisystemic Whipple disease or chronic localized disease).

Acute infection can manifest as a gastroenteritis, bacteremia, or an acute pneumonia and is typically self-limited. This can be followed by seroconversion and cure, chronic carriage, or a chronic infection. The presentation of chronic infection consists of constitutional symptoms (fevers, weight loss), gastrointestinal (GI) symptoms (malabsorptive diarrhea, abdominal pain), polyarthralgia or polyarthritis (nonerosive, often misdiagnosed or mistreated as an inflammatory arthritis), lymphadenopathy, and central nervous system (CNS) disturbances such as memory problems (cognitive impairment), cerebellar signs (ataxia), and psychiatric manifestations. Rarely, one can see cardiac involvement ("culture-negative" endocarditis, pericarditis, myocarditis), ocular manifestations (uveitis, supranuclear ophthalmoplegia with pathognomonic oculomasticatory or oculofacial myorhythmia), and skin hyperpigmentation. A triad of dementia, supranuclear ophthalmoplegia, and myoclonus is highly suggestive. The various manifestations of Whipple disease are summarized in Table 30.1.

Laboratory testing can show anemia of chronic disease, leukocytosis with occasional eosinophilia, thrombocytopenia or thrombocytosis, elevated inflammatory markers, and evidence of malabsorption (hypoalbuminemia, vitamin and mineral deficiencies, etc.).

Table 30.1 – Manifestations of Whipple Disease

Acute Whipple Disease	Classic Whipple Disease	Chronic Localized Whipple Disease	Carrier
• Gastroenteritis • Bacteremia • Pneumonia	• Constitutional symptoms and lymphadenopathy • Gastrointestinal symptoms • Joint involvement (may be the earliest sign) • Neurologic symptoms • Cardiac involvement	• Endocarditis • Encephalitis	• Asymptomatic • Can be detected in saliva or stool

General imaging may show lymphadenopathy, whereas CNS MRI imaging may show high midline T2 signal intensity in the subcortical regions (brainstem, hypothalamus, mesial temporal lobes), without diffusion restriction. Echocardiogram (options A and B) may show valvular lesions suggestive of endocarditis, but none of these tests are conclusive.

The definitive diagnosis of Whipple disease can be challenging. Alternative differential diagnoses including (but not limited to) HIV, tuberculosis, inflammatory diseases, and malignancy should be ruled out first. In general, when evaluating for Whipple disease, one should test the involved (symptomatic) areas to avoid potential false-negatives that can happen if testing a site that is not actually involved clinically. The common diagnostic tests include biopsy with histopathologic evaluation (periodic acid Schiff [PAS] staining), immunohistochemistry (IHC), and PCR. Duodenal biopsy is the initial test of choice, especially if presenting with GI symptoms (classic Whipple disease), but some will use this test regardless of symptoms. Several biopsies should be taken, as the disease can be patchy in nature. PCR testing of the stool, urine, and/or saliva can be done, but is not definitive. PCR testing on the blood is considered insensitive. If there are no GI symptoms, or if endoscopic evaluation is inconclusive, then tissue from involved sites (i.e., synovial tissue, lymph node, etc.) should be obtained for PAS staining and PCR, with or without IHC. Whipple disease is confirmed if two separate tests (i.e., PAS, PCR, or IHC) are positive. This requirement exists to avoid misdiagnosis in the case of asymptomatic carriage and to ensure appropriate diagnosis prior to condemning a patient to a long-term course of antimicrobial therapy. Culturing the organism (option E) may be difficult due to its fastidious nature, but it can be useful for susceptibility testing. The evaluation of suspected Whipple disease is summarized in Fig. 30.1.

Management is somewhat complicated and typically prolonged. Before starting treatment, CNS involvement should be ruled out (even if there are no suggestive symptoms) with cerebrospinal fluid PCR. Treatment should involve an antibiotic with good CNS penetration. Initial treatment phase consists of either ceftriaxone or meropenem for at least 2 weeks (4 weeks for endocarditis or CNS infection). This is followed by prolonged maintenance therapy. Trimethoprim/sulfamethoxazole (TMP/SMX) used to be the first choice based on a small randomized trial where patients received 2 weeks of induction therapy with ceftriaxone or meropenem followed by 1 year of TMP/SMX or tetracycline. TMP/SMX was superior to tetracycline in this trial, but recent data show that TMP/SMX is probably less effective, due to development of resistance. Recently, it has been found that the most active and bactericidal regimen is doxycycline plus hydroxychloroquine (based on a retrospective analysis). The duration of maintenance therapy is typically at least 1 year in most cases, and some consider

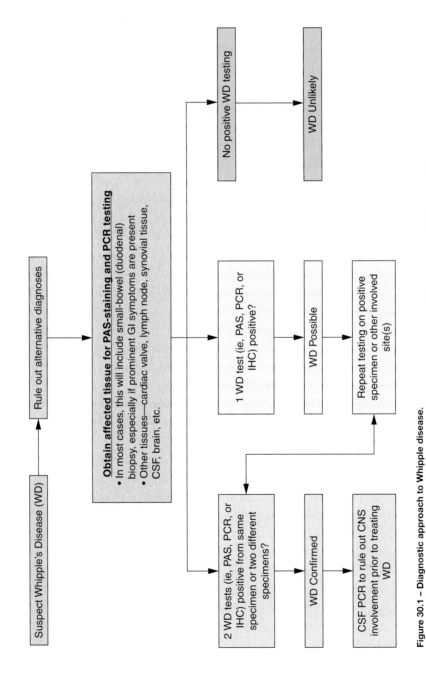

Figure 30.1 – Diagnostic approach to Whipple disease.
CNS, Central nervous system; *CSF*, cerebrospinal fluid; *IHC*, immunohistochemistry; *PAS*, periodic acid Schiff stain; *PCR*, polymerase chain reaction.

The flowchart contains the following elements:

- Suspect Whipple's Disease (WD)
- Rule out alternative diagnoses
- **Obtain affected tissue for PAS-staining and PCR testing**
  - In most cases, this will include small-bowel (duodenal) biopsy, especially if prominent GI symptoms are present
  - Other tissues—cardiac valve, lymph node, synovial tissue, CSF, brain, etc.
- No positive WD testing → WD Unlikely
- 1 WD test (ie, PAS, PCR, or IHC) positive? → WD Possible → Repeat testing on positive specimen or other involved site(s)
- 2 WD tests (ie, PAS, PCR, or IHC) positive from same specimen or two different specimens? → WD Confirmed → CSF PCR to rule out CNS involvement prior to treating WD

long-term doxycycline suppression thereafter. Treatment response is typically seen after a week or two. Follow-up includes repeat duodenal biopsies (at 6-month intervals during treatment) with PAS staining and PCR. The PAS staining may be positive for years, but the PCR should revert to negative with successful therapy. If the diagnosis was made in an extraintestinal location, then testing (usually PCR) relevant to this location should be monitored serially.

Treatment may be complicated by development of immune reconstitution inflammatory syndrome (IRIS), especially if the patient was on immune suppression prior to presentation. Treatment for IRIS may involve corticosteroids or thalidomide, similar to the treatment of leprosy-related inflammatory reactions. In addition, patients may develop a Jarisch–Herxheimer reaction. The most dreaded complication is disease relapse after stopping antibiotic therapy, and this can occur many years after stopping therapy.

KEY LEARNING POINT

The best initial test to diagnose classic Whipple disease (caused by Tropheryma whipplei*) is duodenal biopsy.*

REFERENCES AND FURTHER READING

- Dolmans RA, Boel CH, Lacle MM, Kusters JG. Clinical manifestations, treatment, and diagnosis of *Tropheryma whipplei* infections. *Clin Microbiol Rev.* 2017;30(2):529–555. https://doi.org/10.1128/CMR.00033-16. PMID: 28298472; PMCID: PMC5355640.
- El-Abassi R, Soliman MY, Williams F, England JD. Whipple's disease. *J Neurol Sci.* 2017;377:197–206. https://doi.org/10.1016/j.jns.2017.01.048. PMID: 28477696.
- Marth T, Moos V, Müller C, Biagi F, Schneider T. *Tropheryma whipplei* infection and Whipple's disease. *Lancet Infect Dis.* 2016;16(3):e13–e22. https://doi.org/10.1016/S1473-3099(15)00537-X. PMID: 26856775.
- Marth T, et al. *Whipple disease. Mandell, Douglas, and Bennett's Principles and Practice of Infectious Diseases.* 9th ed. Elsevier; 2020:2578–2584.

A 40-year-old male is admitted to the hospital with fevers and a suspected abscess of the left lower cervical region. He has a history of autoimmune hepatitis, for which he underwent an orthotopic liver transplant at the age of 35 years. Current medications include tacrolimus, mycophenolate, and low-dose prednisone. About 2 weeks ago, he had a left lower cervical lymph node excised as part of an evaluation for unexplained lymphadenopathy. The biopsy results showed a reactive lymph node. He did well after the procedure. Approximately 3 days prior to this admission, he started experiencing fevers along with pain and swelling in the area of the excision. Upon presentation, he had a temperature of 101 ° F, and the remainder of his vital signs were within normal limits. Examination showed an area of swelling in the left lower cervical region measuring 2 cm in diameter. There was tenderness, erythema, warmth, and fluctuance associated with the swelling. He underwent incision and drainage (I&D), and purulent material was sent for routine aerobic and anaerobic culture. He was started on vancomycin and piperacillin/tazobactam after the procedure. The gram stain from the I&D is showing many polymorphonuclear cells, but there are no organisms visible. After 3 days of incubation, the aerobic culture is growing an acid-fast bacillus species. Which of the following organisms is the most likely cause of this patient's presentation?

A. *Mycobacterium xenopi.*
B. *Mycobacterium haemophilum.*
C. *Mycobacterium chelonae.*
D. *Mycobacterium ulcerans.*
E. *Mycobacterium scrofulaceum.*

The most likely cause is *Mycobacterium chelonae* (**option C**). There are several different organisms that can stain acid-fast, as shown in Fig. 31.1. The *Mycobacteria* are the quintessential example, and most are environmental organisms (certain animals, soil, medical devices, water sources, etc.). *Mycobacteria* are gram-positive rods that contain mycolic acids in their cell wall, which makes them resistant to decolorization with acid alcohol; thus, they are called acid-fast. In addition, many of the *nontuberculous mycobacteria (NTM)* are capable of forming biofilms, which makes them difficult to treat and eradicate. Infections due to NTM may be difficult to diagnose, because isolation of NTM can represent colonization, contamination, or true infection. Therefore, one should always consider the clinical context and the specific species when interpreting these results.

The concept to recognize in this case is the difference between rapid-growing NTM (RG-NTM; Table 31.1) and slow-growing NTM (SG-NTM; Table 31.2). RG-NTM typically grow within 7 days on solid media, including standard blood agar (as seen in this case). SG-NTM take more than 7 days to grow under the same circumstances. There are only three major groups of RG-NTM that cause disease in humans. These include *M. abscessus complex*, *M. fortuitum complex*, and *M. chelonae complex*. There are numerous different species of SG-NTM (including **options A, B, D, and E**), and some of the most notable examples are shown in Fig. 31.1. Important clinical associations are discussed in the tables.

In general, the spectrum of illness due to NTM includes skin and soft-tissue infections and bone/joint infections (often via direct inoculation), lymphadenitis, pulmonary infection, and disseminated disease. The manifestation is dependent on the species, as certain species have a predilection for certain manifestations (i.e., RG-NTM more commonly cause skin/soft tissue infections). Risk factors for dissemination include immune compromise and genetic disturbances, such as Mendelian susceptibility to mycobacterial disease, and defects in the interferon-gamma and interleukin-12 pathway (which can include autoantibodies to the pathway components, as seen mainly in people of southeast Asian descent). In addition, most NTM infections require multidrug therapy for prolonged periods of time and appropriate source control (i.e., removal of devices, debridement, resection, etc.). Unfortunately, such long courses of therapy are usually associated with various adverse effects, as noted in Table 31.3.

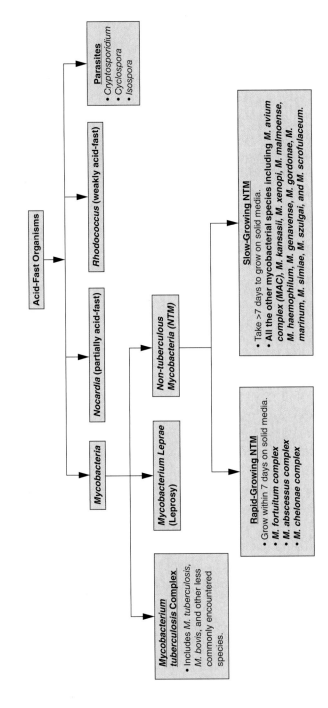

Figure 31.1 – Overview of acid-fast organisms of clinical relevance.

Table 31.1 – Rapid-Growing Nontuberculous Mycobacteria

Rapid-Growing Nontuberculous Mycobacteria Species	Clinically Relevant Associations
Mycobacterium abscessus group	• Considered the most pathogenic and antimicrobial resistant species of RG-NTM • Subspecies include *M. abscessus* subspecies *abscessus, M. abscessus* subspecies *bolletii,* and *M. abscessus* subspecies *massiliense* • **M. abscessus subspecies abscessus and M. abscessus subspecies bolletii possess an inducible erm(41) gene that is associated with inducible macrolide resistance. M. abscessus subspecies massiliense has a nonfunctional erm(41) gene, so macrolide therapy is effective.** Therefore, one should always attempt to identify the subspecies and assess for the presence of the *erm(41)* gene when treating infections due to *M. abscessus* complex. This identification can be done by incubation for 14 days or by specialized sequencing • Resistance to macrolides can also develop in all subspecies through mutations in the *rrl* gene and is referred to as mutational resistance. This feature can be assessed for as well; if resistance is present, macrolides are considered ineffective • Spectrum of illness includes skin and soft-tissue infections, bone/joint infections, pulmonary infections (classically elderly white female patients with no predisposing factor or patients with underlying chronic lung disease) and disseminated infections • Management consists of surgical resection/debridement (often required in most cases) and multidrug antimicrobial therapy. Agents that are active *in vitro* include macrolides (considered highly active if *erm(41)* gene negative/nonfunctional and no mutational macrolide resistance), amikacin, cefoxitin, imipenem, and tigecycline
M. chelonae group	• Several subspecies as well, but not necessary to differentiate in most cases. This group lacks the *erm(41)* gene • Commonly associated with skin and soft-tissue infections and bone infections due to infected piercings, contaminated tattoo ink, or plastic surgery. May also causes a keratitis in association with contact lenses and ophthalmologic surgery. Rarely, can cause disseminated disease (immune-compromised patients) and pulmonary infection • Treatment typically consists of multidrug therapy. Antimicrobial agents with *in vitro* activity include tobramycin (more active than amikacin), clarithromycin, imipenem, tetracyclines (doxycycline or minocycline), fluoroquinolones (ciprofloxacin or moxifloxacin), linezolid, and clofazimine
M. fortuitum group	• Several subspecies as well. Most have an inducible *erm(41)* gene (and thus are macrolide-resistant), except for *M. fortuitum* subspecies *peregrinum* and *M. fortuitum* subspecies *senegalense* • Commonly associated with skin and soft-tissue or bone infections after traumatic inoculation, cosmetic procedures, or cardiac surgery (sternal wound infection). Foot baths (pedicure salons) have been associated with *M. fortuitum* furunculosis. Rarely, this species can cause pulmonary infection in cases of lipoid pneumonia, acid reflux, or disseminated infection • Treatment typically consists of a two-drug regimen. Agents with *in vitro* activity include fluoroquinolones, doxycycline, cefoxitin, imipenem, amikacin, and sulfonamides

Table 31.2 – Slow-Growing Nontuberculous Mycobacteria

Slow-Growing Nontuberculous Mycobacteria Species	Clinically Relevant Associations
Mycobacterium ulcerans	• Causes Buruli ulcer (African name) or Bairnsdale ulcer (Australian name). This disease commonly affects children and manifests as an ulcerative or nodular cutaneous infection that can involve osteomyelitis, limb deformities, contractures, and scarring • May be acquired or transmitted via cutaneous inoculation from contaminated environmental sources (soil, water) • Pathogenesis involves a macrolide toxin called mycolactone that causes tissue damage and inhibits the immune response • Difficult to grow, as requires a temperature of 29°C–33°C and a low oxygen concentration (2.5%). Therefore, diagnosis is made by PCR • Treatment consists of 8 weeks of rifampin + streptomycin or rifampin + clarithromycin, or rifampin + moxifloxacin.
M. avium-intracellulare complex (MAC)	• Several species, with most notable species/subspecies discussed later • Susceptibility testing in MAC infections is only meaningful for macrolides (*rrl* gene mutations) and amikacin (*rrs* gene mutations). *In vitro* susceptibilities for the other agents discussed later do not correlate with clinical response • *M. avium* and *M. intracellulare* can cause pulmonary manifestations. These can occur in immune-competent individuals and include **pulmonary infection (cavitary vs. nodular/bronchiectatic, typically tall, slender patients who are elderly and have acid reflux or pectus deformities) and hypersensitivity pneumonitis ("hot-tub lung" from contaminated spas and showers)**. These species can also cause cervical lymphadenitis and disseminated disease (more likely with *M. avium*) in immune-compromised patients (i.e., HIV with CD4 cell count <50 cells/uL) • **M. chimaera is associated with the use of contaminated heater-cooler devices (HCDs) in patients who have had open cardiac surgery**. These HCDs may still be in use, and cases can occur up to 6 years after index exposure. Most of these infections have involved prosthetic material or heart transplantation. Dissemination is common, so acid-fast bacillus blood cultures are always recommended. These infections are incredibly difficult to cure, and repeated surgical intervention and debridement is often necessary. • Treatment of pulmonary MAC consists of at least three drugs, including a macrolide (if susceptible), ethambutol, and rifampin. For nodular or bronchiectatic disease, therapy is given intermittently (i.e., three times weekly). For severe disease and/or cavitary disease, therapy is given daily, and IV amikacin (if susceptible) three times weekly is added. Duration of treatment is typically at least 12 months after cultures become negative (respiratory cultures are recommended to be done once every 1–3 months). For refractory disease (failure to clear cultures after 6 months of treatment), inhaled amikacin is beneficial if isolate is susceptible • Treatment of disseminated disease (typically patients with advanced HIV) includes multidrug therapy consisting of at least two drugs: a macrolide if susceptible (clarithromycin or azithromycin) and ethambutol. A third or fourth agent (rifabutin, fluoroquinolone, or injectable aminoglycoside) can be added if high mycobacterial load or not on effective antiretroviral therapy. Antiretroviral therapy should be initiated as well. Treatment can be stopped once the patient has completed at least 12 months of treatment, is asymptomatic, and has had a CD4 count >100 cells/uL for >6 months

(Continued)

Table 31.2 – Slow-Growing Nontuberculous Mycobacteria *(Cont'd)*

Slow-Growing Nontuberculous Mycobacteria Species	Clinically Relevant Associations
M. kansasii	• **Almost always considered pathogenic when isolated and can cause a positive tuberculosis interferon gamma release assay (IGRA)** • Rifampin and clarithromycin susceptibility testing are meaningful, but susceptibility testing for other agents is of unclear significance. Notably, *M. kansasii* is intrinsically resistant to pyrazinamide • **Presentation is very similar to that of pulmonary tuberculosis (TB)**, and in the immune-compromised, extrapulmonary and disseminated disease can occur • Treatment consists of rifampin and ethambutol plus either isoniazid or a macrolide. Alternative (second-line) agents include fluroquinolones and amikacin. Treatment duration is a fixed 12 months (from when treatment was started, as it is not necessary to start from day of culture conversion)
M. genavense	• Grows best at an acidic pH (pH 5.5) and may require incubation for 8–12 weeks to grow • *M. genavense* is associated with disseminated infection similar to MAC in immune-suppressed patients (usually HIV/AIDS) • Treatment involves at least two agents for at least 12 months. These may be macrolides (clarithromycin most effective), ethambutol, rifamycin, fluoroquinolones, and aminoglycosides (amikacin)
M. marinum	• Cause of **"fish-tank granuloma,"** which is a sporotrichoid-like skin and soft tissue infection that is acquired classically by cleaning out fish tanks or via soft tissue injury in saltwater, brackish water, or freshwater. This infection may extend deeper to cause deep soft tissue infections and bone/joint infections • Resistant to azithromycin, isoniazid, and pyrazinamide • *M. marinum* **can also cause a positive TB IGRA** • Management includes surgical debridement and at least two active agents (ethambutol + rifampin or clarithromycin). All three of these drugs are used for deeper infections. The regimen is given for 1–2 months after the skin lesions resolve
M. xenopi	• Depending on immune status, may present as cavitary disease resembling TB (pre-existing lung disease patients), nodular disease (immune-competent patients), or an infiltrate form (immune-suppressed patients) • Treatment of pulmonary disease includes at least three drugs, including rifampin, ethambutol, and either macrolide or fluoroquinolone. An IV aminoglycoside should be added if severe bronchiectatic disease or cavitary disease. Treatment duration is at least 12 months after culture conversion
M. malmoense	• Typically recovered from sputum or cervical nodes of patients in certain locations (North Europe, Japan, Congo) with chronic, often cavitary, pulmonary disease • Treatment includes isoniazid, rifampin, and ethambutol +/- macrolide and fluoroquinolone
M. haemophilum	• Grows at cooler temperatures (28°C–33°C) and requires iron (ferric ammonium citrate, hemin, or hemoglobin) to grow. If suspecting this pathogen, then consider notifying the microbiology lab so appropriate evaluation can be done • Classically associated with skin and soft tissue infections of the extremities (given preference for cooler temperatures) • Treatment includes multidrug therapy including macrolide, rifamycin, and fluoroquinolone for at least 6 months

(Continued)

Table 31.2 – Slow-Growing Nontuberculous Mycobacteria *(Cont'd)*

Slow-Growing Nontuberculous Mycobacteria Species	Clinically Relevant Associations
M. szulgai	• Almost always considered pathogenic when isolated and classically affects middle-aged male smokers who have chronic obstructive pulmonary disease or a history of alcohol abuse • Typically causes a pulmonary infection but can have extrapulmonary manifestations as well. Pulmonary presentation is very similar to pulmonary TB. ***M. szulgai* can also cause a positive TB IGRA** • Treatment consists of three drugs (macrolide, rifamycin, and ethambutol) for at least 12 months
M. scrofulaceum	• A causative agent of **scrofula** (cervical lymphadenitis due to mycobacterial infection). This organism can also cause pulmonary and disseminated infections • Treatment of choice for localized infections is surgical. Medical therapy is used in systemic or nonlocalized infections and consists of clarithromycin, ethambutol, and rifampin. Treatment should be continued for at least 12 months
M. celatum	• Typically causes pulmonary infection resembling TB in immune-compromised patients (usually AIDS). ***M. celatum* can also cause a false-positive test on *M. tuberculosis* DNA testing** • Management consists of multidrug therapy including macrolides, ethambutol, ciprofloxacin, rifabutin, pyrazinamide, amikacin, and clofazimine. *M. celatum* is often resistant to rifampin
M. gordonae	• **Identification of this organism most often represents contamination or colonization and not actual infection** • One of the least pathogenic NTM species, but may rarely cause disease in severely immune compromised patients
M. simiae complex	• An uncommon cause of infection that is typically resistant to first-line TB drugs. Agents with activity include clarithromycin, fluoroquinolones, clofazimine, amikacin, and trimethoprim/sulfamethoxazole (TMP/SMX)
M. terrae complex	• Spectrum of disease includes chronic tenosynovitis of the hand, skin/soft tissue infections, and bone/joint infections • Treatment consists of multidrug therapy. Active agents include clarithromycin, ethambutol, rifabutin, and TMP/SMX

Table 31.3 – Notable Adverse Effects of Antimycobacterial Drugs Used to Treat Nontuberculous Mycobacteria

Medication	Adverse Effects
Macrolides	• Hepatotoxicity, gastrointestinal (GI) upset, reversible dose-dependent ototoxicity (with long-term use), neuromuscular blockade (exacerbation of myasthenia gravis), QT-interval prolongation, and increased cardiovascular mortality
Ethambutol	• Peripheral and optic neuropathy
Rifamycin	• Drug-drug interactions, red-orange discoloration of bodily fluids, hepatotoxicity
Fluoroquinolones	• Central nervous system disturbances, QT prolongation, tendinopathy, neuromuscular blockade (exacerbation of myasthenia gravis), glucose disturbances, and potentially aortic aneurysm formation
Aminoglycosides	• Nephrotoxicity, irreversible ototoxicity (vestibular and cochlear), and neuromuscular blockade (exacerbation of myasthenia). Inhaled formulations can cause dysphonia and bronchospasm
Linezolid	• Serotonin syndrome (typically with other serotonergic agents) and with prolonged use, bone marrow suppression (cytopenia), and neuropathy (peripheral and optic). Tedizolid may be less toxic
Isoniazid	• Hepatotoxicity and peripheral neuropathy (mitigated by pyridoxine supplementation)
Tetracyclines	• Pill-esophagitis, photosensitivity, idiopathic intracranial hypertension (pseudotumor cerebri), tinnitus or vertigo, hyperpigmentation/skin discoloration with minocycline, and GI upset and pancreatitis with tigecycline
Imipenem	• Seizures, rashes, bone marrow suppression (cytopenia), and nephrotoxicity
Trimethoprim/ sulfamethoxazole	• Elevated creatinine (can be benign or pathologic), drug rashes, hyperkalemia, GI upset, aseptic meningitis, photosensitivity, and bone marrow suppression
Clofazimine	• QT prolongation, hepatotoxicity, and dermatologic (dry skin, bronze discoloration)
Bedaquiline	• QT prolongation, hepatotoxicity, and increased risk of death

KEY LEARNING POINT

Rapid-growing nontuberculous mycobacteria (RG-NTM) typically grow within 7 days on solid media, including standard blood agar. The RG-NTM include M. abscessus *group,* M. fortuitum *complex, and* M. chelonae *complex.*

REFERENCES AND FURTHER READING

- Bennet JE, Dolin R, Blaser MJ, eds. *Mandell, Douglas, and Bennett's Principles and Practice of Infectious Diseases.* 9th ed. Elsevier; 2020.
- Daley CL, Iaccarino JM, Lange C, et al. Treatment of nontuberculous mycobacterial pulmonary disease: an official ATS/ERS/ESCMID/IDSA clinical practice guideline. *CID.* 2020;71(4):e1–e36. https://doi.org/10.1093/cid/ciaa241.

- Chavarria M, Lutwick L, Dickinson BL. TB or not TB? *Mycobacterium celatum* mimicking *Mycobacterium tuberculosis*: A case of mistaken identity. *IDCases*. 2018;11:83–87. https://doi.org/10.1016/j.idcr.2018.01.015.
- Coolen-Allou N, Touron T, Belmonte O, et al. Clinical, radiological, and microbiological characteristics of Mycobacterium simiae infection in 97 patients. *Antimicrob Agents Chemother*. 2018;62(7):e00395–e00418. https://doi.org/10.1128/AAC.00395-18.
- Forbes BA, Hall GS, Miller MB, et al. Practice guidelines for clinical microbiology laboratories: mycobacteria. *Clin Microbiol Rev*. 2018;31(2):e00038–e00117. https://doi.org/10.1128/CMR.00038-17.
- Jabbour J-F, Hamieh A, Sharara SL, Kanj SS. *Mycobacterium simiae*: harmless colonizer or deadly pathogen? *PLoS Pathog*. 2020;16(4):e1008418. https://doi.org/10.1371/journal.ppat.1008418.
- Longworth SA, Daly JS, Infectious AST. Diseases Community of Practice. Management of infections due to nontuberculous mycobacteria in solid organ transplant recipients—guidelines from the American Society of Transplantation Infectious Diseases Community of Practice. *Clin Transplant*. 2019;33(9):e13588 https://doi.org/10.1111/ctr.13588.
- Mahmood M, Ajmal S, Abu Saleh OM, Bryson A, Marcelin JR, Wilson JW. *Mycobacterium genavense* infections in non-HIV immunocompromised hosts: a systematic review. *Infect Dis (Lond)*. 2018;50(5):329–339. https://doi.org/10.1080/23744235.2017.1404630.
- Misch EA, Saddler C, Davis JM. Skin and soft tissue infections due to nontuberculous mycobacteria. *Curr Infect Dis Rep*. 2018;20(6). https://doi.org/10.1007/s11908-018-0611-3.
- Nookeu P, Angkasekwinai N, Foongladda S, et al. Clinical characteristics and treatment outcomes for patients infected with *Mycobacterium haemophilum*. *Emerg Infect Dis*. 2019;25(9):1648–1652. https://doi.org/10.3201/eid2509.190430.
- Panel on Guidelines for the Prevention and Treatment of Opportunistic Infections in Adults and Adolescents with HIV. Guidelines for the Prevention and Treatment of Opportunistic Infections in HIV-infected Adults and Adolescents: Recommendations from the Centers for Disease Control and Prevention, the National Institutes of Health, and the HIV Medicine Association of the Infectious Diseases Society of America. https://clinicalinfo.hiv.gov/sites/default/files/inline-files/adult_oi.pdf. Accessed November 8, 2020.
- Takemoto Y, Tokuyasu H, Ikeuchi T, et al. Disseminated *Mycobacterium scrofulaceum* infection in an immunocompetent host. *Intern Med*. 2017;56(14):1931–1935. https://doi.org/10.2169/internalmedicine.56.8181.

A 50-year-old male is admitted to the hospital with a 1-day history of fevers and chills. He has a history of poorly controlled type 2 diabetes mellitus complicated by peripheral neuropathy. Medications include insulin and metformin. Vital signs show temperature 101° F, heart rate 105 beats per minute, blood pressure 100/60 mmHg, respiratory rate 18, and oxygen saturation 94% on room air. Physical examination shows rigors and a generally ill appearance. There is a shallow ulceration over the plantar aspect of the right great toe with surrounding erythema, warmth, and swelling. There is no tenderness present. Blood cultures are drawn and eventually turn positive for gram-positive cocci in chains. You review the case with the microbiology laboratory. The lab tech tells you that the isolate shows a clear area of hemolysis on the blood agar plate. The isolate appears to grow in the presence of a bacitracin disc added to the agar. A pyrrolidonyl arylamidase (PYR) test is reported as negative. Based on the information provided by the microbiology lab, which of the following organisms is the most likely cause of this patient's bacteremia?

A. *Streptococcus pyogenes*.

B. *Streptococcus agalactiae*.

C. *Streptococcus pneumonia*.

D. Viridans group *Streptococcus*.

E. *Enterococcus faecalis*.

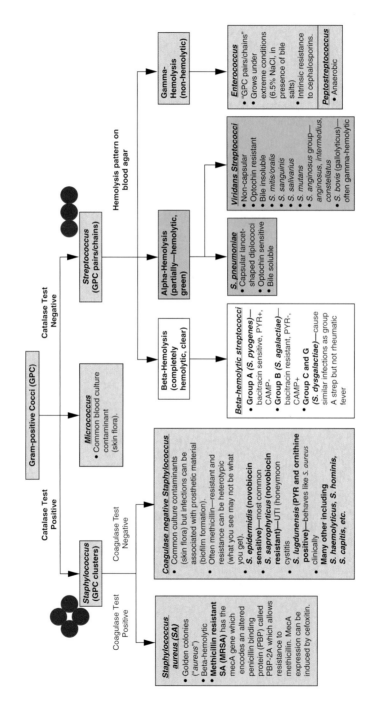

Figure 32.1 – Approach to the identification of common gram-positive cocci (GPC).
CAMP, Christie-Atkins-Munch-Peterson; PYR, pyrrolidonyl arylamidase.

Gram-positive Cocci (GPC)

Catalase Test Positive

Catalase Test Negative

Staphylococcus (GPC clusters)

Coagulase Test Positive

Coagulase Test Negative

Micrococcus
• Common blood culture contaminant (skin flora).

Streptococcus (GPC pairs/chains)

Hemolysis pattern on blood agar

Beta-Hemolysis (completely hemolytic, clear)

Alpha-Hemolysis (partially—hemolytic, green)

Gamma-Hemolysis (non-hemolytic)

Coagulase Test Positive

Staphylococcus aureus (SA)
• Golden colonies ("aureus")
• Beta-hemolytic
• **Methicillin resistant SA (MRSA)** has the mecA gene which encodes an altered penicillin binding protein (PBP) called PBP-2A which allows resistance to methicillin. MecA expression can be induced by cefoxitin.

Coagulase Test Negative

Coagulase negative Staphylococcus
• Common culture contaminants (skin flora) but infections can be associated with prosthetic material (biofilm formation).
• Often methicillin—resistant and resistance can be heterotypic (what you see may not be what you get).
• *S. epidermidis* (novobiocin sensitive)—most common
• *S. saprophyticus* (novobiocin resistant)—UTI (honeymoon cystitis)
• *S. lugdunensis* (PYR and ornithine positive)—behaves like S. aureus clinically
• **Many other including *S. haemolyticus, S. hominis, S. capitis, etc.***

Beta-hemolytic streptococci
• **Group A (*S. pyogenes*)**—bacitracin sensitive, PYR+, CAMP-
• **Group B (*S. agalactiae*)**—bacitracin resistant, PYR-, CAMP+
• **Group C and G (*S. dysgalactiae*)**—cause similar infections as group A strep but not rheumatic fever

S. pneumoniae
• Capsular lancet-shaped diplococci
• Optochin sensitive
• Bile soluble

Viridans Streptococci
• Non-capsular
• Optochin resistant
• Bile insoluble
• *S. mitis/oralis*
• *S. sanguinis*
• *S. salivarius*
• *S. mutans*
• *S. anginosus* group—anginosus, intermedius, constellatus
• *S. bovis* (gallolyticus)—often gamma-hemolytic

Enterococcus
• "GPC pairs/chains"
• Grows under extreme conditions (6.5% NaCl, in presence of bile salts)
• Intrinsic resistance to cephalosporins.

Peptostreptococcus
• Anaerobic

The most likely causative organism is *S. agalactiae* (**option B**). The first step in identifying gram-positive cocci (GPC) is to look at the Gram stain morphology and perform a catalase test (Fig. 32.1). A positive catalase test and GPC in clusters morphology suggests *Staphylococcus* spp. GPC in chains with a negative catalase test suggests *Streptococcus* spp. The hemolysis pattern on the blood agar plate can be used to differentiate the *Streptococcus* spp. into *alpha-hemolytic streptococci* (partial hemolysis with resultant greenish color), *beta-hemolytic streptococci* (complete hemolysis resulting in clear appearance), and *gamma-hemolytic streptococci* (no hemolysis). *S. agalactiae* is a Lancefield group B streptococcus species that is beta-hemolytic on blood agar, resistant to bacitracin (i.e., will grow when a bacitracin disc is added to the agar), PYR test–negative, and CAMP test–positive (Table 32.1). *S. pyogenes* (**option A**) is a Lancefield group A streptococcus that is beta-hemolytic on blood agar, bacitracin-sensitive, PYR test–positive, and CAMP test–negative. *S. pneumoniae* (**option C**) is typically described as a lancet-shaped diplococcus that is alpha-hemolytic. Viridans group streptococci (**option D**) are a heterogeneous group of mainly alpha-hemolytic streptococci. *S. pneumoniae* and viridans streptococci can be differentiated by the optochin disc test, where *S. pneumoniae* is optochin-sensitive and viridans streptococci are optochin-resistant. *Enterococcus* (**option E**) is typically described as "GPC in pairs and chains" and is gamma-hemolytic (nonhemolytic). *Enterococci* can grow under rather harsh conditions, including 6.5% NaCl or in the presence of bile. *S. bovis* is a viridans group streptococci that is typically included in the gamma-hemolytic streptococci. It can be differentiated from *Enterococci* by the fact that it does not grow in 6.5% NaCl.

Table 32.1 – Common Microbiologic Tests for Identification of Gram-Positive Cocci

Test	Utility	Positive Result
Catalase test	• Differentiation of staphylococci from streptococci and enterococci	• Production of bubbles (hydrogen peroxide split into oxygen and water by catalase enzyme) on the slide suggests presence of staphylococci
Coagulase test	• Differentiation of *Staphylococcus aureus* from coagulase-negative staphylococci	• Formation of fibrin clot (clumping) in the test tube suggests presence of *S. aureus*
PYR hydrolysis test	• Differentiation of beta-hemolytic streptococci	• Development of a red color suggests presence of group A streptococci (*Streptococcus pyogenes*), *Enterococcus*, or nutritionally-variant streptococci
CAMP test	• Identification of group B streptococci (*Staphylococcus agalactiae*)	• CAMP factor made by *S. agalactiae* enhances the beta-hemolysis of *S. aureus* and produces an "arrow" of beta-hemolysis between the streaks. This suggests presence of *S. agalactiae*

(Continued)

Table 32.1 – Common Microbiologic Tests for Identification of Gram-Positive Cocci *(Cont'd)*

Test	Utility	Positive Result
Bile solubility	• Differentiation of *S. pneumoniae* from other alpha-hemolytic streptococci	• Bile solubility (clearing or loss of turbidity in test tube or disintegration of colonies) suggests presence of *S. pneumoniae*
Bile esculin	• Identification of group D streptococci (*Enterococcus* and *S. bovis*)	• Brown-black color means organism can hydrolyze esculin in presence of bile (typical of *Enterococcus*). This test will also be positive with *Streptococcus bovis*
Salt (6.5% NaCl) test	• Differentiation of *Enterococcus* from other group D streptococci (*S. bovis*)	• Growth in 6.5% NaCl suggests presence of *Enterococcus* • *S. bovis* will not grow in 6.5% NaCl
Optochin sensitivity	• Differentiation of *S. pneumoniae* from other alpha-hemolytic streptococci	• Optochin susceptibility (will see a zone of inhibition around the optochin disc) suggests presence of *S. pneumoniae*
Bacitracin sensitivity	• Differentiation of *S. pyogenes* from other beta-hemolytic streptococci	• Bacitracin susceptibility (will see a zone of inhibition) suggests presence of *S. pyogenes*
Novobiocin sensitivity	• Differentiation of coagulase-negative staphylococci	• Novobiocin susceptibility (will see a zone of inhibition) suggests *S. epidermidis* • Novobiocin resistance (no zone of inhibition) suggests *S. saprophyticus*
Hippurate hydrolysis test	• Differentiation of *S. agalactiae* from other beta-hemolytic streptococci	• Blue color in test tube suggests presence of *S. agalactiae*. This test will also be positive with *Campylobacter jejuni* and *Listeria*

KEY LEARNING POINT

*Group B streptococcus (***Streptococcus agalactiae***) is catalase-negative, beta-hemolytic, bacitracin-resistant, PYR test–negative, and CAMP test–positive.*

REFERENCES AND FURTHER READING

- Chapter 7. Clinical microbiology. In: Gomella LG, Haist SA, eds. *Clinician's Pocket Reference: The Scut Monkey.* 11th ed. McGraw-Hill.
- Watson R. General & Medical Microbiology. Summary of biochemical tests. https://www.uwyo.edu/molb2210_lab/info/biochemical_tests.htm#bile. Accessed November 12, 2020.
- Acharya T. Learn Microbiology Online. Tests. https://www.uwyo.edu/molb2210_lab/info/biochemical_tests.htm#bile.
- Centers for Disease Control and Prevention. Chapter 8. Identification and characterization of *Streptococcus pneumoniae*. https://www.cdc.gov/meningitis/lab-manual/chpt08-id-characterization-streppneumo.pdf. Accessed November 12, 2020.

A 35-year-old male is admitted to the hospital with a 1-week history of fevers, chills, headaches, myalgias, nausea, vomiting, cough, and shortness of breath. He is otherwise healthy and does not take any medications. He works for a pest control company. He lives in Phoenix, Arizona. He does not smoke cigarettes or vape. He denies alcohol or drug use. On presentation, his vitals show temperature 101.5° F, heart rate 110 beats per minute, blood pressure 110/60 mmHg, respiratory rate 24, and oxygen saturation 88% on room air. He is placed on 3 L/min oxygen by nasal cannula, which results in improvement of his oxygen saturation to 96%. On examination, he appears ill. Heart is regular, and there are no murmurs. Lung exam shows increased work of breathing and diffuse crackles. Abdomen is diffusely tender, and there is no rebound tenderness. The remainder of the examination is normal. Lab studies show white blood cell count 16,000 cells/uL (12% band forms), hemoglobin 16 g/dL, platelet count 80,000 cells/uL, creatinine 2.5 mg/dL (creatinine clearance 25 mL/min), and alanine aminotransferase 200 U/L. Chest x-ray reveals bilateral diffuse airspace opacities. Blood cultures are drawn, and he is started on ceftriaxone and doxycycline. *Legionella* urine antigen is negative. Influenza A and B nasopharyngeal PCR is negative. HIV antigen/antibody screen is negative. His respiratory failure progresses rapidly, and he is intubated on hospital day 3. What is the most likely diagnosis?

A. Pneumonic plague.

B. Legionnaire disease.

C. Hantavirus pulmonary syndrome.

D. Leptospirosis.

E. Coccidioidomycosis.

The most likely diagnosis is hantavirus pulmonary syndrome (**option C**). Hantavirus infections are acquired via inhalation of aerosolized excrement (urine, feces) or saliva from rodents. This typically occurs with close contact with rodents, especially in poorly ventilated areas (i.e., barns, etc.). Old-world hantaviruses are associated with hemorrhagic fever with renal syndrome (HFRS), while new-world hantaviruses (i.e., Sin Nombre virus) cause hantavirus cardiopulmonary syndrome (HCPS). Person-to-person transmission has only been documented with the Andes virus (a new-world hantavirus found in South America). In the United States, new-world hantavirus infections are classically acquired in the Four Corners region (i.e., Arizona, Colorado, New Mexico, Utah). The presentation depends on which capillary bed is predominantly affected—renal medullary capillaries in HFRS and pulmonary capillaries in HCPS. Both forms of disease start out as a flu-like illness and can develop sequelae of vascular leakage (thrombocytopenia, hemoconcentration, hypotension, and left-shifted leukocytosis). The two forms are compared in Table 33.1, but there is some overlap between the two.

Diagnosis is typically made by serology, as most patients will have IgM and even IgG antibodies at the time of symptom onset. Alternatively, detection of viral RNA by reverse transcriptase PCR can be used. Treatment is mainly supportive. Ribavirin has shown some

Table 33.1 – Hantavirus Syndromes

Characteristic	Hemorrhagic Fever With Renal Syndrome	Hantavirus Cardiopulmonary Syndrome
Incubation	• 2–4 weeks	• 2–3 weeks
Manifestations	• Febrile phase—Lasts up to 1 week. Flu-like symptoms, conjunctival hemorrhages, palatal petechiae • Hypotensive phase—Lasts up to 2 days. Shock, hemorrhagic manifestations • Oliguric phase—Lasts up to 1 week. Acute renal failure with active sediment • Polyuric phase—Can last days to weeks. Onset associated with good prognosis • Convalescent phase—Recovery. Can last for months	• Prodromal phase—Lasts up to 1 week. Flu-like symptoms • Cardiopulmonary phase—Noncardiogenic pulmonary edema, myocardial depression, and shock. Can last up to 1 week • Convalescent phase—Slow, but patients often recover completely
Long-term complications	• Chronic renal failure • Hypertension	• Typically none
Mortality	• Lower (<20%) • Severity/mortality depends on the strain	• Higher—30%–50%

benefit in HFRS if given early (within 5 days), but not in HCPS. In addition, there is no benefit to corticosteroids.

Pneumonic plague (**option A**) is caused by *Yersinia pestis*, which is transmitted by rodent fleas. This infection can present similar to hantavirus infection, but the presentation is typically more acute. In addition, the lack of improvement with doxycycline argues against pneumonic plague. Legionnaire disease (**option B**) is a pneumonia syndrome typically caused by a water-loving bacterium called *Legionella pneumophila*. *Legionella* classically affects elderly smokers, patients with structural lung disease, or immune-compromised individuals. The presentation classically also includes confusion, gastrointestinal upset, and hyponatremia. The *Legionella* urine antigen test will be positive if the infection is caused by L1-serotype of *L. pneumophila* (the most common cause of *Legionella* infection). This test does not detect *Legionella* infections due to other species, so the negative antigen test in this case does not completely rule out *Legionella* infection, but it does make it less likely. In addition, the lack of improvement with doxycycline argues against *Legionella* infection. Leptospirosis (**option D**) is caused by a spirochete bacterium called *Leptospira* (classically *Leptospira interrogans*, but other species exist). It is a zoonotic illness acquired by exposure to contaminated bodily fluids (especially urine) of various infected animals, including domestic animals (dogs, cats, etc.) and rodents. In the United States, the highest incidence of leptospirosis is actually in Hawaii. The presentation can be similar to hantavirus infection, but tip-offs for leptospirosis (not seen in this case) include conjunctival suffusion, calf pain, and retroorbital headache. Severe disease presentations include Weil disease (triad of bleeding, renal failure, and jaundice), pulmonary hemorrhage, and acute respiratory distress syndrome. As with the other illnesses mentioned above, lack of improvement with doxycycline argues against this diagnosis. Lastly, coccidioidomycosis (**option E**) is an endemic mycosis caused most commonly by *Coccidioides immitis*. This infection is endemic to desert regions in the southwest United States as well, and it is typically acquired by inhalation of the environmental form (arthroconidia) of the fungus. The presentation can include asymptomatic illness, acute pneumonia, chronic pneumonia, or extrapulmonary disease such as meningitis, bone/joint involvement ("desert rheumatism"), and cutaneous manifestations (erythema nodosum classically). Eosinophilic leukocytosis may be seen, but thrombocytopenia and transaminase elevations are not common findings.

KEY LEARNING POINT

Hantavirus pulmonary syndrome should be considered in patients who present with an acute severe pneumonia, hemoconcentration, and thrombocytopenia in the setting of potential rodent exposure.

REFERENCES AND FURTHER READING

- Avšič-Županc T, Saksida A, Korva M. Hantavirus infections. *Clin Microbiol Infect.* 2019;21S:e6–e16. https://doi.org/10.1111/1469-0691.12291.
- Dheerasekara K, Sumathipala S, Muthugala R. Hantavirus infections-treatment and prevention. *Curr Treat Options Infect Dis.* 2020;12(4):410–421. https://doi.org/10.1007/s40506-020-00236-3.
- Vial PA, Valdivieso F, Ferres M, et al. High-dose intravenous methylprednisolone for hantavirus cardiopulmonary syndrome in Chile: a double-blind, randomized controlled clinical trial. *Clin Infect Dis.* 2013;57(7):943–951. https://doi.org/10.1093/cid/cit394.

A 25-year-old female is admitted to the hospital with a 1-month history of fevers, abdominal pain, and diarrhea. She is otherwise healthy and takes no medications. Vital signs are within normal limits except for low-grade fevers up to 101 ° F. Examination shows oral mucosal aphthous ulceration and abdominal tenderness most prominent over the right lower quadrant. Rectal examination shows a fissure at the 12 o'clock position, and stool guaiac is positive. Labs show white blood cell count 14,000 cells/uL, hemoglobin 10 g/dL, creatinine 1.0 mg/dL (creatinine clearance 90 mL/min), serum albumin 3 g/dL, and otherwise normal liver function testing. C-reactive protein is 15 mg/L (normal <1.0 mg/L). *Clostridioides difficile* stool testing and an enteric pathogen panel (stool film-array) test are negative. Abdominal CT scan reveals enterocolitis with prominent terminal ileal thickening. A colonoscopy shows deep fissuring and areas of mucosal ulceration with intervening normal-appearing mucosa. The patient is started on high-dose steroids. Eventually, the biopsy results return with findings suggestive of Crohn disease and immunohistochemical (IHC) staining showing cytomegalovirus (CMV) in all five biopsy specimens, with up to 10 nuclei per field. What is the next best step in management?

A. Ganciclovir.

B. Valganciclovir.

C. Foscarnet.

D. Cidofovir.

E. Letermovir.

The next best step is ganciclovir (**option A**). This patient is presenting with Crohn disease and CMV colitis. CMV is a common herpes virus with a seroprevalence of greater than 70% in the general community. The infection is acquired by close bodily contact, and primary infection may present as a mononucleosis-like illness. The infection eventually establishes latency and can reactivate in times of immune compromise (e.g., advanced HIV, transplant recipients, etc.). Depending on the host, either primary infection or reactivation may present with certain end-organ manifestations such as encephalitis, retinitis, gastrointestinal (GI) tract inflammation (esophagitis, colitis, etc.), hepatitis, pneumonitis, and various other manifestations. GI CMV reactivation is not uncommon to see in flares of inflammatory bowel disease (IBD), especially in steroid-refractory severe IBD. CMV infection occurs more commonly with ulcerative colitis than Crohn disease.

The diagnosis of GI CMV infections can be challenging. Serology has limited utility. Endoscopy should be done, and the endoscopic findings may resemble IBD fairly closely. Multiple biopsies should be obtained from areas with grossly active inflammation–– the ulcer base/edge may be the highest yield location for biopsy. Identification of CMV inclusions ("owl's eye" inclusions) on histopathologic analysis (H&E staining) is very specific (>90%), but it lacks sensitivity due to the infection being pauciviral in nature and patchy in distribution. The sensitivity can be augmented by utilizing IHC analysis. Serum or blood CMV PCR (quantitative viral load) should also be checked, because it may serve as a useful marker to monitor treatment response. Subsequent CMV PCR tests should be done using the same laboratory and same testing platform, because there is a lot of variability between different labs and testing modalities. The blood or serum PCR may or may not be positive in GI CMV disease, and there is no defined cut-off value at which one should start antiviral therapy based on this test. Another test that can be done is the CMV PCR on GI tissue. This test is highly sensitive and specific, but the downside is that it may be overly sensitive, leading to detection of otherwise clinically insignificant disease. Lastly, a stool PCR can be done, but the utility is rather limited.

Management can be a bit nuanced. It can be difficult to determine if finding CMV in the GI tract in these patients represents true infection or reactivation of latent infection (essentially an innocent bystander). Despite this, finding CMV in this situation is associated with higher rates of colectomy and worse prognosis. Patients with steroid-refractory severe IBD with a high density of CMV involvement (≥5 nuclei per field) are the most likely to benefit from treatment. The drug of choice initially is ganciclovir (intravenous). Once the patient has clinically improved, they can be transitioned to oral valganciclovir to complete at least 2 to 3 weeks of therapy. This duration may need to be extended based on clinical response and the serum/blood CMV PCR response (if available). At completion of therapy, the patient should ideally be clinically resolved (asymptomatic) and have resolution of CMV viremia (if it was present to begin with).

Ganciclovir and valganciclovir (**option B**) are associated with bone marrow suppression (monitor complete blood count with differential), GI upset, rashes, neuropsychiatric effects, and metabolic disturbances (creatinine elevation and, rarely, hepatotoxicity). Alternative agents include foscarnet (**option C**) and cidofovir (**option D**). Foscarnet is associated with nephrotoxicity, electrolyte disturbances, bone marrow suppression, GI upset, and peripheral neuropathy. Cidofovir has a side effect profile similar to that of foscarnet, but it notoriously causes dose-dependent nephrotoxicity and has been associated with ocular abnormalities (uveitis). Reduction of the immune suppression should be considered, especially in severe cases of CMV colitis. Lastly, letermovir (**option E**) is typically used for CMV prophylaxis in high-risk (CMV-seropositive) patients who have undergone allogeneic hematopoietic stem cell transplant.

KEY LEARNING POINT

Cytomegalovirus (CMV) colitis can be seen with flares of inflammatory bowel disease, especially ulcerative colitis. Treatment is most likely to be beneficial in those with severe, steroid-refractory disease with a high burden of CMV infection (≥5 nuclei per field on intestinal biopsy). The drug of choice is ganciclovir, with transition to valganciclovir once improved, to complete at least 2 to 3 weeks of therapy.

REFERENCES AND FURTHER READING

- Beswick L, Ye B, van Langenberg DR. Toward an algorithm for the diagnosis and management of CMV in patients with colitis. *Inflamm Bowel Dis.* 2016;22(12):2966–2976. https://doi.org/10.1097/MIB.0000000000000958.
- Goodman AL, Murray CD, Watkins J, Griffiths PD, Webster DP. CMV in the gut: a critical review of CMV detection in the immunocompetent host with colitis. *Eur J Clin Microbiol Infect Dis.* 2015;34(1):13–18. https://doi.org/10.1007/s10096-014-2212-x.

A 40-year-old male is admitted to the hospital with a 2-week history of fevers, headaches, and confusion. He has a history of HIV-1 infection that was diagnosed 10 years ago. He decided not to take any antiretroviral therapy for this, for "religious reasons." He has no medication allergies and does not take any medications routinely. Vital signs show temperature 101° F, heart rate 75 beats per minute, blood pressure 150/90 mmHg, respiratory rate 18, and oxygen saturation 96% on room air. Examination shows temporal wasting, papilledema, and white patches on the oral mucosa, and he does not cooperate with the neurologic examination. The remainder of the examination is unremarkable. Laboratory studies show white blood cell count 3,500 cells/uL, hemoglobin 10 g/dL, platelets 100,000 cells/uL, creatinine 1.0 mg/dL (creatinine clearance >60 mL/min), HIV viral load (RNA) of 120,000 copies/mL, and CD4 lymphocyte count of 10 cells/uL (2%). Toxoplasma IgG is positive. Glucose-6-phosphate dehydrogenase level is normal. Serum cryptococcal antigen is negative. MRI of the brain is shown in Fig. 35.1.

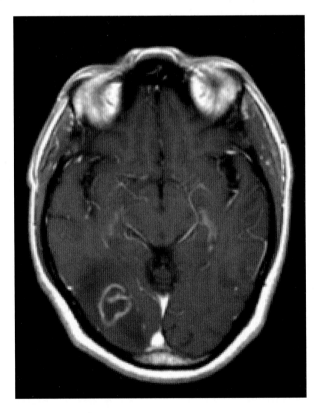

Figure 35.1 – Magnetic resonance image of the brain
Dibble EH, Boxerman JL, Baird GL, Donahue JE, Rogg JM. Toxoplasmosis versus lymphoma: cerebral lesion characterization using DSC-MRI revisited. *Clin Neurol Neurosurg.* 2017;152:84–89.

What is the next best step in the management of this patient?

A. Request brain biopsy.

B. Start antiretroviral therapy.

C. Start sulfadiazine, pyrimethamine, and leucovorin.

D. Obtain lumbar puncture.

E. Start amphotericin-B and flucytosine empirically.

The best next step in management is starting sulfadiazine, pyrimethamine, and leucovorin (**option C**). This patient's presentation is most consistent with cerebral toxoplasmosis. This illness is caused by a protozoan parasite known as *Toxoplasma gondii*. Primary infection with this organism is acquired by ingestion of contaminated raw or undercooked meat or oocysts that are shed in cat feces (i.e., changing litter boxes). Rarely, this infection can be acquired vertically (*in utero*), via transfusion, or during organ transplantation (especially cardiac transplant). Primary infection is often asymptomatic or may manifest as a mononucleosis-like illness. Reactivation of an established latent infection is seen in the immune-compromised population, including patients with advanced HIV (classically CD4 count <100 cells/uL) or transplant patients. In fact, HIV patients with CD4 count less than 100 cells/uL and positive toxoplasma IgG should receive primary prophylaxis for toxoplasmosis (usually trimethoprim/sulfamethoxazole).

In patients with advanced HIV (such as the patient in this case), the presentation usually consists of cerebral toxoplasmosis (*Toxoplasma* encephalitis). There can be a wide array of symptoms, including constitutional symptoms, headaches, confusion, ocular symptoms, or focal neurologic deficits. Rarely, patients can develop disseminated infection resulting in pneumonia/pneumonitis, and myocarditis. Central nervous system (CNS) imaging (usually brain MRI) may show the characteristic multiple ring-enhancing lesions that are usually found in the basal ganglia region. Interestingly, the CNS imaging may also show a solitary lesion (see Fig 35.1) or diffuse encephalitis without any lesions. Almost all patients will be *Toxoplasma* IgG–positive, but if the presentation is due to primary infection, the IgG may be negative. A definitive diagnosis can be established by brain biopsy (**option A**) with appropriate staining. A biopsy is very invasive and is not necessary to do in a patient with a compatible presentation, typical radiographic findings, and a positive *Toxoplasma* IgG (presumptive diagnosis). If a lumbar puncture can be done (**option D**, may not be safe to do in this case due to evidence of raised intracranial pressure), then cerebrospinal fluid (CSF) *Toxoplasma* PCR can be sent, as it is highly specific (96%–100%). Unfortunately, CSF PCR is not very sensitive (~50%), especially if obtained after initiation of therapy. The differential for this type of presentation in advanced HIV patients includes primary CNS lymphoma (PCNSL; related to Epstein–Barr virus [EBV]), and progressive multifocal leukoencephalopathy (PML; related to JC virus reactivation). PCNSL can be very difficult to distinguish from toxoplasmosis clinically, but these patients may have prominent constitutional symptoms and a positive EBV PCR in the CSF. In addition, CSF cytology and flow cytometry may be helpful. PML is easier to distinguish because it is often associated with periventricular white matter lesions that are nonenhancing, and there is usually no mass effect. A positive CSF JC virus PCR test is highly suggestive of PML. Additional differential diagnoses include cytomegalovirus encephalitis (classically CD4 count <50 cells/uL), HIV encephalopathy, CNS tuberculosis (tuberculomas), fungal infections such as CNS cryptococcosis (cryptococcomas), neurologic syphilis (gummas), parasitic infections (neurocysticercosis, Chagas disease reactivation), and pyogenic brain abscesses.

Treatment should be initiated in patients with a consistent presentation (clinically and radiographically), positive *Toxoplasma* IgG, and no alternative explanation for the illness. The first-line regimen is a combination of sulfadiazine, pyrimethamine, and leucovorin. This regimen provides prophylaxis for *Pneumocystis jirovecii* pneumonia (PJP) as well. Alternative regimens include pyrimethamine, leucovorin, and clindamycin (does not provide prophylaxis for PJP) or trimethoprim/sulfamethoxazole monotherapy (provides prophylaxis for PJP). Clinical response occurs in approximately 90% of patients after 2 weeks of treatment. Therefore, a repeat evaluation (clinical and radiographic) should be done at 2 weeks. If there is improvement, then treatment is continued for at least 6 weeks and potentially longer if unsatisfactory response occurs by 6 weeks. If there is no improvement at 2 weeks, then brain biopsy should be pursued. Adjunctive corticosteroids should only be used to treat mass effect and/or cerebral edema. One caveat to be aware of is that steroids may lead to radiographic and clinical improvement in patients with PCNSL, so improvement may not completely rule out the possibility of PCNSL. Most clinicians wait at least 2 weeks after the diagnosis of cerebral toxoplasmosis to start antiretroviral therapy (ART; **option B**). Eventually, after completing the treatment course, patients are placed on long-term suppressive therapy (usually pyrimethamine, sulfadiazine, and leucovorin), and this regimen is continued until asymptomatic and CD4 count is greater than 200 cells/uL for more than 6 months in response to ART. Starting amphotericin-B and flucytosine empirically (**option E**) can be considered if cryptococcal infection is suspected. Cryptococcal infection can present somewhat similarly, and evaluation would include serum cryptococcal antigen and lumbar puncture for CSF analysis. The negative serum antigen in this case makes cryptococcus very unlikely.

KEY LEARNING POINT

The diagnosis of cerebral toxoplasmosis in patients with HIV can be made presumptively based on a consistent clinical and radiographic presentation, a positive Toxoplasma *IgG, and clinical improvement with directed treatment. First-line therapy is sulfadiazine, pyrimethamine, and leucovorin.*

REFERENCES AND FURTHER READING

- CDC. Guidelines for the Prevention and Treatment of Opportunistic Infections in HIV-Infected Adults and Adolescents: Recommendations from the Centers for Disease Control and Prevention, the National Institutes of Health, and the HIV Medicine Association of the Infectious Diseases Society of America. https://clinicalinfo.hiv.gov/sites/default/files/inline-files/adult_oi.pdf. Accessed November 11, 2020.
- Dibble E, Boxerman JL, Baird GL, Donahue JE, Rogg FM. Toxoplasmosis versus lymphoma: cerebral lesion characterization using DSC-MRI revisited. *Clin Neurol Neurosurg.* 2017;152:84–89. https://doi.org/10.1016/j.clineuro.2016.11.023.

A 40-year-old female is admitted to the hospital with a new diagnosis of acute myelogenous leukemia. She received induction chemotherapy, which resulted in complete remission. She then underwent consolidation with an allogeneic hematopoietic stem cell transplant 14 days ago. Current medications include acyclovir, cefepime, and fluconazole. Over the past week, she has had low-grade fevers, a dry cough, shortness of breath, and chest pain. Vital signs reveal temperature 100.8° F, heart rate 95 beats per minute, blood pressure 110/70 mmHg, respiratory rate 18, and oxygen saturation 93% on room air. Examination is fairly unremarkable. She has a peripherally inserted central catheter (PICC) in her right brachial region that appears normal (no outward signs of infection). Laboratory studies show white blood cells 0 cells/uL, hemoglobin 7.5 g/dL, platelets 11,000 cells/uL, creatinine 1.0 mg/dL (creatinine clearance >60 mL/min), and normal liver function tests. Serum galactomannan is positive. Chest CT is shown in Fig. 36.1. The primary team starts the patient on amphotericin-B and stops the fluconazole. Further work-up is pending.

What is the next best step in the management of this patient?

A. Continue amphotericin-B.

B. Change to caspofungin.

C. Change back to fluconazole.

D. Change to voriconazole.

E. Add caspofungin.

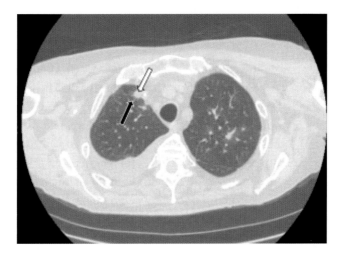

Figure 36.1 – CT scan of the chest
Bays DJ, Thompson GR 3rd. Fungal infections of the stem cell transplant recipient and hematologic malignancy patients. *Infect Dis Clin North Am*. 2019;33(2):545–566. https://doi.org/10.1016/j.idc.2019.02.006.

The best next step here is to change amphotericin-B to voriconazole (**option D**). This patient's presentation is concerning for invasive fungal infection, most likely due to *Aspergillus* spp. Invasive aspergillosis is the most common invasive mold infection (IMI) in the stem cell transplant population. It usually presents like a pneumonia with fevers, cough, chest pain, and shortness of breath. Rarely, patients may develop hemoptysis. Extrapulmonary manifestations include central nervous system (CNS) infection (very high mortality), sinusitis (often will see eschar endoscopically), bone/joint infection, and cutaneous disease (necrotic skin lesions). Lung imaging classically shows a "halo sign" which is a nodular lesion (often >1 cm in size) with surrounding ground-glass opacification (see Fig. 36.1).

Diagnosis of IMIs can be somewhat challenging. Definitive diagnosis of IMI requires direct visualization of fungal forms on histopathologic, cytopathologic, or microscopic evaluation of tissue obtained from a sterile site, or positive cultures from a normally sterile site obtained via sterile procedure. Obtaining tissue in these patients often is not possible due to risk of complications in setting of thrombocytopenia and neutropenia. Therefore, most diagnoses are made by less invasive, albeit less definitive, means. These tests include 1,3-beta-D-glucan (BDG; Fungitell assay) and galactomannan assay. BDG may be elevated in many fungal infections, including invasive aspergillosis, but is not typically elevated in *Mucorales* or *Cryptococcus* infections. BDG is not very specific. Galactomannan can be detected in the serum and bronchoalveolar lavage (BAL). Compared to the serum galactomannan test, the BAL galactomannan test is more sensitive but less specific for the diagnosis of invasive aspergillosis (mainly because *Aspergillus* can colonize the respiratory tract).

Management of invasive aspergillosis is relatively straightforward. The drug of choice for *Aspergillus* infections is voriconazole (**option D**). Voriconazole is associated with improved survival compared with amphotericin-B (**option A**). Isavuconazole is considered noninferior to voriconazole for invasive aspergillosis based on a randomized trial published in 2016. In those with severe disease, combination therapy with voriconazole and an echinocandin (i.e., caspofungin, **option E**) may be considered. If invasive aspergillosis occurs while on appropriate fungal prophylaxis, then consideration should be given to using alternative therapy and/or checking drug levels if appropriate. Surgical intervention should be considered for sinusitis, CNS infections, bone/joint infections, and cutaneous infections. Outcomes are better in those with recovery of neutrophil counts. Any immune suppression that the patient is receiving should be reduced as much as possible. The typical duration of treatment is at least 6 to 12 weeks, but this may be prolonged depending on clinical course, results of serial galactomannan tests, and serial imaging (caveat: imaging may initially appear worse as neutrophil count improves). Secondary prophylaxis should be considered for those with repeated or ongoing immune suppression.

Amphotericin-B (**option A**) has activity against most species of *Aspergillus* (excluding *A. terreus*) but is considered to be less effective than voriconazole. Caspofungin monotherapy (**option B**) is considered a salvage option and is much less likely to be effective than voriconazole. Fluconazole (**option C**) is not a mold-active antifungal, so it would not provide any reliable coverage for *Aspergillus* infection.

KEY LEARNING POINT

The drug of choice for **Aspergillus** *infection is voriconazole.*

REFERENCES AND FURTHER READING

- Bays DJ, Thompson GR 3rd. Fungal infections of the stem cell transplant recipient and hematologic malignancy patients. *Infect Dis Clin North Am*. 2019;33(2):545–566. https://doi.org/10.1016/j.idc.2019.02.006.
- Herbrecht R, Denning DW, Patterson TF, et al. Voriconazole versus amphotericin B for primary therapy of invasive aspergillosis. *N Engl J Med*. 2002;347(6):408–415. https://doi.org/10.1056/NEJMoa020191.
- Maertens JA, Raad II, Marr KA, et al. Isavuconazole versus voriconazole for primary treatment of invasive mould disease caused by *Aspergillus* and other filamentous fungi (SECURE): a phase 3, randomised-controlled, non-inferiority trial. *Lancet*. 2016;387(10020):760–769. https://doi.org/10.1016/S0140-6736(15)01159-9.
- Marr KA, Schlamm HT, Herbrecht R, et al. Combination antifungal therapy for invasive aspergillosis: a randomized trial. *Ann Intern Med*. 2015;162(2):81–89. https://doi.org/10.7326/M13-2508. Erratum in: *Ann Intern Med*. 2015;162(6):463. Erratum in: *Ann Intern Med*. 2019;170(3):220.

A 50-year-old male is admitted to the hospital with a 2-day history of fevers and chills. He has a history of short-gut syndrome related to extensive resections for prior abdominal gunshot wound injuries. He is on total parenteral nutrition via a peripherally inserted central catheter (PICC). Vital signs show temperature 101° F, heart rate 105 beats per minute, blood pressure 110/70 mmHg, respiratory rate 16, and oxygen saturation 96% on room air. Examination shows a PICC line in the right brachial region with no insertion site erythema or tenderness. Blood cultures are obtained from the PICC line and the peripheral circulation. Eventually, the PICC line blood culture returns positive with the microbiologic report showing "yeast resembling bowling pins" on gram stain, but no growth. Consequently, the microbiology technologist decides to culture the isolate on Sabouraud's dextrose agar (SDA) overlaid with olive oil. Which of the following is the most likely organism responsible for this patient's illness?

A. *Malassezia* spp.
B. *Candida* spp.
C. *Cryptococcus* spp.
D. *Histoplasma capsulatum.*
E. *Aspergillus fumigatus.*

The most likely causative organism is *Malassezia* spp. (**option A**). There are various medically relevant fungal organisms that medical practitioners should be aware of. They are summarized in Fig. 37.1 (the most important organisms are bolded).

Fungi can exist as yeasts (unicellular forms), molds (multicellular forms with hyphae), or both (dimorphic fungi—yeasts at body temperature and molds in the environment). The microbiologic diagnosis of fungal infections can involve various tests, including microscopy with specialized staining, culture-based methods, serology, antigen-based testing, and molecular analysis (PCR and sequencing). Microscopy and culture-based methods will be discussed here.

Microscopy involves use of potassium hydroxide to digest tissue cells and allow visualization of fungal cell walls. Visualization is improved by adding calcofluor white stain, which stains fungal cell walls and can be visualized with fluorescent light. Interestingly, most fungi actually stain gram-positive (purple/blue color) on routine gram stain. In pathologic specimens (formalin-fixed), several stains can be employed. Routine hematoxylin and eosin stain will stain most fungal organisms, but the more useful stains are Grocott–Gomori methenamine silver (GMS) and periodic acid Schiff (PAS) stain. GMS will stain fungal organisms "black" (with greenish background), while PAS will stain fungal organisms pink/red. The mucicarmine stain is typically useful to demonstrate the capsular polysaccharide of *Cryptococcus*, which stains red/pink. The usual culture medium used, which is called SDA, supports fungal growth but inhibits bacterial growth. *Candida* spp. can be differentiated using specialized media (CHROMagar). Interestingly, many fungal organisms will grow on routine blood cultures, most commonly *Candida* spp., *Cryptococcus*, and *Fusarium*. The highest-yield microbiologic characteristics of the various fungal organisms are discussed in Table 37.1.

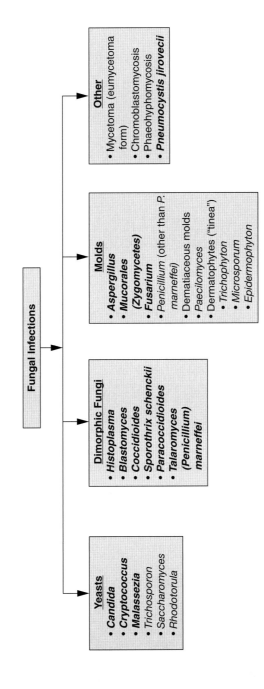

Fungal Infections

Yeasts
- *Candida*
- *Cryptococcus*
- *Malassezia*
- Trichosporon
- Saccharomyces
- Rhodotorula

Dimorphic Fungi
- *Histoplasma*
- *Blastomyces*
- *Coccidioides*
- *Sporothrix schenckii*
- *Paracoccidioides*
- *Talaromyces (Penicillium) marneffei*

Molds
- *Aspergillus*
- *Mucorales (Zygomycetes)*
- *Fusarium*
- Penicillium (other than P. marneffei)
- Dematiaceous molds
- Paecilomyces
- Dermatophytes ("tinea")
  - Trichophyton
  - Microsporum
  - Epidermophyton

Other
- Mycetoma (eumycetoma form)
- Chromoblastomycosis
- Phaeohyphomycosis
- ***Pneumocystis jirovecii***

Figure 37.1 – Overview of medically important fungal organisms

Table 37.1 – Microbiologic Characteristics of Selected Fungal Organisms

Fungus	Microbiologic Characteristics
Candida spp.	• Budding yeast with pseudohyphae (*C. glabrata* does not form pseudohyphae). *C albicans* also forms true hyphae (germ tube test) • CHROMagar pattern—*C. albicans* is green, *C. auris* and *C. tropicalis* are blue, *C. krusei* is pink, *C. glabrata* is purple
Cryptococcus spp.	• Yeast with thick polysaccharide capsule (can be visualized with India ink staining) and narrow-based budding
Malassezia spp.	• Yeast with bowling pin appearance. Require fatty acids for growth (typically use olive oil laid over solid media). Potassium hydroxide preparation may show a "spaghetti and meatballs" appearance
Histoplasma	• Tissue form—small intracellular yeasts within macrophages
Blastomyces	• Tissue form—large yeasts with broad-based budding and thick double-refractile walls
Coccidioides	• Tissue form—large spherules with endospores and thick double-refractile walls
Paracoccidioides	• Tissue form—large yeasts with multiple budding ("ship-wheel" formation)
Sporothrix schenkii	• Tissue form—small yeasts with "cigar shape"
Penicillium (Talaromyces) marneffei	• Tissue form—small yeasts dividing by fission (may see dividing wall)
Aspergillus	• Septate hyphae with acute-angle branching (45 degrees). Septate hyphae can also be seen in *Fusarium* and *Scedosporium*
Mucorales	• Broad ribbon-like nonparallel aseptate hyphae with right-angle branching (90 degrees)
Pneumocystis jirovecii	• Trophozoite and cyst forms in lung specimens that can be stained with Giemsa, Grocott–Gomori methenamine silver, calcofluor, or toluidine blue • Can also be detected via direct fluorescent antibody or PCR

KEY LEARNING POINT

Malassezia spp. can rarely cause line-associated infections, usually in patients on total parenteral nutrition. Malassezia requires fatty acids (olive oil is typically used) for growth.

REFERENCES AND FURTHER READING

- Riedel S, Hobden JA, Miller S, et al. Medical mycology. In: *Jawetz, Melnick, & Adelberg's Medical Microbiology*. 28th ed. McGraw-Hill.
- Ryan KJ, In: eds. Pathogenesis and diagnosis of fungal infections. *Sherris Medical Microbiology*. 7th ed. McGraw-Hill.
- Tragiannidis A, Bisping G, Koehler G, Groll AH. Minireview: *Malassezia* infections in immunocompromised patients. *Mycoses*. 2010;53(3):187–195. https://doi.org/10.1111/j.1439-0507.2009.01814.x.

A 50-year-old female is admitted to the hospital with new-onset acute myelogenous leukemia. She is initiated on induction chemotherapy with cytarabine and daunorubicin. She achieves complete remission followed by consolidation with allogeneic hematopoietic stem cell transplantation. On the 10th day after her stem cell transplant, she develops fevers and rigors. She has no other localizing symptoms. Current antimicrobial medications include acyclovir, fluconazole, and ciprofloxacin. Vital signs show temperature 101° F, heart rate 110 beats per minute, blood pressure 105/60 mmHg, respiratory rate 18, and oxygen saturation 96% on room air. Physical examination shows extensive oral mucosal ulceration. There is a peripheral-inserted central catheter (PICC) line in the right brachial region that has no tenderness or insertion-site redness. The remainder of the exam is unremarkable. Laboratory evaluation shows white blood cell count 0 cells/uL, hemoglobin 7.2 g/dL, platelets 12,000 cells/uL, creatinine 0.9 mg/dL (creatinine clearance >60 mL/min), and normal liver function testing. Blood cultures are obtained from the PICC line and the periphery. The patient's antimicrobial regimen is changed to acyclovir, cefepime, and posaconazole. Eventually, the blood cultures return with both sets growing *Candida glabrata*. Which of the following best describes the mechanism of action of the antifungal drug that is most likely to be effective for this infection?

A. Binds ergosterol to induce pore formation.

B. Inhibition of ergosterol synthesis.

C. Inhibition of beta-D-glucan synthesis.

D. Inhibition of microtubule formation and mitosis.

E. Inhibition of nucleic acid synthesis.

The most effective antifungal is an echinocandin, so the correct answer is inhibition of beta-D-glucan synthesis (**option C**). The polyenes (amphotericin-B and nystatin) bind ergosterol to induce pore formation and fungal cell death (**option A**). The azole antifungals act by inhibiting synthesis of ergosterol via inhibition of the P-450 dependent 14-alpha-demethylase enzyme (**option B**). Griseofulvin is a microtubule inhibitor (**option D**). Lastly, flucytosine acts by inhibiting synthesis of nucleic acids (**option E**). The mechanism of action of the various commonly used antifungals is portrayed in Fig. 38.1.

Candidemia refers to the presence of *Candida* spp. in the bloodstream. In general, *Candida* in a blood culture should not be regarded as a blood culture contaminant, as there is a significant mortality associated with candidemia. Risk factors for development of candidemia include prolonged intensive care unit stays, presence of invasive lines (i.e., central venous catheters), immune compromise, recent surgical procedures (especially abdominal surgeries), use of broad-spectrum antibiotics, necrotizing pancreatitis, and total parenteral nutrition. When a patient develops candidemia, there are several steps that should be taken. First, the infectious disease team should generally be involved in the case. Blood cultures should be repeated to document clearance of the bloodstream, because the treatment duration is typically counted from the date of clearance. Because *Candida* readily grows on routine blood cultures, there is

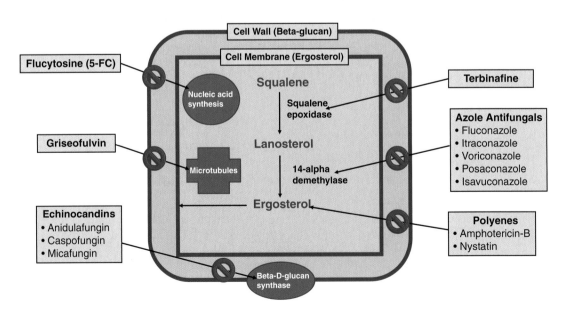

Figure 38.1 – Antifungal mechanisms of action

generally no need to obtain fungal blood cultures. A source of the infection should be sought out by utilizing the clinical history and examination as a guide. Common sources of infection include line infections, urinary tract infections, and intra-abdominal infection/translocation (especially in neutropenic patients). All patients should have a dilated ophthalmologic examination performed within the first week of the diagnosis to rule out ocular infection (i.e., endophthalmitis, chorioretinitis, etc.), which occurs in 15% to 20% of patients. In neutropenic patients, this examination should be done within the first week after recovery of neutrophil count because neutrophils are necessary to generate the clinical manifestations of these ocular infections. Persistent candidemia in the face of appropriate antifungal therapy should prompt a more in-depth investigation for potential sources of infection (i.e., echocardiogram, visceral imaging, etc.).

There is a mortality benefit for those who receive early antifungal therapy and appropriate source control, so these goals should always be strived for. Indwelling vascular devices (i.e., central lines) should be removed as soon as possible in most cases, but especially if the line is considered the source of the infection blood cultures fail to clear, or if the infection is due to *C. parapsilosis* (a species associated with line infections). This recommendation is a bit more lenient in neutropenic patients, who are often somewhat "line-dependent." The choice of empiric therapy will depend on prior antifungal (azole or echinocandin) exposure, the infecting *Candida* species (if known), the clinical status (degree of illness) of the patient, and the location of the infection. The echinocandins are considered the best initial empiric therapy, as they are fungicidal, have broader *Candida* coverage, are better tolerated, and are associated with better outcomes than azole antifungals. Azole antifungals (typically fluconazole) can be used empirically if the patient is hemodynamically stable and unlikely to have an azole-resistant species (i.e., does not have prior azole exposure or certain conditions such as diabetes or malignancy). The echinocandins do not have reliable penetration into the central nervous system (CNS), the eye, and the urine, so the echinocandins should not be used to treat infections in these areas. Targeted therapy is guided by susceptibility testing. Azole susceptibility testing should be done for all bloodstream isolates, while echinocandin susceptibility testing should be done for those with prior echinocandin exposure or if the infection is due to *C. glabrata* or *C. parapsilosis*. Treatment duration for uncomplicated candidemia (i.e., no metastatic site of infection) is typically 2 weeks (14 days) from the day of blood culture clearance and resolution of signs and symptoms. In neutropenic patients, neutrophil recovery is associated with better outcomes; therefore, some providers continue treatment until the neutrophil count recovers. There are various agents that can be used for candidemia, and these are discussed in Table 38.1.

Table 38.1 – Antifungals for Candidemia

Drug	Clinical Considerations	Adverse Effects
Amphotericin-B (Amp-B)	• Three forms—liposomal, deoxycholate, and lipid-complex • Lipid formulations preferred due to better tolerance and less toxicity • Lipid formulations have limited renal excretion, and thus cannot be used for urinary infections • Drug of choice for *Candida* infections in pregnancy • Most species of *C. lusitaniae* are resistant, and many *C. auris* species are resistant as well	• Infusion reactions and phlebitis • Nephrotoxicity—limited by pre- and postdose saline infusion • Metabolic disturbances— hypomagnesemia, hypokalemia, hypophosphatemia, metabolic acidosis (bicarbonaturia → renal tubular acidosis) • Erythropoietin suppression (normocytic anemia)
Fluconazole (Diflucan)	• Highly bioavailable when given orally (no food or pH dependence). No drug level monitoring necessary • Renal dose adjustment (RDA) required once glomerular filtration rate <50 mL/min • Penetrates most tissues, including urinary tract (>10 times the serum concentration), central nervous system (CNS), and eye • *C. krusei* is intrinsically resistant to fluconazole • *C. auris* is often resistant to fluconazole • *C. glabrata* may be either resistant or susceptible dose–dependent (SDD). SDD *C. glabrata* can be treated with higher doses of fluconazole (12 mg/kg), because resistance is related to increased drug efflux	• Classic—gastrointestinal (GI) upset, drug-drug interactions (CYP enzyme inhibition → potential elevation of serum concentration of other CYP metabolized drugs), hepatotoxicity, prolonged QT interval, teratogenic • Alopecia and xerosis (reversible)
Itraconazole (Sporanox)	• Not very well studied for candidemia • Poor CNS penetration due to high serum protein binding. • Bioavailability depends on the formulation used • Capsule form is less well-absorbed. This can be augmented if taken with food and an acidic beverage. Antacid medications (H2 antagonists, proton pump inhibitors, etc.) impair absorption • Solution form has better absorption and should be taken on an empty stomach • Therapeutic drug monitoring (TDM) often used in more severe infections. Typically check drug levels (measure levels of itraconazole and hydroxy-itraconazole via high-performance liquid chromatography) ~2 weeks after starting treatment. The level is calculated by adding these two levels together. Goal level is >1 ug/mL	• Similar to classic fluconazole adverse effects (AEs) • Heart failure (negative inotropic effect) • Inhibition of 11-beta-hydroxysteroid dehydrogenase → hypertension, hypokalemia, and edema (mineralocorticoid excess)
Voriconazole (Vfend)	• Excellent oral bioavailability (take on empty stomach) with no RDA necessary for oral formulation. • IV formulation has cyclodextrin vehicle that may accumulate in renal dysfunction and cause nephrotoxicity (controversial) • Excellent penetration into CNS and eye, but poor urinary penetration	• Similar to classic fluconazole AEs • Nonlinear kinetics—change in dose results in disproportionate change in serum level, which may lead to toxic levels • Visual disturbances (~20% incidence) – onset within 1 hour of last dose

(Continued)

Table 38.1 – Antifungals for Candidemia *(Cont'd)*

Drug	Clinical Considerations	Adverse Effects
	• Efficacious for fluconazole-resistant species such as *C. krusei, C. guilliermondii*, and *C. glabrata*, if susceptibility testing reveals they are susceptible to voriconazole • TDM often done for severe infections. Goal trough concentration is 1–5.5 micrograms/mL (typically checked ~1 week after starting)	• Encephalopathy and hallucinations (at toxic levels) • Photosensitivity • Long-term use associated with skin cancer and reversible periostitis (↑ fluoride level)
Posaconazole (Noxafil)	• Not very well studied for invasive *Candida* infections, but anti-*Candida* spectrum/activity is similar to that of voriconazole	• Similar to classic fluconazole AEs
Isavuconazole (Cresemba)	• Did not meet noninferiority when compared with caspofungin for treatment of candidemia (ACTIVE trial)	• Similar to classic fluconazole AEs, except will SHORTEN the QT interval
Echinocandins	• Three IV drugs (all given once daily)—caspofungin, micafungin, and anidulafungin. Rezafungin is under investigation as a new echinocandin agent • No RDA necessary for any of these agents • Poor penetration into CNS, eye, and urine (although there are reports of successful treatment of *Candida* urinary tract infection with these drugs). • *C. parapsiolosis* has higher minimum inhibitory concentrations for echinocandins (may be less effective for *C. parapsilosis* infections)	• Typically well-tolerated • Hepatotoxicity may occur. Only caspofungin requires dose adjustment with significant hepatic dysfunction • Potentially teratogenic
Flucytosine (5-FC)	• Excellent oral bioavailability and requires RDA • Penetrates well into CNS, eye, and urine • *C. krusei* is intrinsically resistant to 5-FC. • Resistance may develop if used as monotherapy	• GI upset—nausea, vomiting, diarrhea • Bone marrow suppression (cytopenia) • Hepatitis • Teratogenic

KEY LEARNING POINT

Echinocandins are the best initial therapy for invasive Candida *infections (not involving the eye, central nervous system, or urinary tract). They function by inhibiting the synthesis of beta-D-glucan.*

REFERENCES AND FURTHER READING

• Bennet JE, Dolin R, Blaser MJ. *Mandell, Douglas, and Bennett's Principles and Practice of Infectious Diseases*. 9th ed. Elsevier; 2020.
• Pappas PG, Kauffman CA, Andes DR, et al. Clinical practice guideline for the management of candidiasis: 2016 update by the Infectious Diseases Society of America. *Clin Infect Dis.* 2016;62(4):e1–e50. https://doi.org/10.1093/cid/civ933.

A 50-year-old male is admitted with several days of fevers and abdominal pain. He has a history of appendiceal carcinoma with metastases to the liver. He is currently receiving palliative chemotherapy (5-fluorouracil and oxaliplatin), which he last received 7 days prior to admission. Medications include ondansetron, oxycodone, acetaminophen, and a probiotic supplement. Vital signs reveal temperature 101° F, heart rate 100 beats per minute, blood pressure 105/60 mmHg, respiratory rate 18, and oxygen saturation 98% on room air. Examination reveals right lower quadrant tenderness with mild rebound tenderness. He has a port catheter in place that appears normal. Laboratory work-up reveals white blood cell count 100 cells/uL and creatinine 1.0 mg/dL (creatinine clearance >60 mL/min). Blood cultures are drawn. The patient is started on cefepime and metronidazole. CT of the abdomen reveals a 3 × 4 cm abscess in the right lower quadrant. A percutaneous drain is placed into the abscess, and purulent-appearing fluid is sent for gram stain and culture. Gram stain reveals gram-positive rods, gram-positive cocci, and gram-negative rods. After 2 days, the culture is only growing *Lactobacillus rhamnosus*. The patient's abdominal pain has improved, but he continues to have low-grade fevers. The drain is functioning well and putting out 50 cc/day of purulent-appearing fluid. In addition to stopping the probiotic supplement, what is the next best step in management?

A. Add vancomycin.

B. Stop cefepime and metronidazole. Start piperacillin/tazobactam.

C. Stop cefepime and metronidazole. Start clindamycin.

D. Stop cefepime and metronidazole. Start ampicillin/sulbactam.

E. Add intravenous penicillin-G.

The best answer is to stop cefepime and metronidazole and start piperacillin/tazobactam (**option B**). This patient has febrile neutropenia and a polymicrobial intraabdominal abscess (likely related to the underlying malignancy and gastrointestinal translocation in the setting of neutropenia). The abscess involves *L. rhamnosus* and various other anaerobic organisms, as suggested by a positive gram stain (gram-negative rods and gram-positive cocci) with no growth on culture. Anaerobic organisms are difficult to grow in general, but the growth becomes even more difficult in patients with prior antimicrobial exposure, as in this patient. *Lactobacillus* spp. are facultative anaerobic gram-positive rods that are a normal part of the flora in the gastrointestinal tract and even the vagina. They are often seen in polymicrobial intra-abdominal abscesses and are usually considered nonpathogenic. However, *Lactobacillus* spp. have rarely been associated with invasive infections, including bacteremia, endocarditis, and intra-abdominal infections. Probiotics may contain *Lactobacillus* spp. that may contribute to infections in the appropriate setting. The initial antibiotic regimen in this patient (cefepime and metronidazole) provides adequate coverage for the febrile neutropenia and most intra-abdominal pathogens. The regimen does not reliably cover *Lactobacillus* spp., which should probably be covered in this patient, who has ongoing fevers despite adequate source control. Agents with reliable activity against *Lactobacillus* include penicillin, ampicillin, piperacillin/tazobactam, clindamycin, and carbapenems. Switching this patient to piperacillin/tazobactam (**option B**) would provide adequate coverage for febrile neutropenia and various intra-abdominal pathogens, including *Lactobacillus*. Adding vancomycin (**option A**) would likely be ineffective, because most *Lactobacillus* spp. are intrinsically resistant to vancomycin. As a side note, there are several other gram-positive bacteria that are typically resistant to vancomycin, and these include *Clostridium innocuum, Enterococcus gallinarum, Enterococcus casseliflavus, Erysipelothrix rhusiopathiae, Leuconostoc,* and *Pediococcus*. Switching to clindamycin (**option C**) would provide coverage for the *Lactobacillus* and some anaerobes, but not for febrile neutropenia and various other intra-abdominal pathogens (many gram-negative organisms and *Bacteroides fragilis*). Switching to ampicillin/sulbactam (**option D**) would cover the intra-abdominal infection, including *Lactobacillus*, but would provide inadequate coverage for febrile neutropenia. Lastly, adding penicillin-G (**option E**) would add better coverage for the *Lactobacillus* spp., but this option would not be ideal, as it would create an odd regimen with dual beta-lactam therapy that could predispose the patient to more adverse effects.

KEY LEARNING POINT

*Most **Lactobacillus spp**. are intrinsically resistant to vancomycin. The most reliable agents are penicillin, ampicillin, piperacillin/tazobactam, clindamycin, and carbapenems.*

REFERENCES AND FURTHER READING

- Bennet JE, Dolin R, Blaser MJMandell. *Douglas, and Bennett's Principles and Practice of Infectious Diseases*. 9th ed. Elsevier; 2020.
- Spec A, Escota G, Chrisler C, Davies B, eds. *Comprehensive Review of Infectious Diseases*. 1st ed. Elsevier; 2019.

A 60-year-old male presents to the emergency room with a 1-day history of fevers, chills, confusion, and scrotal pain, redness, and swelling. He denies any recent injuries to the genital region. He is allergic to penicillin, which caused a rash when he was a child. His medical history is notable for type 2 diabetes mellitus complicated by peripheral neuropathy, retinopathy, chronic kidney disease, and peripheral vascular disease. Medications include baby aspirin, metformin, insulin, gabapentin, lisinopril, furosemide, and atorvastatin. He is not sexually active. Vital signs show temperature 102.5° F, heart rate 120 beats per minute, blood pressure 95/55 mmHg, respiratory rate 22, and oxygen saturation 90% on room air. Examination reveals an obese man with panscrotal erythema, warmth, and swelling. The scrotum is exquisitely tender to palpation, but there is no obvious crepitus palpable. He is a bit combative on examination. Laboratory evaluation shows white blood cell count 20,000 cells/uL (85% neutrophils), creatinine 1.5 mg/dL (creatinine clearance 40 mL/min), and hemoglobin A1c 12%. Blood cultures are obtained. What is the next best step in the management of this patient?

A. Start vancomycin and piperacillin/tazobactam.

B. Start vancomycin, cefepime, and metronidazole.

C. Start vancomycin, cefepime, metronidazole, and clindamycin.

D. Start daptomycin, cefepime, metronidazole, and clindamycin.

E. Urologic consultation.

The best next step would be to consult a urologist (**option E**). This patient's presentation is highly concerning for a necrotizing skin and soft tissue infection (NSSTI). NSSTI is a general term used to describe several different types of high-mortality infections that involve the deeper soft tissues (fascia, subcutaneous fat, and potentially even muscle), spread rapidly, and are associated with significant systemic toxicity. These infections classically occur in patients with certain risk factors including obesity, poorly-controlled diabetes mellitus, peripheral arterial or venous disease, immune compromise, or intravenous (IV) drug abuse, or as a sequela of skin trauma/injury (may be minor) or surgery.

NSSTI can be polymicrobial (type I NSSTI) or monomicrobial (type II NSSTI) Fig. 40.1. Type I infections are often caused by mixed aerobic-anaerobic organisms, whereas type II infections are due to either *beta-hemolytic streptococci* (classically *Streptococcus pyogenes*) or *Staphylococcus aureus*. The latter two organisms may cause toxic-shock syndrome as well. Rarely, *Aeromonas* can be a cause in those exposed to fresh or brackish water. Furthermore, *Vibrio* spp. (classically *V. vulnificus* and *V. parahaemolyticus*) can cause NSSTI in patients (classically those with chronic liver disease) who have been exposed to salt water or brackish water or have consumed shellfish. NSSTIs most commonly involve the extremities, but in certain body regions they have been given specific names. For example, this patient likely has Fournier's gangrene, which is NSSTI of the male genitalia or male/female perineum. Another example is Ludwig's angina, which is a sequela of an odontogenic infection that manifests as submandibular (deep neck space) NSSTI.

The diagnosis can be challenging and may require a high degree of clinical suspicion. Patients will often be toxic-appearing, with high fevers, hypotension, tachycardia, leukocytosis, and end-organ damage (i.e., encephalopathy, acute kidney injury, etc.). They will have classic inflammatory signs (erythema, warmth, edema, pain/tenderness), but the pain is classically "out of proportion." In addition, there may be hard, "woody" induration, crepitus (subcutaneous gas/emphysema), lack of sensation (anesthesia), bullae, and skin discoloration (even necrosis). These findings will not be present in every patient and will depend on causative organism(s), host immune status, and stage of illness. Failure to clinically improve or progression on seemingly appropriate antimicrobial therapy suggests NSSTI as well. Blood cultures should be obtained, but definitive microbiologic diagnosis is obtained via gram stain and culture of deep tissue specimens at the time of surgical intervention. Imaging (CT or MRI) may show nonspecific findings including subcutaneous swelling/edema and gas, but imaging does not make the diagnosis and should not delay appropriate evaluation and management.

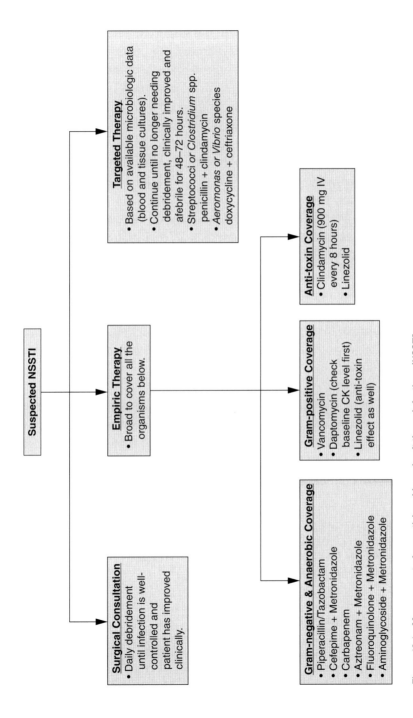

Suspected NSSTI

Surgical Consultation
• Daily debridement until infection is well-controlled and patient has improved clinically.

Targeted Therapy
• Based on available microbiologic data (blood and tissue cultures).
• Continue until no longer needing debridement, clinically improved and afebrile for 48–72 hours.
• Streptococci or *Clostridium* spp. penicillin + clindamycin
• *Aeromonas* or *Vibrio* species doxycycline + ceftriaxone

Empiric Therapy
• Broad to cover all the organisms below.

Anti-toxin Coverage
• Clindamycin (900 mg IV every 8 hours)
• Linezolid

Gram-positive Coverage
• Vancomycin
• Daptomycin (check baseline CK level first)
• Linezolid (anti-toxin effect as well)

Gram-negative & Anaerobic Coverage
• Piperacillin/Tazobactam
• Cefepime + Metronidazole
• Carbapenem
• Aztreonam + Metronidazole
• Fluoroquinolone + Metronidazole
• Aminoglycoside + Metronidazole

Figure 40.1 – Management of necrotizing skin and soft tissue infections (NSSTI).

Management is relatively straightforward. If NSSTI is suspected, the most important next step is to involve a surgeon, because these patients will need debridement for successful control of infection. In fact, they typically receive repeated debridement until the surgeon feels the infection has been well-controlled. Empiric antimicrobial therapy is typically broad, to cover gram-positive organisms such as *streptococci* and *staphylococci* (including methicillin-resistant *S. aureus*), gram-negative organisms (often including coverage for *Pseudomonas*, although it is not a common pathogen), anaerobic organisms, and toxin-producing organisms. Gram-positive coverage can be achieved with vancomycin, daptomycin, or linezolid. Gram-negative and anaerobic coverage can be achieved via piperacillin/tazobactam, cefepime plus metronidazole, or a carbapenem such as meropenem. In patients with severe penicillin allergies, aztreonam, an aminoglycoside, or a fluoroquinolone (ciprofloxacin or levofloxacin) plus metronidazole can be used. Drugs with antitoxin effect include clindamycin (dosed 900 mg IV every 8 hours) and linezolid. The coverage can be de-escalated based on results of available microbiologic data and clinical trajectory. For infections due to *Streptococci* or *Clostridium*, the regimen of choice is penicillin plus clindamycin. For *Aeromonas* and *Vibrio* spp., the regimen of choice is doxycycline plus ceftriaxone. In general, the antitoxin drug is limited to no more than 5 days' duration. The antimicrobial therapy is given until debridement is no longer needed and the patient has clinically improved and has been afebrile for 48 to 72 hours.

Option A (vancomycin and piperacillin/tazobactam) would provide broad coverage but would not provide any antitoxin effect and may be a bit risky in someone with a history of a mild penicillin allergy (cross-reactivity with piperacillin/tazobactam). **Option B** would be a suitable alternative to option A but still does not provide any antitoxin effect. **Options C and D** would both be valid options, but surgical consultation takes precedence.

KEY LEARNING POINT

The best initial step in the management of a patient with suspected necrotizing skin and soft tissue infection is an urgent surgical consultation.

REFERENCES AND FURTHER READING

- Stevens DL, Bisno AL, Chambers HF, et al. Practice guidelines for the diagnosis and management of skin and soft tissue infections: 2014 update by the Infectious Diseases Society of America. *Clin Infect Dis.* 2014;59(2):e10–e52. https://doi.org/10.1093/cid/ciu296.
- Bennet JE, Dolin R, Blaser MJ, eds. *Mandell, Douglas, and Bennett's Principles and Practice of Infectious Diseases.* 9th ed. Elsevier; 2020.

A 35-year-old male presents to the emergency room in Tennessee with a 2-day history of fevers, chills, malaise, myalgias, nausea, vomiting, and headaches. He is otherwise healthy and does not take any medications. He has no medication allergies. He is an avid outdoorsman who goes on frequent hikes with his dog. He regularly finds ticks on himself and his dog. He is in a monogamous marriage and is sexually active with his wife. They do not use condoms regularly. He works as a kindergarten teacher. He denies any substance use or recent travel out of the Tennessee area where he lives. Vital signs reveal temperature 102° F, heart rate 110 beats per minute, blood pressure 100/60 mmHg, respiratory rate 18, and oxygen saturation 96% on room air. Examination shows an ill-appearing man. There is no icterus or conjunctival injection. Oral mucosa is dry and without mucosal ulceration. Heart is tachycardic, regular, and without murmur. Lungs are clear, and abdomen is soft and nontender. There is no palpable hepatosplenomegaly or skin rash. Laboratory evaluation shows white blood cell count 14,000 cells/uL (80% neutrophils), hemoglobin 12 g/dL, platelet count 90,000 cells/uL, creatinine 1.2 mg/dL (creatinine clearance >60 mL/min), sodium 128 mEq/L, AST 95 U/L, and ALT 110 U/L. Peripheral smear shows neutrophilia and thrombocytopenia, but no intracellular abnormalities. Blood cultures are drawn. Which of the following is the best next step in management?

A. Obtain serologic testing.
B. Start doxycycline.
C. Supportive care and discharge.
D. Start atovaquone and azithromycin.
E. Start clindamycin and quinine.

The best next step would be to start doxycycline (**option B**). This patient's presentation is concerning for Rocky Mountain spotted fever (RMSF). RMSF is a tickborne illness caused by *Rickettsia rickettsii* that carries a high mortality if left untreated. The disease occurs during the warmer months and can be acquired anywhere in the United States, but most commonly in the southeast United States (contrary to what the name suggests). The incubation period is 3 to 12 days. Early symptoms include fevers, headache, confusion, malaise, myalgias, and gastrointestinal symptoms (nausea, vomiting, and loss of appetite). The characteristic RMSF rash (Fig. 41.1) typically shows up 2 to 5 days after symptom onset, but one in 10 patients

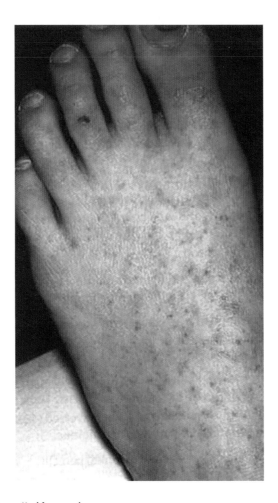

Figure 41.1 – Rocky Mountain spotted fever rash
McGinley-Smith DE, Tsao SS. Dermatoses from ticks. *J Am Acad Dermatol*. 2003 Sep;49(3):363–392; quiz 393–396.
https://doi.org/10.1067/s0190-9622(03)01868-1. PMID:12963900.

do not develop a rash. The rash starts as a maculopapular eruption involving the wrists and ankles and then spreads to the trunk and palms/soles. Eventually, the rash becomes petechial (vasculitis) after approximately 1 week, which signifies severe illness.

In addition, patients may develop encephalopathy, respiratory compromise (acute respiratory distress syndrome, pulmonary edema), renal failure, and ischemic complications requiring amputation. Labs may be relatively normal early on, but with time patients develop thrombocytopenia, transaminase elevations, and hyponatremia. Patients may have leukocytosis or leukopenia as well. The diagnosis is often clinical in nature, and therapy should not be delayed while awaiting diagnostic confirmation. Serologic testing (**option A**) can be obtained, but antibodies take 7 to 10 days to develop, and definitive diagnosis can only be established by showing a four-fold rise in IgG-specific antibody titer by indirect immunofluorescence antibody assay in paired serum samples (separate by 2–4 weeks). Alternatively, a skin biopsy can be sent for PCR or immunohistochemical staining. If RMSF is clinically suspected, the patient should be started on doxycycline as soon as possible, because delays in therapy are associated with increased mortality. Treatment should be given for a least 1 week and continued for 3 days after resolution of fever and clinical improvement. A 14 day course of doxycycline is often given in clinical practice as it will cover for most the doxycycline-treatable illnesses that can present in a similar fashion.

Providing supportive care and discharging the patient (**option C**) would result in devastating consequences. **Option D** (atovaquone and azithromycin) and **option E** (clindamycin and quinine) are regimens that are used for the treatment of babesiosis. Babesiosis can present similarly, but these patients typically have clinical evidence of hemolytic anemia and intraerythrocytic inclusions on peripheral smear, which are not seen in this patient.

Most of the illnesses listed in Table 41.1 present similarly with a nonspecific "viral-like" prodrome, with disturbances in liver function and cell counts. There are certain characteristics that can be used to help narrow the differential, including incubation period, geographic location (epidemiology), and certain distinguishing clinical features. The list below is not an exhaustive one, but it includes the more common tickborne illnesses, especially the ones we can do something about. Note: the *Ixodes* tick is a common vector for transmission of Lyme disease, anaplasmosis, and babesiosis (classic coinfection association).

Table 41.1 – Tickborne Diseases *(Cont'd)*

Disease	Distinguishing Features	Diagnosis	Treatment
Rocky Mountain spotted fever (RMSF) (*Rickettsia rickettsii*)	• Centripetal maculopapular rash starting on wrists and ankles and spreading to trunk and palms/soles. Eventually, evolves into petechial rash • Incubation—3–12 days • Epidemiologic (epi) tip-off—Southeast and South Central United States	• Labs—thrombocytopenia, transaminase elevation, hyponatremia • ≥4-fold rise in IgG antibody between acute and convalescent samples • Skin biopsy for PCR or immunohistochemistry	Doxycycline for at least 1 week and continued for 3 days after resolution of fever and clinical improvement
Anaplasmosis (*Anaplasma phagocytophilum*)	• Incubation—5–14 days • Epi tip-off—upper midwest and northeast United States (similar to Lyme due to similar vector—*Ixodes* tick)	• Labs—leukopenia (lymphopenia), thrombocytopenia, transaminase elevation • Peripheral blood smear showing morulae in granulocyte cytoplasm (negative smear does not rule out anaplasmosis) • Blood PCR—first week of illness, decreased sensitivity postantibiotics • ≥4-fold rise in IgG antibody between acute and convalescent samples	Doxycycline for 10–14 days
Ehrlichiosis (various *Ehrlichia* species)	• Severe illness and rash more common than with anaplasmosis • Incubation—5–14 days • Epi tip-off—southeast and south-central United States	• Same as for anaplasmosis • Morulae in 20% (less than with anaplasmosis)—*E. chaffeensis* (monocytes), *E. ewingii* (granulocytes)	Doxycycline × 7–14 days (similar to RMSF)
Babesiosis (*Babesia microti* and others)	• Severe illness in immune-compromised (classically asplenia) • Hemolytic anemia • Incubation—1 week to several weeks. • Epi tip-off—upper midwest and northeast United States (similar to Lyme due to similar vector—*Ixodes* tick)	• Labs—hemolytic anemia, azotemia • Peripheral blood smear showing intraerythrocytic *Babesia* parasites (classic Maltese cross formation) • Blood PCR—allows species identification	First line—atovaquone + azithromycin × 7–10 days Alternative—clindamycin + quinine × 7–10 days. Severe or >10% parasitemia) → consider exchange transfusion

(Continued)

Table 41.1 – Tickborne Diseases

Disease	Distinguishing Features	Diagnosis	Treatment
Lyme disease (*Borrelia burgdorferi* and *Borrelia mayonii*)	• Erythema migrans (EM) rash—80%, classically bull's eye appearance, but various morphologies exist • Cardiac manifestations—atrioventricular block, carditis • Various neurologic manifestations • Incubation—3–30 days • Epi tip-off—upper midwest and northeast United States	• Early localized stage—clinical diagnosis • Later stages—serology (two-tier testing) • CNS disease—serology (CSF Lyme Index—ratio of CSF to serum antibody)	Depends on the manifestation Drugs used include doxycycline, amoxicillin, and ceftriaxone Duration ranges from 10 days to 28 days
Southern tick-associated rash illness (STARI)	• Similar to early Lyme (EM, flu-like illness) but no long-term sequelae • Epi tip-off—southern United States (lone star ticks)	• Diagnosis of exclusion • Looks like early Lyme but diagnosed in an area where Lyme disease is not prevalent	Most treat like early Lyme, but unclear if antibiotic therapy is even needed
Rickettsia parkeri rickettsiosis (spotted fever)	• Presents similar to RMSF but has eschar lesion ("tache noire") at site of tick bite (Gulf coast tick) • Incubation—2–10 days • Epi tip-off—southeast and mid-Atlantic United States (Gulf Coast) and south Arizona	• PCR of eschar swab, whole blood or skin biopsy • ≥4-fold rise in IgG antibody between acute and convalescent samples	Similar to RMSF
Tickborne relapsing fever (*Borrelia spp.*)	• Febrile syndrome every 7–10 days • Epi tip-off—southwest United States	• Blood smear obtained during febrile episode showing spirochetes	Tetracycline × 10 days Ceftriaxone × 10–14 days if CNS involvement

KEY LEARNING POINT

If Rocky Mountain spotted fever is clinically suspected, the best initial step is to start doxycycline as soon as possible to decrease mortality.

REFERENCES AND FURTHER READING

• Centers for Disease Control and Prevention. *Tickborne Disease of the United Status: A Reference Manual for Healthcare Providers.* 5th ed. 2018. https://www.cdc.gov/ticks/tickbornediseases/TickborneDiseases-P.pdf.
• McGinley-Smith DE, Tsao SS. Dermatoses from ticks. *J Am Acad Dermatol.* 2003;49(3):363–392, quiz 393–396. https://doi.org/10.1067/s0190-9622(03)01868-1.
• Spec A, Escota G, Chrisler C, Davies B, eds. *Comprehensive Review of Infectious Diseases.* 1st ed. Elsevier; 2019.

A 40-year-old female is admitted to the hospital in December with a 4-day history of fevers, chills, headache, nausea, myalgias, arthralgias, and a skin rash. She has no medication allergies. She has a history of eczema, for which she uses a topical corticosteroid and emollient cream. She works with mice in a research laboratory at the local university. She is sexually active and is currently in a monogamous relationship. She does not use condoms consistently during sexual activity. She lives in Iowa. She has not traveled anywhere recently and denies substance use. She has a dog at home and denies any other animal exposures. Vital signs show temperature 101.5° F, heart rate 90 beats per minute, blood pressure 110/60 mmHg, respiratory rate 16, and oxygen saturation 98% on room air. Examination reveals a maculopapular rash predominantly involving the extremities, including palms and soles. There is tenderness, swelling, and reduced range of motion in the left ankle, right knee, and right elbow. There is no evidence of nuchal rigidity, oral mucosal lesions, or genital lesions. The remainder of the examination including pelvic exam is unremarkable. Laboratory evaluation reveals white blood cell count 20,000 cells/uL (85% neutrophils), hemoglobin 13 g/dL, platelet count 250,000 cells/uL, creatinine 1.0 mg/dL (creatinine clearance >60 mL/min), and normal liver function testing. Blood cultures are obtained. Which of the following organisms is the most likely cause of this patient's illness?

A. *Treponema pallidum.*
B. *Rickettsia rickettsii.*
C. *Spirillum minus.*
D. *Streptobacillus moniliformis.*
E. *Neisseria gonorrhoeae.*

The most likely cause is *S. moniliformis* (**option D**). This presentation is most consistent with rat-bite fever (RBF). RBF is caused by two species of gram-negative bacteria found in rodent nasopharyngeal and oral flora—*S. moniliformis* (United States and Europe) and *S. minus* (Asia, **option C**). The disease can be seen in laboratory workers who work with rodents or in crowded rodent-infested urban areas. Haverhill fever is a rare form of this infection caused by oral ingestion of the organisms in contaminated foods. Most patients present within 1 to 2 weeks of the bite with abrupt onset of fevers, chills, headaches, nausea, vomiting, myalgias, migratory arthralgias, and polyarthritis (even septic arthritis). A nonpruritic maculopapular (morbilliform) or petechial rash may develop after a couple days that predominantly involves the extremities (including palms and soles). Compared with *S. moniliformis*, *S. minus* is associated with more regional lymphadenopathy and bite-site ulceration and eschar. Patients may have striking leukocytosis and false-positive nontreponemal syphilis serologic testing. Even without treatment, most patients will improve, but they may go on to develop relapsing fevers and chronic arthritis. The diagnosis is often clinical. The organism can also be directly visualized by stained smears of blood, purulent fluid, or synovial fluid. Culturing the organism can be difficult, due to specific growth requirements, so the microbiology laboratory should be notified if this organism is suspected. Management is relatively straightforward. The drug of choice is penicillin (PCN), which is typically given IV initially and then transitioned to oral PCN after approximately 1 week to complete a 14-day total course. Tetracycline is an alternative treatment that can be used in PCN-allergic patients. Longer durations may be necessary in more complicated cases (i.e., endocarditis). Patients may experience symptomatic worsening after treatment (Jarisch–Herxheimer reaction), and counseling regarding this reaction should be provided. The bite wound should be thoroughly cleansed, and appropriate tetanus prophylaxis should be provided. Rabies prophylaxis is not necessary for rat bites.

T. pallidum (**option A**) causes syphilis. The secondary form of syphilis can present similar to RBF with influenza-like symptoms and a bronze-colored, diffuse maculopapular rash involving the palms and soles. This patient's low-risk sexual history and polyarthritis are not typical of secondary syphilis. Rocky Mountain spotted fever (RMSF), caused by *R. rickettsii* (**option B**), also presents like RBF, but RMSF would be more likely to cause transaminase elevations and thrombocytopenia. In addition, polyarthritis is not a prominent feature of RMSF. Disseminated gonococcal infection (DGI) is caused by *N. gonorrhoeae* (**option E**) and can present with fevers, skin rash (usually pustular-appearing), tenosynovitis, and migratory polyarthritis. The low-risk sexual history and normal pelvic examination make DGI less likely.

KEY LEARNING POINT

Rat-bite fever is caused by either Streptobacillus moniliformis *(United States and Europe) or* Spirillum minus *(Asia). The treatment of choice is penicillin.*

REFERENCES AND FURTHER READING

• Mekala V, Washburn R. Rat-bite fever: *Streptobacillus moniliformis* and *Spirillum minus. Mandell, Douglas, and Bennett's Principles and Practice of Infectious Diseases.* 9th ed. Elsevier; 2020:2803–2806.

A 40-year-old African American male is admitted with an abrupt onset of fevers, chills, and confusion. He has no medication allergies. He has a history of sickle cell disease. Medications include hydroxyurea, acetaminophen, morphine as needed, and folic acid. He lives in an apartment and owns two dogs. He denies alcohol or drug abuse. Vital signs on presentation reveal temperature 102° F, heart rate 120 beats per minute, blood pressure 80/40 mmHg, respiratory rate 20, and oxygen saturation 94% on room air. Examination reveals an ill-appearing man with conjunctival pallor and mild scleral icterus. He is confused and combative. There is no nuchal rigidity. Heart is tachycardic and regular. There is a soft early systolic murmur at the left upper sternal border. Lungs are clear. Abdomen is soft, and there is no hepatosplenomegaly palpable. Skin is dry, and there are scattered excoriations. Laboratory evaluation reveals white blood cell count 20,000 cells/uL, hemoglobin 8 g/dL, platelet count 90,000 cells/uL, creatinine 1.5 mg/dL (creatinine clearance 40 mL/min), total bilirubin 4 mg/dL, indirect (unconjugated) bilirubin 3 mg/dL, and ALT 100 U/L. Peripheral smear shows Howell–Jolly bodies and sickled red blood cells. Blood cultures are drawn. Which of the following is the best initial therapy?

A. Atovaquone and azithromycin.

B. Vancomycin.

C. Ceftriaxone.

D. Vancomycin plus ceftriaxone.

E. Vancomycin plus meropenem.

The best initial therapy in this patient with overwhelming postsplenectomy infection (OPSI) is vancomycin and meropenem (**option E**). OPSI is considered a medical emergency because it carries a high mortality. OPSI occurs in patients with functional or anatomic asplenia. The typical organisms that cause OPSI are encapsulated bacteria, classically *Neisseria meningitidis*, *Haemophilus influenzae*, and *Streptococcus pneumoniae*. *S. pneumoniae* is the most common pathogen. Less common causes include *Capnocytophaga spp.* (acquired by dog bite or scratch— suggested by the excoriations in this patient), *Escherichia coli*, *Staphylococcus aureus*, *Bordetella holmesii*, *Salmonella spp.* (especially in sickle cell disease), *Babesia spp.*, and *Plasmodium falciparum*.

The presentation is often severe, including high fevers, chills, shock, disseminated intravascular coagulation (DIC), and multiorgan dysfunction. The most important diagnostic test to obtain is blood cultures, ideally before administering antibiotics. A peripheral blood smear should be obtained if *Babesia* or malaria are suspected. Coagulation parameters and a complete blood count with differential should be done to evaluate for evidence of DIC. Metabolic testing (i.e., hepatic and renal function) should be obtained to evaluate for end-organ damage. Additional evaluation should be obtained based on clinical suspicion (i.e., lumbar puncture if meningitis is expected).

Patients should be counseled to seek medical attention at the first sign of infection and to notify medical personnel of their asplenic status. These patients should be prescribed "prophylactic antibiotics" that can be taken at the first sign of infection. Typical options include amoxicillin/clavulanic acid, cefuroxime, or fluoroquinolones. Intramuscular ceftriaxone can be used for this purpose in an urgent care or outpatient (office) setting. Upon hospital presentation, the typical empiric regimen that is started is vancomycin and either a third-generation cephalosporin (usually ceftriaxone, **option D**) or a fluoroquinolone (levofloxacin or ciprofloxacin). This regimen will cover the majority of the pathogens listed above. If meningitis is suspected, then dexamethasone should be added. If there is concern for *Capnocytophaga* (as in this patient), then the initial therapy should be vancomycin plus either piperacillin/tazobactam or meropenem (option E). **Options B and C** will not cover *Capnocytophaga*. If *Babesia* is suspected, then the regimen of choice is atovaquone and azithromycin (**option A**). The regimen can eventually be tailored based on clinical response and available culture data. Preventative strategies include patient education, provision of a prescription for prophylactic antibiotics, and immunization (pneumococcal, *H. influenzae*, and meningococcal) (Fig. 43.1).

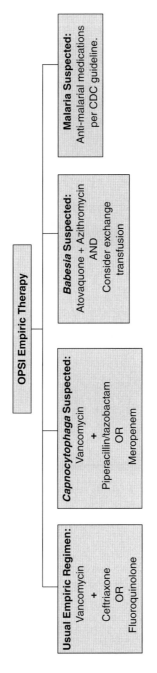

Figure 43.1 – Management of overwhelming postsplenectomy infection (*OPSI*). *CDC*, US Centers for Disease Control and Prevention.

KEY LEARNING POINT

Overwhelming postsplenectomy infection in a patient with a potential for Capnocytophaga *infection (i.e., dog bite or scratch) can be empirically treated with vancomycin (covers resistant gram-positives such as* Streptococcus pneumoniae *and potentially methicillin-resistant* Staphylococcus aureus) *and either piperacillin/tazobactam or meropenem (to cover* Capnocytophaga Haemophilus influenzae, Neisseria meningitidis, Salmonella, *and* Escherichia coli).

REFERENCES AND FURTHER READING

- Bennet JE, Dolin R, Blaser MJ. *Mandell, Douglas, and Bennett's Principles and Practice of Infectious Diseases.* 9th ed. Elsevier Inc; 2020.
- O'Neal HR Jr, Niven AS, Karam GH. Critical illness in patients with asplenia. *Chest.* 2016;150(6):1394–1402. https://doi.org/10.1016/j.chest.2016.03.044.

A 50-year-old male presents to the emergency room with a 5-day history of fevers, cough, red and watery eyes, and a skin rash. He initially thought he had a cold or influenza, but the rash worried him enough to come in for evaluation. He notes that the rash started on his face and neck and is now on his chest, back, upper arms, and abdomen. He has no medication allergies. He is otherwise healthy and does not take any medications. He works as a pharmaceutical representative, which requires constant travel all over the United States. He is not sexually active. He denies any animal or tick exposures. Vitals show temperature 103° F, heart rate 100 beats per minute, blood pressure 110/70 mmHg, respiratory rate 18, and oxygen saturation 96% on room air. Physical examination reveals bilateral conjunctival injection and tearing, but no icterus. There is pharyngeal erythema and gray-blue–colored lesions over the buccal mucosa. Skin examination reveals an erythematous maculopapular rash involving the face, neck, trunk, and proximal extremities. The erythema is confluent in some regions and blanchable. The eruption does not involve the palms and soles. The remainder of the examination is unremarkable. What is the next best step in management?

A. Airborne isolation/precaution.

B. Contact isolation/precaution.

C. Standard isolation/precaution.

D. Start vitamin A.

E. Start ribavirin.

The best next step is placing the patient on airborne isolation/precaution (**option A**).

This patient's presentation is most concerning for measles (rubeola) virus infection. Measles is a very contagious viral infection that is spread by direct contact with respiratory droplets and via the airborne route. Risk factors for acquiring this infection include lack of immunization (either never immunized or waning of immunity in some people) and travel to areas with higher incidence of measles. Natural infection seems to be associated with lifelong immunity, as seen in those born before 1957. After an incubation period of 10 to 14 days, patients initially present with fever, influenza-like symptoms, and the three Cs (cough, coryza, conjunctivitis). They may also have grayish-blue spots on an erythematous base in the oral mucosa that are called Koplik spots (Fig. 44.1). These oral findings are pathognomonic of

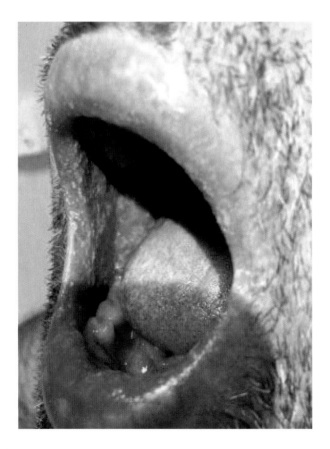

Figure 44.1 – Koplik spots
Famularo G. Koplik's spots and measles. *Am J Med*. 2018;131(6):e249–e250. https://doi.org/10.1016/j.amjmed.2018.01.030.

measles virus infection and herald the rash. The rash starts on the face (classically behind the ears) and spreads downward to involve the trunk and extremities, including palms/soles. It is described as erythematous, maculopapular ("morbilliform"), and coalescent/confluent as it progresses (Fig. 44.2). The rash is considered a manifestation of a cell-mediated immune response to the virus. Patients are considered infectious for the 4 days preceding the rash until 4 days after the rash onset. Uncomplicated infection typically lasts 1 to 2 weeks.

Complications of measles infection include primary viral pneumonia (giant cell or Hecht pneumonia), secondary bacterial infections (otitis media, pneumonia), diarrhea, acute encephalitis (primary acute measles encephalitis or an immune-mediated encephalitis), or chronic encephalitis (inclusion body encephalitis or subacute sclerosing panencephalitis). Severe and/or complicated illness is more likely to occur in patients with cell-mediated immune deficiency (including pregnancy), in young children (<5 years age), or in adult-onset cases (>20 years of age). Measles during pregnancy has been associated with spontaneous abortion and premature birth. There are certain variants to be aware of. Modified measles is a milder form of infection seen in those who received passive immunization to measles

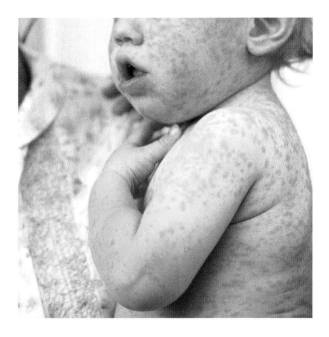

Figure 44.2 – Measles rash
Reprinted with permission from Elsevier. From Kremer JR, Muller CP. Measles in Europe—there is room for improvement. *Lancet.* 2009;373:356–358.

(i.e., postexposure immune globulin [IG]). Atypical measles is a more severe form that occurs in those who have received inactivated (killed) measles vaccination but are then exposed to the wild-type virus (natural infection). It is felt to be a hypersensitivity reaction that typically manifests with a pneumonitis, edema, and an atypical (nonclassical) measles rash.

The diagnosis is often clinical and based on the presentation described. The diagnosis can be confirmed with serology by showing a positive serum IgM antibody or a four-fold rise in serum IgG antibody between acute and convalescent samples. Serology may not be useful in immune-compromised patients and may be negative prior to the onset of the rash. In addition, the IgM antibody may persist for up to 1 month, which limits the utility. Detection of measles RNA in respiratory or urinary samples by reverse transcriptase PCR can also be used. Lastly, the virus can by isolated by viral culture.

The management of measles infection is largely supportive. Patients with suspected measles infection should be placed on airborne isolation, and the appropriate public health authorities should be notified (Table 44.1). Vitamin A (**option D**) may reduce mortality in children with measles. Data on the use of ribavirin (**option E**) are limited. Prevention measures include vaccination and postexposure prophylaxis (PEP). The immunization is provided in the measles, mumps, rubella (MMR) vaccine, which is typically given as a two-dose series at a very young age (12–15 months and at school entry [4–6 years of age]). This vaccine is a live vaccine, which is contraindicated in people with cell-mediated immunity defects (including pregnancy). Notably, this vaccine has not been found to cause (or even have an association with) autism. The primary immunization is very effective, but immunity may wane over time in some individuals, which puts them at risk for acquiring measles infection. Booster immunization should be given to patients without evidence of immunity (born 1957 or later, lack of written documentation of immunity, lack of serologic titers showing immunity, or lack of laboratory evidence of measles infection). PEP should be given to patients who have been exposed to a measles-infected individual and are unable to readily provide definitive evidence of immunity to measles. If within 72 hours of exposure and there are no contraindications, then an MMR vaccine should be given as PEP. If within 6 days of exposure and no contraindications, then IG should be given. The vaccine and IG should NOT be administered together, as the antibodies in the IG will neutralize the vaccine. Importantly, in those receiving IG, the vaccination should be given at least 6 months afterward, because the effect of the IG will disappear (Fig. 44.3).

Table 44.1 – Summary of Important Isolation Recommendations[a]

Precaution	Definition	Empirically Consider if	Recommended for These Diseases
Contact	• Patient in private room • Providers wear gown and gloves when entering the room	• Draining wound that cannot be covered • Acute diarrhea that is likely infectious • History of multidrug-resistant gram-negative infection (MDR-GNI)	• Localized varicella zoster virus(VZV)—until lesions all crusted • Scabies/lice—until 24 hours of effective therapy • MDR-GNI or *Candida auris*—for duration of hospitalization • *Clostridioides difficile*—for duration of illness, wash hands with soap and water (preferred to alcohol-based modalities) • Norovirus—until 48 hours after resolution of symptoms
Droplet	• Patient in private room and should wear surgical mask when leaving the room • Providers should wear a surgical mask when entering the room	• Meningitis or disseminated meningococcemia-like illness • Influenza-like respiratory illness	• Most respiratory viral illnesses • Pertussis (whooping cough)—until 5 days after initiation of effective therapy • Mumps—until 5 days after onset of swelling • Rubella—until 7 days after onset of rash • *Neisseria meningitidis*—until 24 hours after starting effective antibiotic therapy • Epiglottitis or meningitis due to *Haemophilus influenzae* type B—until 24 hours after starting effective antibiotic therapy • Pneumonia due to *Mycoplasma*—for duration of illness • Pneumonia due to group A *Streptococcus*—until 24 hours after initiation of effective antibiotic therapy • Pneumonic plague (*Yersinia pestis*)—until 48 hours after initiation of effective antibiotic therapy
Airborne	• Patient in private, negative-pressure room with door always closed. Must wear a surgical mask when leaving the room • Providers should wear N-95 respirator or powered air purifying respirator when entering the room	• Vesicular eruption of unclear etiology • Measles-like illness • Tuberculosis-like presentation (i.e., cavitary, upper-lobe pneumonia)	• Measles—until 4 days after onset of rash (or for duration of illness if immune-compromised) • Pulmonary or laryngeal tuberculosis (suspected)—isolation can be discontinued if tuberculosis deemed unlikely (or alternative diagnosis established) and either three negative acid-fast bacilli smears or two negative tuberculosis PCR (nucleic acid amplification) tests • Pulmonary or laryngeal tuberculosis (confirmed)—isolation can be discontinued after patient has clinically improved on AT LEAST 2 weeks of anti-tuberculosis therapy and there are three negative acid-fast bacillus smears • Disseminated VZV or VZV in immune-compromised—duration of illness (also contact isolation) • Chickenpox (primary varicella)—until lesions dry and crusted (also contact isolation) • MERS-CoV—for duration of illness (also contact and eye precautions) • SARS-CoV—until 10 days after resolution of fever (also contact and eye precautions) • SARS-CoV-2 (COVID-19)—isolation precautions depend on various factors including location of patient, severity of illness, and immune status of patient • Monkeypox—until diagnosis confirmed and smallpox excluded, also contact isolation until lesions crusted • Smallpox—for duration of illness (also contact isolation)

[a]Standard precautions apply to all patients. These include hand hygiene, safe needle practices, and appropriate use of personal protective equipment.

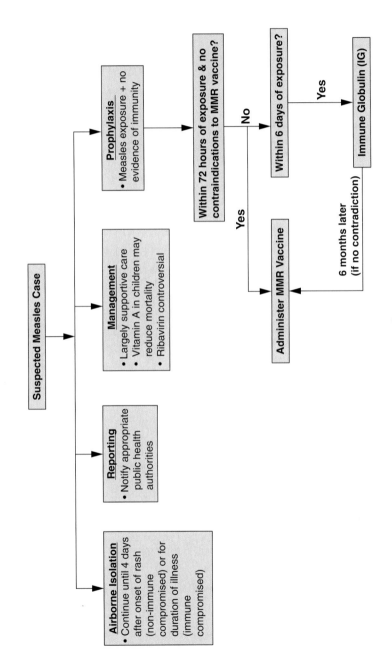

Figure 44.3 – Management of measles. *MMR*, Measles, mumps, and rubella.

KEY LEARNING POINT

If a patient is suspected to have measles infection, airborne isolation/precaution should be instituted.

REFERENCES AND FURTHER READING

- Famularo G. Koplik's spots and measles. *Am J Med*. 2018;131(6):e249–e250. https://doi.org/10.1016/j.amjmed.2018.01.030.
- Gershon A. Measles virus (rubeola). In: Bennet JE, Dolin R, Blaser MJ, eds. *Mandell, Douglas, and Bennett's Principles and Practice of Infectious Diseases*. 9th ed. Elsevier; 2020:2110–2116.
- Siegel JD, Rhinehart E, Jackson M, Chiarello L; Healthcare Infection Control Practices Advisory Committee. 2007 Guidelines for isolation precautions: preventing transmission of infectious agents in healthcare settings. https://www.ajicjournal.org/article/S0196-6553(07)00740-7/fulltext.
- Spec A, Escota G, Chrisler C, Davies B. *Comprehensive Review of Infectious Diseases*. 1st ed. Elsevier; 2019.

A 20-year-old male is admitted to the hospital with fevers, cough, chest pain, and shortness of breath for the past 3 days. He has a history of recurrent pneumonias due to *Streptococcus pneumoniae*, bronchiectasis, intestinal giardiasis, and Hashimoto thyroiditis. The only medication he takes is levothyroxine. Vitals signs show temperature 102° F, heart rate 110 beats per minute, blood pressure 100/55 mmHg, respiratory rate 30, and oxygen saturation 92% on 3 L/min oxygen by nasal cannula. Physical examination shows an ill-appearing male. There is no thrush. Heart exam reveals regular tachycardia but no murmurs. Lung exam reveals decreased breath sounds with dullness and crackles over the right-lower lobe posteriorly. The remainder of the exam is unremarkable. Complete blood count shows white blood cell count 14,000 cells/uL (80% neutrophils, 20% lymphocytes), platelet count 350,000 cells/uL, and normal peripheral smear. Creatinine, hemoglobin A1c, and liver function testing are within normal limits. HIV antigen/antibody test is negative. Quantitative immunoglobulins reveal undetectable IgA, IgG, IgM, and IgE. Flow cytometry shows normal levels of B lymphocytes. Which of the following is the most likely diagnosis?

A. X-linked (Bruton) agammaglobulinemia.
B. Common variable immunodeficiency (CVID).
C. IgA deficiency.
D. Hyper-IgM syndrome.
E. Hyper-IgE (Job) syndrome.

The most likely diagnosis is CVID (**option B**). Immunodeficiencies can be daunting to most providers, so in order to appropriately understand the immune deficiency disorders, one should understand some basic "normal" immunology. The structure and function of the immune system can be summarized as shown in Fig. 45.1.

The diagram is a bit oversimplified, but it will suffice for a working understanding of the immune response to an infection. The diagram implies that these processes occur independently, but in reality all of these processes are occurring in concert. In general, the immune response can be categorized into the innate immune response and the adaptive immune response. The innate response is generally the first line of defense and is always (innately) present and active. Innate immunity is rapidly responsive and nonspecific, which means it will defend against any foreign invader. The first line of innate defense against invading pathogens includes the physical barriers (i.e., skin and mucus membranes, etc.) and chemical barriers (i.e., lysozyme, gastric pH, etc.). Once these are breached, the cellular component of the innate immune response kicks in. The cells of the innate immune system (i.e., macrophages, dendritic cells, etc.) contain pathogen recognition receptors (PRRs) such as toll-like receptors that recognize various pathogen-associated molecular patterns (PAMPs) that are found on all sorts of microbial pathogens but not on human cells. The PRR–PAMP interaction results in activation of the acute inflammatory response, which leads to the characteristic signs of inflammation that are related to local vasodilation, hyperemia, fluid extravasation, and various inflammatory mediators (i.e., prostaglandins, interleukins, etc.). These signs include fever, rubor (redness), calor (warmth), dolor (pain), tumor (edema), and impaired function. In addition, various cells are recruited to the area, including neutrophils, macrophages, and natural killer (NK) cells, which aid in the inflammatory response via phagocytosis (neutrophils, macrophages) and killing of cells that are viral-infected or tumor-affected (NK cells stimulated by interferon released by viral-infected cells, interleukin [IL]-12, or lack of major histocompatibility complex [MHC]-1 on tumor-affected cells). The humoral component of the innate immune response consists of various serum proteins that are activated and/or upregulated in response to inflammation. One example is the acute-phase reactants, which can be upregulated (i.e., C-reactive protein, which is an opsonin that aids in phagocytosis, ferritin and hepcidin, which sequester the iron that some microbes need to thrive, etc.) or downregulated (i.e., serum albumin). Another example is the complement system, which is a series of serum proteins that circulate in their inactive state but then become activated in the presence of infection (alternative or mannose-binding lectin pathway) or antigen/antibody (IgG or IgM) complexes (classic pathway). This system "complements" the immune response by enhancing phagocytosis (opsonization), promoting neutrophil

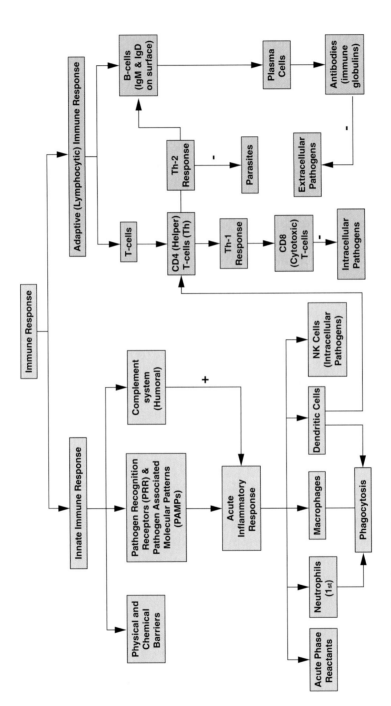

Figure 45.1 – Overview of the normal immune response.
NK, Natural killer.

chemotaxis, promoting anaphylactic response, and eliminating gram-negative pathogens via formation of the membrane-attack complex (formed by terminal complement components C5–C9). The last thing to note is that the majority of the innate immune system is designed to respond to extracellular pathogens, but NK cells and activated macrophages (as part of the Th-1 response—see later) are able to respond to intracellular pathogens.

The adaptive immune response is primarily mediated by T and B lymphocytes (or T-cells and B-cells, for short). This response is slower, because it is much more specific in nature (recognizes a particular antigen only), and this takes time to generate. In addition, the adaptive immune response will generate memory B- and T-cells that will allow for a faster and more robust response when the same antigen is encountered again. Both types of lymphocytes are produced in the bone marrow, but the key distinction is that B-cells mature in the bone marrow (hence the name B-cells), whereas T-cells mature in the thymus (hence the name T-cells). Mature (naïve) B-cells express IgM and IgD on their surfaces, and, when activated, they will become antibody (immunoglobulin)–secreting plasma cells, which mediate the humoral arm of the adaptive immune response. T-cells can be either helper T-cells (Th), which are CD4-positive, or cytotoxic T-cells, which are CD8-positive. Helper T-cells can further be subdivided into Th-1 and Th-2 cells, and the predominant subtype will be determined by the invading pathogen. Mature lymphocytes typically reside in various immunologic tissues, including lymph nodes, spleen, bone marrow, mucosa-associated lymphoid tissue, and even the bloodstream. These are the areas where they will encounter antigens and become activated effector cells. This antigenic encounter is facilitated by the innate immune system, as discussed next.

Certain antigen presenting cells (APCs), such as dendritic cells and macrophages, serve to link the innate immune response to the adaptive immune response (Fig. 45.2). These APCs will express a particular antigen on MHCs and travel to local lymphoid tissues (i.e., lymph node) to present the antigen to naïve T-cells. Intracellular antigens are carried on MHC-I, which is found on all nucleated cells and platelets and binds to the T-cell receptor on CD8+ T-cells. Extracellular antigens are carried on MHC-II, which is only found on APCs and binds to the T-cell receptor on CD4+ T-cells. In order for T-cell activation to occur, a second costimulatory signal is required (CD28–B7 interaction). Activated CD8+ T-cells can then go on to kill cells that are virus-infected or malignant. Activated CD4+ T-cells have several possible fates. In response to TGF-beta, they can become regulatory helper T-cells, which control (regulate) the T-cell response and immune tolerance. In response to TGF-beta and IL-6, they can become Th-17 cells, which secrete IL-17 and IL-22 to regulate neutrophil number and epithelial response to extracellular bacterial and fungal infection (i.e., *Candida*). In addition, in response to interferon-gamma (IFN-γ) and IL-12

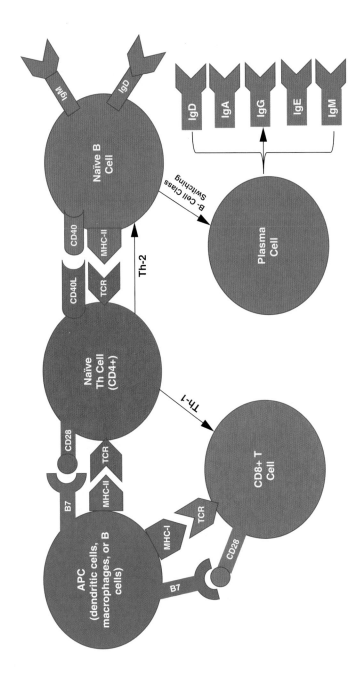

Figure 45.2 – Immune cell interactions.
APC, Antigen-presenting cell; Ig, immunoglobulin; MHC, major histocompatibility complex; TCR, T-cell receptor.

secreted by macrophages, they become Th-1 cells that are geared toward "helping" the immune response to intracellular pathogens ("cell-mediated immunity") by secreting cytokines that promote the activation of macrophages (IFN-γ) and CD8+ T cells (IL-2). On the other hand, Th-2 cells are produced in response to IL-4 and promote the immune response to extracellular pathogens ("humoral" or "antibody-mediated") by "helping" B-cells make additional antibodies (IgG, IgE, IgA) in a process called class switching. This interaction requires a second costimulatory signal (CD40 ligand on Th-2 cell binding to CD40 receptor on B-cell) to activate the B-cell. IgA is necessary for mucosal defense against pathogens. IgG activates complement (classic pathway), promotes opsonization, and mediates antibody-dependent cell-mediated cytotoxicity. IgE is involved in allergic responses and the immune response to parasitic infections. Lastly, Th-2 cells also help with the immune response to parasites by recruiting eosinophils. With all this in mind, it is important to recognize that immunopathology results from defects that arise anywhere in this orchestrated immune response.

Defects in certain components of the immune system are classically associated with particular manifestations, as shown Fig. 45.3.

So when should an immunodeficiency syndrome be suspected? The following list is a useful starting point:

- Recurrent/frequent infections (variable definitions exist for these)
- Infections that are unusually severe (i.e., meningitis, unexplained deep-seated infections)
- Infections that are protracted and poorly responsive to usual therapy
- Infections caused by unusual or opportunistic pathogens (i.e., *Pneumocystis*, nontuberculous mycobacteria)
- Infections caused by common pathogens in unusual locations (i.e., central nervous system infection with *Aspergillus*)
- Infections caused by (that occur following) administration of live vaccines
- Vaccination failures, as identified by development of infections or seronegativity in a previously vaccinated individual
- Presence of certain complications that indicate recurrent infection (i.e., bronchiectasis, malignancy, autoimmunity, lymphadenopathy, hepatosplenomegaly, granulomatous lesions, etc.)
- Family history of immunodeficiency or recurrent infections

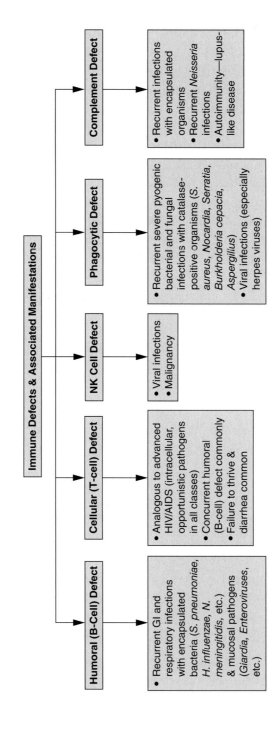

Figure 45.3 – Overview of immune defects and their consequences.
NK, Natural killer.

It can be helpful to have a rational approach to the evaluation of a patient with a suspected immunodeficiency. The first step is always to obtain a thorough history and physical examination. Historical considerations (in addition to the usual medical history) include age of symptom or infection onset, timing of umbilical cord stump separation, detailed infection history (type of infections/organisms, duration of illness, treatments utilized and treatment response, and complications), immunization history (response to vaccination or development of infection following live vaccination), food and drug allergies, and history of consanguinity. Physical examination considerations include gender (X-linked disorders typically seen in males), nutritional status, hair color/sheen, facial features, dentition, presence or absence of tonsils, lymphadenopathy, hepatosplenomegaly, nail clubbing (sign of chronic lung disease), and skin abnormalities such as eczema or telangiectasia.

Prior to diagnosing a patient with a primary deficiency, one should evaluate for and rule out secondary causes of immunodeficiency. The etiologies of secondary immunodeficiency are shown in Table 45.1.

It is important to remember that a primary and secondary immunodeficiency may coexist, so these entities are not mutually exclusive. The evaluation for primary immunodeficiencies will depend largely on the suspected immune defect (which is based on the presentation/infection history). The testing to consider is outlined in Table 45.2.

When evaluating for infection in a patient with a known immunodeficiency, it is important to obtain a direct tissue diagnosis (culture and/or histopathologic), because these patients can have multiple infections at one time, and other methods of diagnosis (i.e., serology) may be unreliable.

There are an ever-increasing number of primary immunodeficiencies, and a discussion of all of these is beyond the scope of this book. The list of immunodeficiencies in Table 45.3 are either fairly common and/or commonly tested, so they are worth knowing about.

MANAGEMENT CONSIDERATIONS

Patients with primary immunodeficiency should be managed by a specialist with training in allergy and immunology. The definitive treatment for cellular or combined immunodeficiency is stem cell transplantation. Ig replacement therapy (intravenous or subcutaneous Ig) should be given to those with impaired antibody formation. The end goal of Ig therapy is to attain

Table 45.1 – Causes of Secondary Immunodeficiency

Cause of Secondary Immunodeficiency	Comments
Medications/toxins	• Review medications. Most immunosuppressing medications will be obvious (i.e., corticosteroids). Some medications can impair physiologic function and predispose to infection (i.e., proton pump inhibitors and *Clostridiodes difficile* infection) • Some toxins can impair immune function (ciliary dysfunction in smokers, bone marrow toxicity in alcoholics)
Anatomic and physiologic defects	• These typically affect the "barriers," including skin, mucus membranes, gastrointestinal tract, genitourinary tract, and respiratory tract • Example: an obstructive lesion causing stasis and organismal overgrowth/infection
Malignancy	• Hematologic malignancies (leukemia, lymphoma, myeloma, etc.) can cause leukopenia and functional leukocyte deficiencies • Thymoma can be associated with hypogammaglobulinemia (Good syndrome)
Metabolic	• Chronic kidney disease (affects lymphocyte function), chronic liver disease (decreased antibody and complement protein production), and poorly-controlled diabetes (hyperglycemia impairs several aspects of immunity)
Protein deficiency	• Inadequate protein intake (malnutrition) or absorption (malabsorption syndromes) • Inadequate protein production—chronic liver disease (cirrhosis) • Protein loss in the urine (nephrotic syndrome) or gastrointestinal tract (protein-losing enteropathy)
HIV/AIDS	• Advanced HIV/AIDS impairs CD4+ T-cell number and function, which causes a mixed cellular and humoral deficiency
Asplenia	• Asplenia can be anatomic (postsplenectomy) or functional (i.e., sickle cell disease) • Opsonized pathogens are typically cleared by the spleen, so patients with asplenia have decreased opsonizing ability, which leads to infections with encapsulated pathogens
Other	• Extremes of age, excessive stress, thymectomy, and pregnancy

Work-up to consider in all patients

• Complete blood count with white blood cell differential

• Metabolic status—serum total protein, serum albumin, urinary protein, renal and hepatic function, HbA1c

• HIV screening with HIV antigen/antibody screening assay

• Peripheral blood smear—can detect certain suggestive abnormalities (i.e., Howell–Jolly bodies in asplenia, malignant cells, etc.)

• Imaging to look for anatomic defects (i.e., shrunken spleen, bronchiectasis, etc.).

Table 45.2 – Testing for Immune Defects

Humoral (B-cell or Ig) Defect	Cellular (T-cell) Defect	Phagocytic Defect	Complement Defect
• Quantitative Igs—IgG (rarely IgG subclasses), IgA, IgM, and IgE • Baseline immunization titers (tetanus, pneumococcal, *Haemophilus influenzae* type B) and response to booster (recheck titers at least 4 weeks after the booster) • Flow cytometry to look at number of B-cells—best done when not ill • Rarely, isohemagglutinins (natural antibodies to blood group antigens, not present in AB blood group)	• Flow cytometry to look at number of CD4+, CD8+ T-cells, and natural killer cells—best done when not ill to avoid confounding due to illness-induced suppression • Cutaneous delayed hypersensitivity or response to mitogens	• Complete blood count with differential • Peripheral smear to look at neutrophil staining and morphology • Dihydrorhodamine test or nitroblue tetrazolium • Flow cytometry for adhesion molecules	• CH-50 (classic pathway) • AH-50 (alternative pathway) • Individual components of complement system
• Genetic testing should be considered in most cases, as it can definitively establish the diagnosis and facilitate genetic counseling.			

a symptom- and infection-free status. Interestingly, chronic rhinosinusitis may not go away with Ig therapy. Prophylactic antimicrobials are indicated in certain disorders, and the choice of agent depends on the defect/disorder. Patients with a history of or risk for recurrent lung infections/disease should have periodic lung imaging and pulmonary function testing. If blood products are necessary for patients with cellular or combined immunodeficiency, then only irradiated, cytomegalovirus-negative, lymphocyte-depleted blood products should be used. Live vaccinations (i.e., oral polio, measles-mumps-rubella, oral typhoid, varicella, yellow fever) should be avoided in many of these disorders, but inactivated (killed) vaccines can still be administered.

Table 45.3 – Primary Immunodeficiencies

Primary Immunodeficiency	Defect and Pathophysiology	Presentation and Diagnosis	Treatment Considerations
Predominant Humoral (B-Cell or Antibody) Immunodeficiency			
X-linked (Bruton) agammaglobulinemia (XLAG)	• Defective Bruton tyrosine kinase (BTK) gene → failure of B-cells to mature and eventually home appropriately • Note: there are other forms of agammaglobulinemia that are due to other gene defects and can be autosomal recessive	• Recurrent humoral defect–type infections starting after waning of maternal antibody (>6 months of life) • Typically male patients • Absent or scant tonsils and lymph nodes • ↓ number of B cells, all Igs, and immunity to vaccination • Molecular testing for BTK protein	• Avoid live vaccinations • Ig replacement • Antimicrobial prophylaxis
Common variable immune deficiency	• Defective B-cell maturation into plasma cells	• Similar presentation to XLAG, but often older patient, and B-cell count is either normal or mildly ↓ • Presentation is "variable," and patients can have malignancies and autoimmune disease	• Similar to XLAG • May require splenectomy, immune modulation, or chemotherapy
Selective IgA deficiency	• Absent or reduced serum IgA	• Often asymptomatic but may have recurrent mucosal infections, autoimmune disorders, atopic disease, or anaphylaxis to IgA-containing blood products (due to IgG antibody against IgA) • Normal number of B-cells and Igs, except ↓ IgA	• If asymptomatic → monitor • Treat infections as they arise • IgA deficiency is not a contraindication to IV immune globulin, if necessary
Predominant Cellular (T-Cell) Immunodeficiency			
DiGeorge syndrome (thymic aplasia)	• 22q11 deletion syndrome → failure of third and fourth pharyngeal pouches to develop	• Lack of thymus (T-cell deficiency, most will have some residual thymus that prevents full-blown T-cell deficiency), parathyroid glands (hypocalcemia), facial and cardiac abnormalities • Absent thymic shadow on imaging, ↓ T-cell numbers and function, positive molecular testing	• Thymic transplant • Avoid live vaccines • Antimicrobial prophylaxis
Mendelian susceptibility to mycobacterial disease	• Defect in interferon-gamma/interleukin-12 pathway or STAT-1 • Could also be classified as a phagocytic deficiency	• Disseminated mycobacterial infections, salmonella infections, and herpes virus infections • Classically, southeast Asian descent	• Avoid live vaccines and exposures associated with the common infections

(Continued)

Table 45.3 – Primary Immunodeficiencies *(Cont'd)*

Primary Immunodeficiency	Defect and Pathophysiology	Presentation and Diagnosis	Treatment Considerations
Combined Humoral and Cellular Immunodeficiency			
Hyper-IgM syndrome	• Various defects, but commonly CD40L or CD40 defect → B-cells unable to class switch • Some forms have defective CD4 T-cell function as well	• Recurrent humoral defect type infections +/- opportunistic infections, ↑ malignancy risk • ↑ or normal IgM and ↓ IgA, IgG, and IgE • Normal number of B, T, and natural killer (NK) cells • ↓ response to vaccination • Flow cytometry for CD40 or CD40L	• Stem cell transplant is curative • Ig and granulocyte-colony stimulating factor (if neutropenic) • *Pneumocystis* prophylaxis • Avoid live vaccines and use irradiated, cytomegalovirus (CMV)-negative blood products
Severe combined immunodeficiency	• Various possible defects → all will have lack of T-cells and may or may not have ↓ B-cells or NK cells • Adenosine deaminase (ADA) deficiency is most severe (lack of T, B, and NK cells)	• Recurrent cellular defect (+/- humoral defect)–type infections • Omenn syndrome—similar to graft-versus-host disease, erythroderma, ↑ IgE and eosinophils • Lack thymus and lymphoid tissues • ↓ T-cells, ↓ T-cell receptor excision circles (newborn screening) • Depending on mutation, may have ↓ or normal B-cells (but all will be functionally B-cell–deficient)	• Stem cell transplant as soon as possible • Gene therapy or enzyme replacement in some types (i.e., ADA deficiency) • Polyethylene glycol modified–ADA replacement (if above not available) • Ig replacement • *Pneumocystis* prophylaxis • Avoid live vaccines and use irradiated, CMV-negative blood products
Wiskott–Aldrich syndrome (WAS)	• X-linked recessive mutation in WAS protein → T-cells cannot reorganize cytoskeleton → defective cell migration and signal transduction	• Recurrent infections (humoral and cellular defect type), eczema, thrombocytopenia (bleeding), ↑ risk of malignancy (esp. Epstein–Barr virus–associated lymphoma) and autoimmune disease • ↓ B- and T-cells, ↑ IgE and IgA, ↓ or normal IgM and IgG, thrombocytopenia with small platelets (low mean platelet volume)	• Stem cell transplant • Gene therapy • Splenectomy if severe thrombocytopenia • Ig replacement • Avoid live vaccines
Ataxia-telangiectasia	• Autosomal recessive defect in *ATM* gene (codes for DNA repair enzymes) → DNA damage → cell cycle arrest → B- and T-cell deficiency	• Ataxia, telangiectasia (oculocutaneous), recurrent infections (humoral and cellular defect type), ↓ growth, ↑ risk of malignancy • Variable lymphocyte and Ig levels, but ↑ alpha-fetoprotein and carcinoembryonic antigen levels in 95%	• Avoid unnecessary radiation (↑ risk of malignancy) • Ig replacement in some

(Continued)

Table 45.3 – Primary Immunodeficiencies *(Cont'd)*

Primary Immunodeficiency	Defect and Pathophysiology	Presentation and Diagnosis	Treatment Considerations
Hyper-IgE (Job) syndrome	• Classically autosomal dominant mutation in *STAT-3* (involved in many immune functions) → ↓ IL-6, ↓ Th-17, ↓ Th-1, ↑ Th-2 (↑ IgE and eosinophilia)	• Abnormal facies, eczema, "cold" (uninflamed) skin abscesses, mucocutaneous candidiasis, recurrent sinopulmonary infections (may see pneumatoceles), and connective tissue and skeletal abnormalities (retained primary teeth) • Eosinophilia and ↑ IgE, but normal number of B-cells, T-cells, and other Igs	• Consider stem cell transplant • Dental care • Prophylactic antimicrobials
Phagocytic Immunodeficiency (Most Will Have Dental Issues)			
Leukocyte adhesion deficiency (LAD)	• Type I—defect in phagocytic cell CD18 integrin (and associated LFA-1 it binds to) • Type II—defect in sialylated Lewis X antigen on neutrophil or endothelial cell selectin • Net effect is ↓ phagocyte adhesion, extravasation, and migration/chemotaxis	• Recurrent skin/soft tissue infections (esp. *Staphylococcus aureus*) with "lack of pus" (no neutrophils) • Neutrophilic leukocytosis (demargination of marginated neutrophil pool due to lack of adherence) • Poor wound healing and delayed umbilical cord separation (due to lack of neutrophils) • Dental issues—gingivitis, periodontitis, etc. • LAD I/II—complete blood count with differential, flow cytometry • LAD III—genetic analysis for *FERMT3* mutation	• Stem cell transplantation is curative for LAD-I and LAD-III • LAD-I—granulocyte transfusion • LAD-II—fucose supplementation • Antimicrobial prophylaxis • Dental care • Avoid live vaccines
Chediak–Higashi syndrome	• Autosomal recessive defect in lysosomal transport gene/protein (regulates synthesis and maintenance of storage or secretory granules in various cells) • Microtubule dysfunction in various cells, which disrupts cell trafficking and results in the myriad of manifestations	• Impaired phagolysosome fusion → recurrent pyogenic bacterial infections (esp. *S. aureus*) • Neutropenia and impaired neutrophil chemotaxis • Partial oculocutaneous albinism (light skin and silvery hair) • Central and peripheral neuropathy (progressive) • Lymphoproliferative phase—often viral-induced (Epstein–Barr virus) and can present like lymphoma • Peripheral smear → giant granules in leukocytes, platelets, melanocytes, nervous system, etc.	• Stem cell transplant—will not correct albinism and neurologic issues

(Continued)

Table 45.3 – Primary Immunodeficiencies *(Cont'd)*

Primary Immunodeficiency	Defect and Pathophysiology	Presentation and Diagnosis	Treatment Considerations
Chronic granulomatous disease	• Defect in NADPH oxidase → cannot convert oxygen to superoxide anion → impaired respiratory burst (oxygen-dependent killing) in phagocytes	• Recurrent granulomatous infections with catalase + organisms (*S. aureus, Burkholderia cepacia, Nocardia, Serratia, Aspergillus*, etc.) • Hepatic abscess due to *Staphylococcus* may be a tip-off, and infection with certain organisms may be pathognomonic (i.e., *Chromobacterium violaceum, B. cepacia*, etc.) • Positive dihydrorhodamine (DHR) test	• IFN-γ replacement • Granulocyte transfusions (last resort in life-threatening infections) • Stem cell transplantation • Antimicrobial prophylaxis (trimethoprim/sulfamethoxazole + itraconazole) • Dental care • Avoid live vaccines
Myeloperoxidase (MPO) deficiency	• Defect in MPO → inability of phagocyte to convert H_2O_2 (hydrogen peroxide) to HOCl (bleach)	• Mostly asymptomatic but can have ↑ risk of *Candida* infections (usually when combined with another immune deficiency like diabetes) • Negative DHR test	• Treat infections as they arise
Complement Immunodeficiency			
Terminal complement deficiency	• Defect in C5–C9, which form the membrane attack complex (needed for gram-negative infections)	• Recurrent *Neisseria* infections (gonorrhea and meningococcus)	• Meningococcal vaccination
Early complement deficiency	• C1, C2, or C4 deficiency	• Infection with encapsulated organisms and lupus-like syndrome	• Pneumococcal vaccination
C3 deficiency	• C3 deficiency	• Infection with encapsulated organisms, but NO lupus-like syndrome	• Pneumococcal vaccination
Other Immunodeficiency Syndromes			
Granulocyte-macrophage colony-stimulating factor (GM-CSF)	• Anti–GM-CSF autoantibodies	• Cryptococcal meningitis and pulmonary alveolar proteinosis	• Replace missing component • Immune modulation —rituximab, plasmapheresis
Interferon-gamma (IFN-γ)	• Anti–IFN-γ autoantibodies	• ↑ risk of infections with *Mycobacteria, Salmonella*, fungal infections, and varicella-zoster virus	• •

(Continued)

Table 45.3 – Primary Immunodeficiencies *(Cont'd)*

Primary Immunodeficiency	Defect and Pathophysiology	Presentation and Diagnosis	Treatment Considerations
GATA-2 deficiency (MonoMAC syndrome)	• GATA-2 deficiency	• Recurrent mycobacterial, fungal, and viral (esp. papilloma and herpesviruses) infections • ↓ lymphocytes (esp. B-cells and NK cells), dendritic cells, and monocytes. Normal Ig	• Stem cell transplant can be curative
Chronic mucocutaneous candidiasis	• Various mutations, including of IL-17 and STAT-1	• Recurrent mucocutaneous *Candida* infections • Rarely, invasive *Candida* (and other fungal) infections.	• Targeted antifungal therapy

KEY LEARNING POINT

Common variable immunodeficiency occurs when B-cells are unable to mature into plasma cells, so the levels of immune globulins will be low, but B-cell number is typically preserved.

REFERENCES AND FURTHER READING

- Bennet JE, Dolin R, Blaser MJ, eds. *Mandell, Douglas, and Bennett's Principles and Practice of Infectious Diseases*. 9th ed. Elsevier; 2020.
- Bonilla FA, Khan DA, Ballas ZK, et al. Practice parameter for the diagnosis and management of primary immunodeficiency. *J Allergy Clin Immunol*. 2015;136(5):1186–2105, e1–e78. https://doi.org/10.1016/j.jaci.2015.04.049.
- Grammatikos A, Bright P, Bhatnagar R, Johnston S. How to investigate a suspected immune deficiency in adults. *Respir Med*. 2020;171:106100 https://doi.org/10.1016/j.rmed.2020.106100.
- Spec A, Escota G, Chrisler C, Davies B, eds. *Comprehensive Review of Infectious Diseases*. 1st ed. Elsevier; 2019.

A 30-year-old male presents to the HIV clinic for routine follow-up. He is currently on Biktarvy (bictegravir, tenofovir alafenamide fumarate, and emtricitabine) but wishes to switch to an alternative agent due to issues with insomnia and gastrointestinal upset. He is otherwise healthy and takes no other medications. He has no allergies. Physical examination is within normal limits. Previous HIV genotype testing revealed the presence of a K103N mutation. This mutation is most likely to confer resistance to which of the following antiretroviral agents?

A. Tenofovir.

B. Emtricitabine.

C. Abacavir.

D. Efavirenz.

E. Rilpivirine.

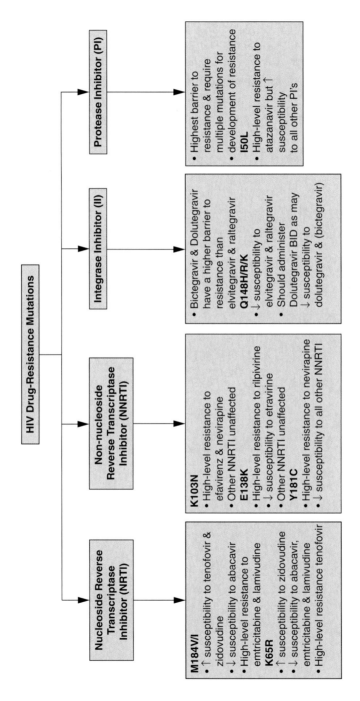

Figure 46.1 – HIV resistance mutations

The best answer here is efavirenz (**option D**). The K103N mutation confers resistance to the early-generation non-nucleoside reverse transcriptase inhibitors (NNRTIs) such as efavirenz and nevirapine. The newer NNRTIs such as rilpivirine (**option E**) and etravirine are unaffected by this mutation. In addition, the other drugs listed (**options A, B, and C**) are likely to be unaffected by this mutation as well.

It is important to recognize that HIV resistance can be transmitted or acquired. This resistance can be identified by resistance testing, which usually involves obtaining a HIV-genotype test. This test can only be done in patients with viremia (requires at least 500–1000 copies/mL for successful performance) because mutations only arise in an actively replicating HIV. Genotype (resistance) testing should be obtained upon entry into care (prior to starting antiretroviral therapy [ART]), but the initiation of ART should not be delayed while awaiting genotype results. For those already on ART, resistance testing should be obtained if virologic failure occurs despite optimization of other causes of virologic failure (i.e., adherence, drug interactions, etc.). In these cases, the resistance will only become evident under selective pressure (i.e., in the presence of the drug). Therefore, resistance testing is best done while the patient is still taking the failing drug regimen or within 4 weeks of discontinuing the regimen (i.e., before the virus can revert back to the wild-type strain, where the mutation may not be evident). In addition, routine genotypic testing only looks for mutations that confer resistance to nucleoside reverse transcriptase inhibitors, NNRTIs, and protease inhibitors. Resistance testing for integrase inhibitors is not routinely done, but if integrase inhibitor resistance is suspected then specific testing should be requested. Lastly, when constructing a new regimen for a patient, one should consider all prior drug-resistance tests and their relation to the ART the patient was taking at the time.

There are many different HIV drug-resistance mutations, so committing all of these to memory is not very practical. Fig. 46.1 shows the mutations that are either fairly common or easily testable.

KEY LEARNING POINT

The K103N HIV mutation confers high-level resistance to earlier-generation non-nucleoside reverse transcriptase inhibitors (efavirenz and nevirapine).

REFERENCE AND FURTHER READING

• Spec A, Escota G, Chrisler C, Davies B, eds. *Comprehensive Review of Infectious Diseases*. 1st ed. Elsevier; 2019.

A 40-year-old female presents to the HIV clinic to initiate antiretroviral therapy following a recent diagnosis of HIV during routine screening. She feels well and has no complaints. She has no medication allergies. Her medical history includes asymptomatic cholelithiasis, Gilbert disease, gastroesophageal reflux disease, and nephrolithiasis. Her only medication is omeprazole. Surgical history includes a prior lithotripsy. Vital signs are within normal limits. Body mass index is 35 kg/m². Physical examination reveals mild scleral icterus but is otherwise unremarkable. Basic laboratory work-up is significant for creatinine 1.2 mg/dL (creatinine clearance >60 mL/min), total bilirubin 3 mg/dL, alkaline phosphatase 70 U/L, and alanine aminotransferase 30 U/L. Baseline HIV viral load is 120,000 copies/mL, and CD4 cell count is 540 cells/uL. HIV genotype test is pending, and urine pregnancy test is negative. Hepatitis B virus (HBV) testing shows negative HBV surface antigen, negative HBV core antibody (IgM and IgG), and positive HBV surface antibody. HLA-B*5701 testing is negative. Based on the available information, it would be best to avoid which of the following antiretroviral agents?

A. Atazanavir (ATV).

B. Darunavir.

C. Efavirenz.

D. Abacavir.

E. Dolutegravir.

The best antiretroviral therapy (ART) to avoid would be ATV (**option A**). ATV is a poor option for this patient for various reasons. First, ATV requires an acidic environment for absorption, so using this medication may be difficult for someone (such as this patient) on a proton-pump inhibitor. Second, ATV reversibly inhibits the hepatic UDP-glucuronosyltransferase (bilirubin conjugation) enzyme, which results in indirect (unconjugated) hyperbilirubinemia. This consequence may result in worsening of cholelithiasis and hyperbilirubinemia in a patient with Gilbert disease. Lastly, ATV may cause kidney stones as well, and, given this patient's history of kidney stones, ATV should be avoided if possible. Darunavir (**option B**) is associated with a rash in patients with a history of sulfa allergy. Efavirenz (**option C**) is associated with neuropsychiatric adverse events (i.e., vivid dreams, depression, suicidality, etc.), rash, and prolonged QT interval, and may be teratogenic (teratogenic potential is controversial). Abacavir (**option D**) is typically well tolerated but may cause a hypersensitivity reaction (in patients with HLA-B*5701 positivity) and has been associated with increased risk of myocardial infarction (although studies are mixed). Dolutegravir (**option E**) may raise serum creatinine by impairing the tubular secretion of creatinine, cause myopathy, and weight gain (common to all integrase inhibitors). Common ART adverse effects and considerations are summarized in Table 47.1.

Table 47.1 – Adverse Effects of Antiretroviral Therapy

Adverse Effect	Common Causes
Reduction in bone mineral density	• Can be seen after starting any antiretroviral therapy (ART), but tenofovir is the most problematic (disoproxil fumarate [DF] formulation more problematic than alafenamide [AF] formulation)
Bone marrow suppression (cytopenia)	• Zidovudine
Cardiovascular	• Efavirenz and rilpivirine associated with prolonged QT interval • Atazanavir associated with prolonged PR interval • Abacavir associated with increased risk of myocardial infarction (controversial but best to avoid in patients at high cardiovascular risk)
Dyslipidemia	• Tenofovir adverse effects (AF) (DF formulation actually improves lipids), zidovudine, abacavir, efavirenz, elvitegravir, and various protease inhibitors (PIs)
Nephrotoxicity	• Tenofovir (DF > AF) associated with ↑ serum creatinine and proximal tubulopathy (Fanconi-like syndrome). Avoid tenofovir DF if creatinine clearance (CrCl) <50 mL/min and avoid tenofovir AF if CrCl <15 mL/min. • Atazanavir associated with crystalluria nephrolithiasis • ↑ serum creatinine (related to decreased tubular secretion and not a true kidney injury) associated with cobicistat, dolutegravir, bictegravir, and rilpivirine

(Continued)

Table 47.1 – Adverse Effects of Antiretroviral Therapy *(Cont'd)*

Adverse Effect	Common Causes
Hepatotoxicity	• Exacerbation of hepatitis B when discontinuing tenofovir, emtricitabine, or lamivudine in patients with chronic hepatitis B virus infection • Atazanavir associated with indirect (unconjugated) hyperbilirubinemia (reversible inhibition of hepatic UGT enzyme) and cholelithiasis. • Hepatotoxicity associated with nevirapine, efavirenz, and all PIs.
Neurologic	• Nonnucleoside reverse transcriptase inhibitors (NNRTIs; especially efavirenz) associated with various neuropsychiatric AEs • Integrase inhibitors associated with insomnia, depression, and suicidality
Dermatologic	• Emtricitabine can cause skin hyperpigmentation • NNRTIs (esp. nevirapine and efavirenz) are associated with Stevens–Johnson syndrome/toxic epidermal necrolysis • Darunavir is associated with a skin rash in patients with a history of sulfa allergy
Other AEs and considerations	• Weight gain has been associated with initiation of ART and subsequent viral suppression (most pronounced with integrase inhibitors) • Myopathy can be seen with zidovudine, dolutegravir, and raltegravir • Hypersensitivity reaction seen with abacavir in patients with HLA-B*5701 positivity • Atazanavir and rilpivirine require acidic environment for absorption • Rilpivirine requires food (~400 calories) for absorption and should be avoided if viral load is >100,000 and/or CD4 cell count is <200 cells/uL • Boosted PI and NNRTI are often associated with drug-drug interactions

KEY LEARNING POINT

Atazanavir is a protease inhibitor that can cause unconjugated (indirect) hyperbilirubinemia, cholelithiasis, and nephrolithiasis. In addition, an acidic environment is required for appropriate absorption.

REFERENCE AND FURTHER READING

• Panel on Antiretroviral Guidelines for Adults and Adolescents. Guidelines for the Use of Antiretroviral Agents in Adults and Adolescents with HIV. Department of Health and Human Services. https://clinicalinfo.hiv.gov/sites/default/files/inline-files/AdultandAdolescentGL.pdf. Accessed January 8, 2021.

A 45-year-old male is admitted with a 3-day history of fevers, chills, and left-hand pain, redness, and swelling. He has a history of alcoholic cirrhosis complicated by ascites. Medications include lactulose, furosemide, and spironolactone. He notes he quit drinking 3 months ago. He is currently unemployed but enjoys fishing at a small local lake. He denies any animal bites or exposure to fish tanks or shellfish. Vital signs show temperature 101° F, heart rate 110 beats per minute, blood pressure 95/58 mmHg, respiratory rate 18, and oxygen saturation 96% on room air. There is no lymphadenopathy, bullae, vesicles, or subcutaneous emphysema. Skin examination shows scattered telangiectasia and palmar erythema. The dorsal left-hand lesion is shown in Fig. 48.1. The abdomen is distended with ascites, and the remainder of the examination is unremarkable. White blood cell count is 12,000 cells/uL (80% neutrophils). Blood cultures are drawn.

Which of the following organisms is the most likely cause of this patient's illness?

A. *Mycobacterium marinum.*
B. *Vibrio vulnificus.*
C. *Aeromonas hydrophila.*
D. *Erysipelothrix rhusiopathiae.*
E. *Sporothrix schenckii.*

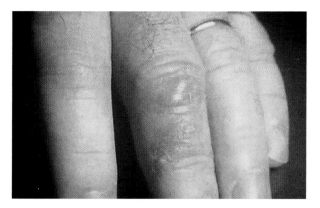

Figure 48.1 – Left-hand skin lesion
Reboli A. *Erysipelothrix rhusiopathiae.* In: Bennet JE, Dolin R, Blaser MJ, eds. *Mandell, Douglas, and Bennett's Principles and Practice of Infectious Diseases.* 9th ed. Elsevier; 2020:2575–2577.

The most likely cause is *E. rhusiopathiae* (**option D**). This organism is a gram-positive rod that is classically found in association with swine and fish (commensal organism for these animals). *E. rhusiopathiae* causes a zoonotic infection in humans through direct contact with animals harboring the organism (usually enters via a break in the skin). Individuals in certain occupations are at high risk, including fishermen, veterinarians, and other people who work with large animals. The infection manifests in one of three ways: a localized erysipelas-like cellulitis, usually on the hand ("erysipeloid"—Fig. 48.1), a diffuse cutaneous eruption with systemic symptoms, and rarely, bacteremia with endocarditis. Diagnosis is established by isolation of the organism from a skin biopsy or sterile bodily fluid (i.e., blood). The organism grows best at 35° C in 5% carbon dioxide. *E. rhusiopathiae* is usually susceptible to penicillins and cephalosporins but is notably resistant to vancomycin and sulfonamides. The localized skin infection is typically treated for 7 to 10 days, usually with penicillin or amoxicillin. Rapid treatment response is a hallmark. The other manifestations often require longer duration, and endocarditis should be ruled out.

M. marinum (**option A**) classically causes a papular or sporothrichoid (lymphangitic) infection of the upper extremity (in setting of minor skin trauma) and is associated with exposure to fish tanks ("fish tank granuloma"), aquariums, or swimming pools. Management may include surgical debridement and combination antimycobacterial drug therapy, often for several weeks.

V. vulnificus (**option B**) and *Vibrio parahaemolyticus* are comma-shaped gram-negative organisms that can cause a severe skin/soft tissue infection resembling necrotizing skin/soft tissue infection (often with hemorrhagic bullae). It is classically associated with exposure to brackish water and salt water (especially Gulf of Mexico region) or handling and/or ingesting shellfish. In addition, patients with chronic liver disease are at highest risk for severe infection. Management includes doxycycline plus a third-generation cephalosporin. Fluoroquinolones are an alternative. Duration is contingent upon clinical response.

A. hydrophila (**option C**) can also cause a severe skin/soft tissue infection, often in association with exposure to fresh or brackish water or leeches. Empiric therapy consists of doxycycline plus either ciprofloxacin or ceftriaxone.

S. schenckii (**option E**) is a dimorphic fungus that causes sporotrichosis ("rose-gardener's disease"). This can be acquired by traumatic inoculation (often in an extremity) in patients who work with soil or vegetation (e.g., gardeners). Sporotrichosis presents as an indolent infection, initially with a papule/nodule at the site of inoculation followed by a sporotrichoid (lymphangitic) spread. Treatment consists of itraconazole for several weeks, until all lesions have resolved.

KEY LEARNING POINT

Erysipelothrix rhusiopathiae infection classically manifests as an erysipelas-like cellulitis of the hand in patients with certain exposures (fishermen, etc.).

REFERENCES AND FURTHER READING

- Reboli A. *Erysipelothrix rhusiopathiae*. In: Bennet JE, Dolin R, Blaser MJ, eds. *Mandell, Douglas, and Bennett's Principles and Practice of Infectious Diseases*. 9th ed. Elsevier; 2020:2575–2577.
- Spec A, Escota G, Chrisler C, Davies B, eds. *Comprehensive Review of Infectious Diseases*. 1st ed. Elsevier; 2019.

A 55-year-old male presents to the emergency room in November with a 2-day history of fevers, cough, chest pain, and shortness of breath. Approximately 1 week prior he was diagnosed with influenza A virus infection and elected for symptomatic management (i.e., no antivirals were prescribed). He notes he initially improved after a few days and was slowly feeling better up until about 2 days ago when his current symptoms started. He has no medication allergies. Medical history is significant for chronic obstructive pulmonary disease (COPD), hypertension, and type 2 diabetes mellitus. Medications include albuterol as needed, metformin, atorvastatin, and lisinopril. He smokes one pack of cigarettes a day. Vital signs reveal temperature 102.5° F, heart rate 135 beats per minute, blood pressure 80/50 mmHg, respiratory rate 32, and oxygen saturation 85% on room air with improvement to 92% on 4 L/min oxygen by nasal cannula. Physical examination reveals an ill-appearing male with rapid, shallow breathing and accessory muscle use. Heart is tachycardic and irregular with no murmurs. Lung exam reveals decreased breath sounds and crackles over the right lower lung field posteriorly. The skin is diffusely erythematous, and the erythema blanches when the skin is compressed. There is no jugular venous distension or peripheral edema. Laboratory studies reveal white blood cell count 25,000 cells/uL (90% neutrophils), platelet count 75,000 cells/uL, creatinine 2.5 mg/dL (creatinine clearance 25 mL/min), and alanine aminotransferase 150 U/L. Chest x-ray reveals a large right-sided pleural effusion. Which of the following is the most appropriate diagnosis for this patient?

A. Primary influenza pneumonia.

B. Acute respiratory distress syndrome (ARDS).

C. Secondary bacterial pneumonia.

D. Acute exacerbation of COPD.

E. Acute systolic heart failure with cardiogenic shock.

The most appropriate diagnosis is secondary bacterial pneumonia (**option C**), with likely complicated parapneumonic effusion and toxic shock syndrome (TSS). This patient initially had influenza A virus infection that lasted several days and was followed by a period of clinical improvement prior to clinical worsening (with prominent lower respiratory tract signs and symptoms). This illness pattern is classic for postinfluenza secondary bacterial pneumonia (PISBP). The most common bacterial etiologies of PISBP are *Staphylococcus aureus* and *Streptococcus pneumoniae*. Less common pathogens include *Streptococcus pyogenes*, various gram-negatives including *Haemophilus influenzae*, and *Aspergillus*. The pneumonia (and associated consolidation) of PISBP is typically more focal in nature than that seen with primary influenza pneumonia (**option A**). In rare cases, patients (such as the one in this case) may develop TSS in the setting of deep-seated infections caused by *S. aureus and S. pyogenes*. These pathogens produce toxins that act as superantigens to cause "hyperactivation" of T-cells and massive cytokine release. This phenomenon is responsible for the manifestations of TSS. A comparison of the subtypes of TSS is shown in Table 49.1.

The presentation of TSS is fairly nonspecific and initially presents as an influenza-like illness. A high degree of clinical suspicion is necessary to make the diagnosis. Helpful features include an unexplained shock state with or without end-organ damage, mucous membrane involvement (especially with staphylococcal TSS), and a skin rash (sunburn-like rash [erythroderma] with staphylococcal TSS or scarlatina-like rash with streptococcal TSS). For additional manifestations, see "clinical features" in Table 49.1. Work-up should include basic metabolic laboratory work-up (i.e., complete blood count with differential, renal function testing, liver function testing, coagulation parameters, urinalysis with microscopy, lactic acid, and creatine kinase), blood cultures (at least two sets), and cultures of any involved site. In addition, imaging of involved areas may be helpful. Lastly, alternative differential diagnoses should be ruled out.

The management of TSS is fairly straightforward. The most important aspects are to manage the shock and the associated complications and to eradicate the source of the infection (i.e., remove a retained tampon, debride area of necrotizing skin infection). Antimicrobial therapy is a bit more nuanced. Empiric therapy will depend on various factors including the suspected organism(s) and source of infection. Initially, coverage may need to be fairly broad to cover all possible pathogens including staphylococci (including methicillin-resistant *S. aureus*), streptococci, gram-negatives, and anaerobes. In addition, if suspecting TSS, an agent with toxin-suppressing activity (i.e., clindamycin or linezolid) should be provided as well. Once a definitive diagnosis is made, targeted therapy can be prescribed. This therapy is summarized

Answer and Explanation

Table 49.1 – Toxic Shock Syndrome Classification

	Staphylococcal Toxic Shock Syndrome	Streptococcal Toxic Shock Syndrome
Causative organisms	• *Staphylococcus aureus* (methicillin-resistant *S. aureus* [MRSA] or methicillin-sensitive *S. aureus* [MSSA])	• Beta-hemolytic streptococci—group A (*Streptococcus pyogenes*) most commonly, but also group B (*Streptococcus agalactiae*), and group C/G (*Streptococcus dysgalactiae*)
Etiologies	• Menstrual (i.e., prolonged tampon use) • Nonmenstrual—deep-seated infections due to *S. aureus* (i.e., postinfluenza secondary bacterial pneumonia), retained nasal packing, etc.	• Invasive streptococcal infections (typically group A streptococci and a skin and soft tissue infection source)
Lab criteria	• Cultures (blood or cerebrospinal fluid) negative for alternative pathogens (blood cultures may be positive for *S. aureus*) • Serologic testing negative for Rocky Mountain spotted fever, leptospirosis, and measles	• Isolation of *Streptococcus* (typically group A) from a normally sterile site (**IA**) or a nonsterile site (**IB**)

Clinical criteria	• **Fever ≥38.9° C (102° F)**
	• **Rash**—diffuse macular erythroderma (similar to a sunburn)
	• **Desquamation**—1–2 weeks after onset
	• **Hypotension**—systolic blood pressure (SBP) ≤90 mmHg
	• **Three or more end organs damaged:**
	  • Gastrointestinal—vomiting and/or diarrhea
	  • Muscular—severe myalgia or creatine kinase level ≥2 times the upper limit of normal (ULN)
	  • Mucous membranes—vaginal, oropharyngeal, or conjunctival hyperemia
	  • Renal—blood urea nitrogen or creatinine ≥2 times the upper limit of normal ULN, or urinary sediment with pyuria (5 or more white blood cells per high-power field) without evidence of urinary tract infection
	  • Hematologic—thrombocytopenia (<100,000 cells/uL)
	  • Hepatic—total bilirubin, aspartate aminotransferase (AST), or alanine aminotransferase (ALT) ≥2 times the ULN
	  • Central nervous system—disorientation or altered consciousness without focal neurologic deficits
		• **Hypotension—SBP ≤90 mmHg, AND**
		• **Two or more end organs damaged:**
		  • Renal—creatinine ≥2 mg/dL or ≥2 times the baseline (if pre-existing renal dysfunction)
		  • Coagulopathy—thrombocytopenia (≤100,000 cells/uL) or disseminated intravascular coagulopathy
		  • Hepatic—total bilirubin, AST, or ALT ≥2 mg/dL or ≥2 times the baseline
		  • Acute respiratory distress syndrome
		  • Generalized macular rash (scarlatina-like) ± desquamation
		  • Soft tissue necrosis

Diagnosis	• Probable—meets lab criteria and four clinical criteria • Confirmed—meets lab criteria and all five clinical criteria	• Probable—meets criteria **IB** and clinical criteria; no other cause is identified • Confirmed—meets criteria **IA** and clinical criteria

(Continued)

Table 49.1 – Toxic Shock Syndrome Classification *(Cont'd)*

	Staphylococcal Toxic Shock Syndrome	Streptococcal Toxic Shock Syndrome

Management	• Management of shock and complications
	• Source control – remove offending agent (i.e., tampon), debride deep-seated infection source, etc.
	• Targeted antimicrobial therapy
	  • **MSSA**—antistaphylococcal penicillin (oxacillin or nafcillin) OR cefazolin
	  • **MRSA**—vancomycin (alternatives are daptomycin and ceftaroline)
	  • **Both MRSA and MSSA**—ADD anti-toxin agent for up to 5 days (clindamycin 900 mg IV q8h [if the isolate is susceptible] or linezolid 600 mg PO/IV q12h [if unable to use clindamycin or resistant to clindamycin])
		• Management of shock and complications
		• Source control—surgical debridement
		• Targeted antimicrobial therapy
		• **Penicillin-G (alternative: ceftriaxone) PLUS**
		• **Antitoxin agent (similar to** *S. aureus***)**
		• Intravenous immune globulin has a mortality benefit in streptococcal TSS

Mortality	• Lower (<5%)	• Higher (30%–50%)

in Table 49.1, but a few points are worth adding. First, clindamycin (at a dose of 900 mg IV every 8 hours) and intravenous immune globulin may be associated with a mortality benefit in patients with streptococcal (mostly group A streptococci) TSS; thus, their use is much more justified for streptococcal TSS (as opposed to staphylococcal TSS, where the data for these agents is sparse). Clindamycin is typically given for 3 to 5 days. Second, penicillin-G has been shown to be less effective at higher streptococcal organism loads. It is postulated that this reduced effectiveness is due to reduced expression of penicillin-binding proteins by bacteria in the stationary phase of growth, which is reached more rapidly with large organism loads. Lastly, the final duration of therapy (and transition to oral therapy) will depend on the source of infection (and the degree of source control) and the clinical trajectory (response to therapy).

Aside from secondary bacterial pneumonia and TSS, other complications of influenza infection include primary influenza pneumonia, tracheobronchitis, ARDS, myositis and rhabdomyolysis, myopericarditis, myocardial infarction, various neurologic manifestations (including Guillain–Barré syndrome), and, rarely, Reye syndrome (typically in children who receive aspirin during influenza infection). Primary influenza pneumonia (**option A**) is a very severe complication that typically presents as a progressive worsening of the infection, without any intervening period of improvement. The pneumonia tends to be bilateral in nature as well. ARDS (**option B**) presents with an acute onset of respiratory failure (within 1 week of the inciting factor), as well as bilateral pulmonary opacities on imaging that are not explained by a different process (i.e., volume overload, heart failure, etc.). ARDS has several potential causes, including infection, but the presentation in this patient is not consistent with ARDS. Acute exacerbation of COPD (**option D**) manifests as an increase in at least one of the following symptoms (compared with the patient's baseline symptoms): cough, shortness of breath, or sputum production. Although this patient may meet the criteria for acute exacerbation of COPD (with the exacerbating factor being viral infection), it would not be the best explanation for all of the symptoms. Acute systolic heart failure with cardiogenic shock (**option E**) could happen in the setting of influenza-induced myocarditis or severe sepsis (septic cardiomyopathy), but the lack of jugular venous distension and peripheral edema make this less likely. In addition, erythroderma is not a manifestation of heart failure.

KEY LEARNING POINT

The diagnosis of toxic shock syndrome (TSS) requires a high degree of clinical suspicion. TSS should be suspected in a patient with unexplained shock associated with dermatologic manifestations in the setting of infections caused by **Staphylococcus aureus** *or beta-hemolytic streptococci.*

REFERENCES AND FURTHER READING

- Elsevier ClinicalKey. Clinical overview: Toxic shock syndrome. https://www.clinicalkey.com/#!/content/clinical_overview/67-s2.0–8106cf2d-7991-4c0f-a2a2–97821ea3d2cf. Updated June 21, 2021. Accessed July 28, 2021.
- Lappin E, Ferguson A. Gram-positive toxic shock syndromes. *Lancet Infect Dis.* 2009;9(5):281–290. https://doi.org/10.1016/S1473-3099(09)70066-0.
- Treanor J. Influenza viruses, including avian influenza and swine influenza. In: *Mandell, Douglas, and Bennett's Principles and Practice of Infectious Diseases.* 9th ed. Elsevier; 2020:2143–2168.

A 22-year-old female presents to the clinic with a 2-day history of sore throat and anterior neck discomfort. She denies nasal discharge, cough, or shortness of breath. She is otherwise healthy and does not take any medications. She has no medication allergies. She denies sexual activity and illicit drug use. HIV screening 1 year ago was negative. Vitals show temperature 99° F, heart rate 90 beats per minute, blood pressure 120/80 mmHg, respiratory rate 16, and oxygen saturation 98% on room air. Physical examination is notable for pharyngeal erythema with tonsillar enlargement and exudate. She has tender anterior cervical lymphadenopathy. The remainder of the examination is unremarkable. Which of the following is the most appropriate next step in management?

A. Rapid streptococcal antigen test.
B. Empiric penicillin therapy.
C. Rapid influenza antigen test.
D. HIV antigen/antibody screen.
E. Symptomatic treatment (i.e., saltwater gargle, lozenges, etc.).

The most appropriate next step would be to perform a rapid streptococcal antigen test (**option A**). This patient's presentation is most consistent with streptococcal (strep) pharyngitis. This infection is most commonly caused by group A streptococcus (GAS; *Streptococcus pyogenes*). The infection typically occurs in the winter and early spring in patients aged 5 to 15 years. Prior (recent) exposure to GAS is also suggestive. Strep pharyngitis presents abruptly with fevers and sore throat (patients may also complain of odynophagia and dysphagia). In addition, many patients will have headache and gastrointestinal upset. Rarely, a scarlatiniform rash (resembles a sunburn and has a sandpaper-like quality) and/or "strawberry tongue" may be seen, which suggest scarlet fever. Viral features (conjunctivitis, cough, rhinorrhea, hoarseness, oral ulcers) are characteristically absent, and their presence actually argues against the diagnosis of streptococcal pharyngitis. Examination may reveal tender anterior cervical lymphadenopathy and exudative tonsillitis with palatal petechiae. The various infectious causes of acute pharyngitis are summarized in Table 50.1.

Complications of GAS pharyngitis can be suppurative and nonsuppurative. Suppurative complications include peritonsillar abscess, parapharyngeal space abscess, otitis media, mastoiditis, lymphadenitis, and sinusitis. Nonsuppurative complications include acute rheumatic fever, poststreptococcal glomerulonephritis (PSGN; more common with GAS skin infections), poststreptococcal reactive arthritis, toxic shock syndrome, scarlet fever, and, in children, pediatric autoimmune neuropsychiatric disorder associated with GAS.

In a patient presenting with a pharyngitis syndrome, emergency etiologies (e.g., retropharyngeal abscess) should be ruled out first. An emergent etiology should be considered in patients with drooling, muffled ("hot potato") voice, trismus, stridor, respiratory distress, neck stiffness, and "tripod" positioning. If any of these symptoms are present, then further work-up (i.e., imaging) may be necessary. If none of these signs or symptoms are present, then evaluation for the "less urgent" etiologies can be done.

If obvious viral features are present (i.e., conjunctivitis, cough, rhinorrhea, oral ulcers, hoarseness), then evaluation for strep pharyngitis is not needed, as the diagnosis is unlikely. If no viral features exist, and the presentation is consistent with GAS pharyngitis, then further evaluation should be pursued. Evaluation of a patient with suspected streptococcal pharyngitis should include rapid antigen detection testing (RADT), because the clinical manifestations and the validated scoring systems (such as Centor criteria) that incorporate these manifestations are not very sensitive or specific. RADT have been shown to be modestly sensitive (70%–90%) and very specific (96%). Thus, false-positive results are very rare, but a

Table 50.1 – Etiologies of Acute Pharyngitis

Etiology	Description and Associations
Bacterial Etiologies	
Group A streptococci (*Streptococcus pyogenes*)	• Causes 5%–15% of acute pharyngitis in adults • Presentations include asymptomatic carriage, acute pharyngotonsillitis, suppurative complications, and nonsuppurative complications (see text)
Group C and G streptococci (*Streptococcus dysgalactiae*)	• Cause acute pharyngotonsillitis similar to *S. pyogenes*, but not associated with rheumatic fever, and very rarely implicated in poststreptococcal glomerulonephritis
Arcanobacterium haemolyticum	• Acute pharyngitis with scarlatiniform rash in an adolescent or young adult • Treatment of choice is a macrolide.
Fusobacterium spp.	• *F. necrophorum* (and other fusobacteria less commonly) are associated with septic thrombophlebitis of the internal jugular vein (Lemierre syndrome)
Neisseria gonorrhoeae	• Tonsillopharyngitis in a sexually active individual (receptive oral intercourse)
Viral Etiologies	
Respiratory viruses	• Adenovirus (pharyngoconjunctival fever), influenza, rhinovirus, coronavirus, respiratory syncytial virus, parainfluenza
Herpes simplex virus (HSV) 1 and 2	• Gingivostomatitis (primary HSV-1 infection) • Tonsillopharyngitis—often severe and may also have concurrent HSV esophagitis
Enteroviruses (coxsackievirus)	• Hand, foot, and mouth disease and herpangina are typically seen in children and are classically caused by coxsackie A virus
Human immunodeficiency virus (HIV)	• Acute retroviral syndrome (acute HIV infection) presents as a mononucleosis-like illness several weeks after initial infection/exposure • Consider if there are risk factors for HIV acquisition—men who have sex with men, IV drug abuse, etc.
Infectious mononucleosis	• Epstein–Barr virus and cytomegalovirus
Other Etiologies	
Rare etiologies	• *Corynebacterium diphtheriae*—diphtheria; gray pharyngeal pseudomembrane, myocarditis, neuropathy, unvaccinated or travel-related • *Yersinia enterocolitica*—enterocolitis syndrome + pharyngitis • *Francisella tularensis*—oropharyngeal tularemia • *Chlamydophila*—*C. pneumoniae* and *C. psittaci* • *Treponema pallidum*—secondary syphilis • *Mycoplasma pneumoniae* • *Toxoplasma gondii*

negative RADT cannot completely rule out GAS pharyngitis. Throat culture, on the other hand, is 90% to 95% sensitive. Reflex throat culture (i.e., follow-up testing after a negative RADT) is not necessary in most adult cases of acute pharyngitis, because the risk of postinfectious complications is very low. Neither of these tests can differentiate a true GAS pharyngitis from an asymptomatic GAS carrier.

The differential diagnosis to consider is outlined in Table 50.1. Testing for all of these entities is not necessary, and clinical suspicion should guide the appropriate testing.

Once GAS pharyngitis is confirmed, treatment should be given, because treatment decreases time to resolution of symptoms, reduces disease transmission, and reduces postinfectious sequelae (especially suppurative complications and rheumatic fever). Treatment does not affect the risk of developing PSGN. The first line therapy is penicillin VK (oral) or amoxicillin for 10 days. Alternative options include benzathine penicillin-G (if compliance with oral therapy is a concern), or, in patients with penicillin allergies, a 10-day course of either clindamycin or a cephalosporin (first-, second-, or third-generation), or a 5-day course of azithromycin. Clinical improvement is expected in 1 to 2 days. Failure to improve should prompt consideration of treatment adherence, improper diagnosis, or development of a complication (i.e., abscess). Supportive therapies include hydration and pain control with acetaminophen, topical agents, and/or nonsteroidal anti-inflammatory drugs. In general, aspirin and corticosteroids should not be given routinely. Follow-up "tests of cure" are not routinely recommended in most cases. Lastly, for asymptomatic household contacts of a patient with GAS pharyngitis, testing and empiric treatment of the household contact is not routinely recommended.

Empiric penicillin therapy (**option B**) in patients meeting all four Centor criteria (i.e., fever, exudative tonsillitis, tender anterior cervical lymphadenopathy, and absence of cough) is no longer recommended. Only patients with proven GAS pharyngitis should be given treatment. Rapid influenza testing (**option C**) can be considered, but the lack of viral features in this case suggests that influenza is less likely than GAS pharyngitis. HIV screening (**option D**) should always be considered in patients presenting with a pharyngitis syndrome, but this patient is at very low risk for acquiring HIV (not sexually active, denies IV drug use, HIV test 1 year ago was negative). Symptomatic treatment (**option E**) should certainly be provided, but it should not take precedence over identifying and treating GAS pharyngitis.

KEY LEARNING POINT

In a patient with suspected group A streptococcus (GAS) pharyngitis (with no features suggestive of viral infection), rapid antigen detection testing should be performed. Empiric treatment is no longer recommended, and only confirmed cases of GAS pharyngitis should receive antibiotic treatment.

REFERENCES AND FURTHER READING

- Flores A, Caserta M. Pharyngitis. In: Bennet JE, Dolin R, Blaser MJ, eds. *Mandell, Douglas, and Bennett's Principles and Practice of Infectious Diseases*. 9th ed. Elsevier; 2020:824–831.
- Shulman ST, Bisno AL, Clegg HW, et al. Clinical practice guideline for the diagnosis and management of group A streptococcal pharyngitis: 2012 update by the Infectious Diseases Society of America. *Clin Infect Dis*. 2012;55(10):e86–e102.

A 35-year-old male is hospitalized with *Staphylococcus aureus* bacteremia complicated by infective endocarditis, valvular heart failure, and a large splenic abscess that is not amenable to drainage. The plan is to perform concurrent valvular repair and splenectomy in the next day or two. He is otherwise healthy and does not know his vaccination history. Consequently, it is deemed that he should receive the following vaccinations: meningococcal, *Haemophilus influenzae* type b, and pneumococcal. When should these vaccines be given?

A. Now.

B. The day after splenectomy.

C. 7 days after splenectomy.

D. 14 days after splenectomy.

E. 3 months after splenectomy.

The vaccinations should be given 14 days after splenectomy (**option D**). Patients with functional or anatomic asplenia are at risk for infection with encapsulated organisms. Infection with these organisms can cause an illness known as overwhelming postsplenectomy infection. One method of prevention is vaccination against certain encapsulated pathogens, namely *H. influenzae* type B, *Streptococcus pneumoniae*, and *Neisseria meningitidis*. The vaccination specifics are shown in Table 51.1. The timing of these vaccinations depends on the urgency of the splenectomy. In patients undergoing elective splenectomy, the vaccinations should be provided at least 14 days prior to the procedure. In patients undergoing emergent splenectomy, the vaccinations can be started 14 days after splenectomy. In patients receiving immune suppression or radiation therapy, the vaccinations should be given at least 3 months (**option E**) after completion of the treatment. The other choices (**options A, B, and C**) are not recommended vaccination timings.

Table 51.1 – Postsplenectomy Vaccinations

Vaccine	Recommendation
Pneumococcal (*Streptococcus pneumoniae*)	• One dose of PCV-13 (Prevnar) followed by PPSV-23 (Pneumovax) at least 8 weeks later • If previously received PPSV-23, then give PCV-13 at least 1 year after the PPSV-23 that was received • PPSV-23 should then be repeated in 5 years and at age 65 years
Haemophilus influenzae type B (HiB)	• One dose of HiB vaccine
Meningococcal (*Neisseria meningitidis*) Quadrivalent (ACWY)	• Primary series—two doses at least 8 weeks apart • If using MenACWY-D (Menactra), PCV13 should be completed first, and MenACWY-D should be given 4 weeks after the PCV13 series is completed • Revaccinate every 5 years
Meningococcal-B	• Can be given as either a two-dose series of MenB-4C (Bexsero) or a three-dose series of MenB-FHbp (Trumenba). The same vaccine product must be used for all doses. • Based on available data and expert opinion, MenB-4C or MenB-FHbp may be administered concomitantly with MenACWY vaccines, but at a different anatomic site, if feasible
Routine vaccines	• Annual inactivated influenza vaccination

KEY LEARNING POINT

*For patients undergoing elective splenectomy, perisplenectomy vaccinations (*Streptococcus pneumoniae, Neisseria meningitidis, *and* Haemophilus influenzae *type B) should be given at least 14 days before the procedure. For patients undergoing emergent splenectomy, these vaccinations should be given 14 days after splenectomy.*

REFERENCES AND FURTHER READING

- Gilsdorf JR, Dawid S. Infections in splenic Patients. In: Bennet JE, Dolin R, Blaser MJ, eds. *Mandell, Douglas, and Bennett's Principles and Practice of Infectious Diseases*. 9th ed. Elsevier; 2020:3713–3722.
- Kroger A, Bahta L, Hunter P. Vaccine recommendations and guidelines of the ACIP: general best practice guidelines for immunization. CDC website. https://www.cdc.gov/vaccines/hcp/acip-recs/general-recs/index.html. Updated May 4, 2021. Accessed June 4, 2021

A 40-year-old zookeeper presents to the emergency room (ER) for evaluation of a monkey bite. Earlier today, while working with one of the macaque monkeys, he was bitten on his right forearm by the monkey. He notes the bite "drew blood." He cleansed the wound with soap and water and was able to stop the bleeding prior to coming to the ER. He is otherwise healthy. He has no medication allergies and does not take any medications. He does not recall when his last tetanus vaccination was. He says he has received a full rabies pre-exposure vaccination series, as this was required for his job. He says follow-up titers have been "adequate." He does not know if the monkey has been immunized against rabies, and the zoo just received the monkey recently from Thailand. He does not want the monkey to be euthanized for rabies testing. Vital signs are within normal limits. Examination reveals a fresh puncture wound over the right forearm with no significant surrounding erythema or fluctuance. Neurologic examination is within normal limits. The remainder of the exam is unremarkable. The wound is thoroughly cleansed and allowed to heal by secondary intention. You discuss postexposure prophylaxis. Which of the following prophylaxis measures is NOT indicated at this time?

A. Rabies vaccination.

B. Rabies immune globulin (RIG).

C. Tetanus vaccination.

D. Valacyclovir.

E. Amoxicillin/clavulanate.

All of the measures listed are indicated except for RIG (**option B**).

The herpes B virus (*Cercopithecine herpesvirus* 1 or "B virus") is a zoonosis that is acquired by exposure (i.e., bites, scratches, bodily fluid exposure, mucous membrane exposure) to macaque monkeys. Similar to herpes simplex virus (HSV), the B virus ascends the peripheral nervous system in a retrograde fashion to reach the central nervous system (CNS). Interestingly, antibody to HSV does not protect humans from B virus infection. The incubation period is 2 days to 5 weeks. Presentation may include an influenza-like illness, vesicular herpetic lesions, lymphadenitis, peripheral nerve symptoms (pain, numbness, etc.) at the site of inoculation, and central nervous system disturbances (including an often-fatal encephalomyelitis).

Diagnostic testing is typically only performed in symptomatic patients, because asymptomatic infection has never been reported. Serologic testing can be done at baseline and 3 to 6 weeks later. Seroconversion or a four-fold rise in the titer is consistent with infection. Other diagnostic options include PCR (highly sensitive and specific) and culture from involved/exposed areas. Furthermore, symptomatic patients should have CNS imaging (MRI typically) and lumbar puncture for cerebrospinal fluid (CSF) analysis, including CSF PCR, serology, and culture. Testing of the nonhuman primate (NHP) may need to be done as well. Further diagnostic and therapeutic guidance can be found at the National B Virus Resource Center (Atlanta, Georgia) webpage.

In the event of an exposure (i.e., macaque monkey bite), providers should strongly consider giving postexposure prophylaxis (PEP) for B virus (Figs. 52.1 and 52.2). PEP is most effective if it is given within 5 days of the exposure. Options include valacyclovir 1-gram PO three times daily (**option D**) or Acyclovir 800 mg PO five times daily. The duration of PEP is 14 days. In addition to B virus PEP, patients should be given the usual bite management, which includes cleansing of the wound and exposed sites (and allowing healing by secondary intention), antibiotic prophylaxis (**option E**, see case 7 for indications for bite wound antibiotic prophylaxis), tetanus prophylaxis (**option C**, Table 51.1), and rabies prophylaxis (**option A**). RIG (**option B**) is not necessary, given this patient's prior rabies vaccination with adequate titers. Rabies from NHP bites is rare, but rabies PEP should be provided for victims of NHP bites where rabies is endemic (e.g., Thailand, as in this case).

Treatment of B virus disease is a bit more involved. The rationale for treatment lies in the fact that untreated herpes B virus carries a high mortality (up to 80%), and antiviral medications

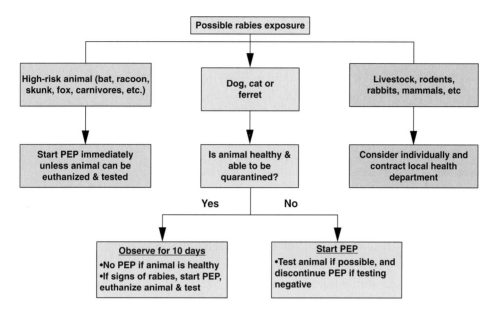

Figure 52.1 – Approach to rabies postexposure prophylaxis (*PEP*).

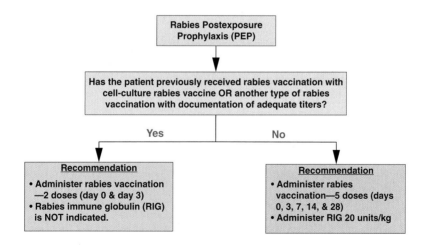

Figure 52.2 – Choosing the appropriate rabies postexposure prophylaxis (*PEP*). *RIG*, Rabies immune globulin.

Table 52.1 – Tetanus Prophylaxis

Number of Prior Tetanus Toxoid Doses	Minor or Clean Wound	All Other Wounds (Dirty Wounds)
<3 doses or unknown	• Tetanus toxoid–containing vaccine[a] only	• Tetanus toxoid–containing vaccine[a] + human tetanus immune globulin
3 or more doses	• Tetanus toxoid–containing vaccine[a] only if last dose was ≥10 years ago	• Tetanus toxoid–containing vaccine[a] only if last dose was ≥5 years ago

[a]Tetanus toxoid–containing vaccines typically include Td (tetanus-diphtheria toxoids absorbed) and Tdap (booster tetanus toxoid-reduced diphtheria toxoid-acellular pertussis). Tdap preferred if patient has not received Tdap previously.

reduce this mortality to 20%. Treatment choice depends on whether or not CNS symptoms are present. If there are no CNS symptoms, then the drug of choice is acyclovir 12.5 to 15 mg/kg IV every 8 hours. An alternative option is ganciclovir 5 mg/kg IV every 12 hours. If CNS symptoms are present, then the treatment should be ganciclovir 5 mg/kg IV every 12 hours. Treatment is continued until symptoms resolve and the results of two cultures are negative for B virus (after being held for 2 weeks). Some authorities advocate for long-term suppressive therapy, but this practice is controversial.

KEY LEARNING POINT

Macaque monkey bites can result in herpes B virus infection, which can be fatal in humans. Consequently, B virus prophylaxis is recommended in most cases. The regimens of choice for B virus prophylaxis are valacyclovir or acyclovir given for 14 days.

REFERENCES AND FURTHER READING

• Cohen J. Herpes B virus. In: Bennet JE, Dolin R, Blaser MJ, eds. *Mandell, Douglas, and Bennett's Principles and Practice of Infectious Diseases*. 9th ed. Elsevier; 2020:1904–1907.
• Cohen JI, Davenport DS, Stewart JA, et al. Recommendations for prevention of and therapy for exposure to B virus (cercopithecine herpesvirus 1). *Clin Infect Dis*. 2002;35(10):1191–1203. https://doi.org/10.1086/344754.
• Johnston W, Yeh J, Neirenburg R, Procopio G. Exposure to macaque monkey bite. *J Emerg Med*. 2015;49(5):634–637.
• Mills L. *Rabies*. In: *Emergency Medicine Clinical Essentials*. 2nd ed. Elsevier; 2013:1511–1517.
• Newton F. United States Armed Forces. Monkey bite exposure treatment protocol. *J Spec Oper Med*. 2010;10(1):48–49.
• Usatine RP, Coates WC. *Laceration and incision repair*. In: *Pfenninger and Fowler's Procedures for Primary Care*. 4th ed. Elsevier; 2020:136–148.
• Wu AC, Rekant SI, Baca ER, et al. Notes from the field: monkey bite in a public park and possible exposure to herpes B virus—Thailand, 2018. *MMWR Morb Mortal Wkly Rep*. 2020;69:247–248. https://doi.org/10.15585/mmwr.mm6909a6.

A 35-year-old male presents to the HIV clinic with a 3-day history of dysphagia and odynophagia. He has a history of poorly-controlled chronic HIV infection due to his decision to not take antiretroviral therapy. When you last saw him 6 months ago, he had a CD4 count of 100 cells/uL (7%). He believes he acquired HIV from having unprotected sex with various male partners. He has not been sexually active since his diagnosis. Vital signs are within normal limits. BMI is 17 kg/m². Physical examination shows cachexia and temporal wasting. Oral mucosa is dry. There are white patches on the buccal mucosa. The remainder of the exam is unremarkable. What is the next best step in the management of this patient?

A. Refer for esophagogastroduodenoscopy.

B. Barium swallow (esophagram).

C. Valacyclovir.

D. Valganciclovir.

E. Fluconazole.

The best next step in management would be a trial of fluconazole (**option E**). This patient with advanced HIV (AIDS) is presenting with esophagitis. The most likely etiology of esophagitis in these patients is *Candida spp.* The diagnosis of *Candida* esophagitis is also supported by the presence of thrush (oropharyngeal candidiasis) in this patient, although patients may have *Candida* esophagitis without thrush. Other infectious etiologies of esophagitis in advanced HIV patients include cytomegalovirus (CMV) and herpes simplex virus (HSV). These organisms cannot be differentiated based on presentation alone.

When an advanced HIV patient presents with esophagitis and there are no alarm features that require urgent endoscopic intervention (i.e., gastrointestinal bleeding), the best initial step in management is a trial of fluconazole (empiric treatment for *Candida* esophagitis). The typical duration of treatment is 14 to 21 days, and most patients should clinically improve within 1 week (Fig. 53.1). Failure to improve suggests either resistant *Candida* infection (very uncommon unless the patient had prior azole exposure) or incorrect diagnosis (it is not uncommon to have more than one etiology in these patients). In this scenario, the next best step is to perform upper endoscopy (**option A**). Based on endoscopic appearance, esophageal

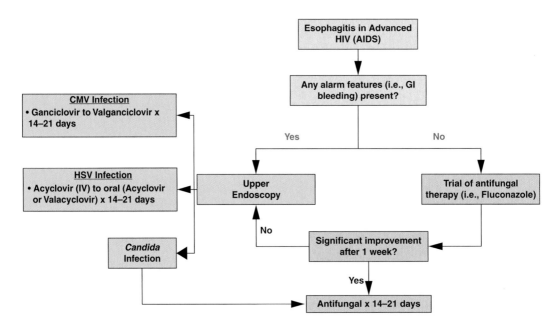

Figure 53.1 – Approach to esophagitis in advanced HIV (AIDS).
CMV, Cytomegalovirus; *GI*, gastrointestinal; *HSV*, herpes simplex virus.

brushings, and esophageal biopsy (histopathology) results, an etiology can be established. If there is evidence of CMV infection, then the treatment should start with ganciclovir, followed by valganciclovir (**option D**) after clinical improvement. If there is evidence of HSV infection, then treatment should start with IV acyclovir followed by transition to oral therapy (acyclovir or valacyclovir [**option C**]) after clinical improvement. The typical minimum duration of treatment for HSV and CMV is 14 to 21 days.

Barium swallow (esophagram, **option B**) is seldom helpful in the diagnosis of esophagitis in advanced HIV patients.

KEY LEARNING POINT

When an advanced HIV patient presents with esophagitis and there are no alarm features that require urgent endoscopic intervention (i.e., gastrointestinal bleeding), the best initial step in management is a trial of fluconazole (empiric treatment for Candida *esophagitis). Failure to improve after 1 week of fluconazole therapy should prompt consideration of upper endoscopy.*

REFERENCE AND FURTHER READING

• Graman P. Esophagitis. In: Bennet JE, Dolin R, Blaser MJ, eds. *Mandell, Douglas, and Bennett's Principles and Practice of Infectious Diseases*. 9th ed. Elsevier; 2020:1340–1345.

54

CASE

A 65-year-old male is admitted to the hospital with a 3-day history of fevers, headache, nausea, vomiting, and confusion. He had been feeling unwell for the week preceding these symptoms and had fallen twice at home. He has a history of alcoholic cirrhosis. Medications include lactulose, furosemide, spironolactone, and a multivitamin. He has no medication allergies. He drinks six pack of beer daily. Vital signs show temperature 102° F, heart rate 95 beats per minute, blood pressure 95/65 mmHg, respiratory rate 18, and oxygen saturation 95% on room air. On examination, he appears ill and confused. There is no nuchal rigidity. His gait is ataxic with a tendency to fall to his right side. Cranial nerve examination is normal. Right-sided dysmetria is noted. Scratching the plantar aspect of the right foot results in dorsiflexion of the great toe. Heart and lung examination are within normal limits. Abdomen is mildly distended with ascites. The remainder of the examination is unremarkable. Blood cultures are obtained. Noncontrast CT scan of the brain is unremarkable. A lumbar puncture shows 50 white blood cells (80% neutrophils), glucose 45 mg/dL, and protein 120 mg/dL. MRI of the brain reveals T2-hyperintesnity in the right cerebellum. What is the most likely organism responsible for this patient's presentation?

A. *Cryptococcus neoformans.*
B. Herpes simplex virus (HSV).
C. JC virus.
D. *Listeria monocytogenes.*
E. *Borrelia burgdorferi.*

The most likely cause is *L. monocytogenes* (**option D**). *L. monocytogenes* is an aerobic gram-positive rod that classically affects immune-compromised patients (in particular, cell-mediated immune compromise). In addition, *Listeria* may affect less severely immune-compromised patients, including the very young, the elderly (typically >65 years of age, but >50 years of age is used in meningitis), alcoholics, patients with chronic liver disease, and pregnant patients. A key microbiologic characteristic is "tumbling motility" in a wet mount or in a semisolid agar slant. Infection is classically acquired via ingestion of "cold foods" such as hot dogs, soft cheeses, and unpasteurized milk. This predilection for cold foods is explained by *Listeria*'s ability to survive at lower temperatures.

Listeria presentations may include a febrile gastroenteritis (often short-lived and occurs in immune-competent individuals), bacteremia, and focal invasive disease, especially central nervous system (CNS) disease. *Listeria* has a tropism for CNS tissue and can cause meningoencephalitis (often acute to subacute), cerebritis, and even brain abscesses. *Listeria* rhombencephalitis (LRE; as portrayed by this case) is a form of meningoencephalitis that involves the brainstem and cerebellum. As a result, patients will present with a meningoencephalitis that is associated with cranial nerve deficits, cerebellar signs, and seizures. Diagnosis is supported by a neutrophilic pleocytosis, which often comes with a mild cerebrospinal fluid (CSF) protein elevation and mildly decreased CSF glucose. In those without preceding antibiotic exposure, blood cultures are positive in approximately 60% of cases, and CSF cultures are positive in up to 40% of cases. In patients with LRE, MRI may show hyperintensity in the brainstem and/or cerebellum. The typical MRI findings in LRE are shown in Fig. 54.1.

Before discussing the management of this case, a review of the general approach to the management of meningoencephalitis is appropriate. Empiric antimicrobial therapy in acute meningoencephalitis is guided by the age of the patient, the severity of illness, and the suspected causative pathogen(s). Empiric therapy should not be delayed to obtain work-up (CSF analysis and imaging). Table 54.1 summarizes empiric therapy in acute meningoencephalitis.

Dexamethasone can be given empirically before or concurrently with antibiotic administration (but not after antibiotics have been given). Dexamethasone has been shown to have a small mortality benefit, mainly in cases of acute bacterial meningitis caused by *Streptococcus pneumoniae*. In addition, dexamethasone may reduce postinfectious neurologic sequelae, especially hearing loss. Therefore, if dexamethasone is started, it should only be continued

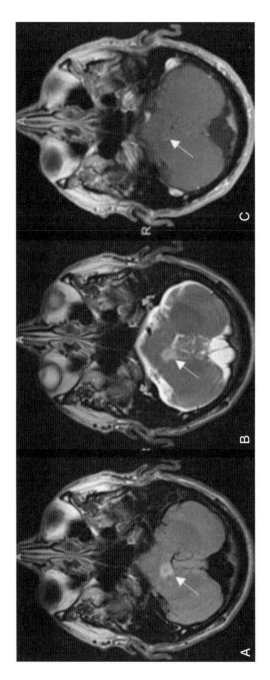

Figure 54.1 – Listeria rhombencephalitis. Axial FLAIR and T2 images show a focus of hyper signal intensity in the right middle cerebellar peduncle (arrows in A and B). The lesion shows classical rim enhancement after contrast injection (arrow in C).

FLAIR, Fluid-attenuated inversion recovery.

Sotouden H, et al. Brainstem encephalitis. The role of imaging in diagnosis. In: *Current Problems in Diagnostic Radiology.* Elsevier; 2020.

Table 54.1 – Acute Meningoencephalitis Empiric Therapy

Scenario	Organisms to Cover	Empiric Therapy	Alternatives and Comments
Age 2–50 years	• *Neisseria meningitidis* • *Streptococcus pneumoniae*	• Vancomycin + third-generation cephalosporin	• Third-generation cephalosporin = ceftriaxone or cefotaxime • Vancomycin is used to cover for potential resistant *S. pneumoniae*
Age >50 years or risk factors for *Listeria*	• *N. meningitidis* • *S. pneumoniae* • *Listeria monocytogenes*	• Vancomycin + third-generation cephalosporin + ampicillin	• Alternative to ampicillin (*Listeria* coverage)—trimethoprim/sulfamethoxazole or meropenem
Hospital-acquired (postneurosurgery, shunt) or penetrating head trauma	• Staphylococci (*S. aureus* and coagulase-negative staphylococci) • Gram-negative rods including *Pseudomonas* • *Cutibacterium acnes* (central nervous system shunt)	• Vancomycin + cefepime	• Alternative for cefepime—meropenem >> aztreonam or fluoroquinolone
Immune-compromised	• *N. meningitidis* • *S. pneumoniae* • *L. monocytogenes* • Gram-negative rods	• Vancomycin + cefepime + ampicillin	• Similar alternatives as per above
Basilar skull fracture or cochlear implant	• *S. pneumoniae* • *Haemophilus influenzae* • Group A *Streptococcus* (*S. pyogenes*)	• Vancomycin + third-generation cephalosporin	• Similar alternatives as per above

- The dosing of antimicrobials for central nervous system (CNS) infections may need to be higher than for other infections (i.e., ceftriaxone is typically given 2 grams IV every 12 hours). Providers need to be cognizant of this when treating patients with CNS infections.
- The use of dexamethasone and acyclovir is discussed further later.

(duration 4 days) if *S. pneumoniae* is isolated. Some authorities will use dexamethasone for *Haemophilus influenzae* meningitis as well, as pediatric *H. influenzae* meningitis studies have shown improved neurologic outcomes with dexamethasone. The Infectious Diseases Society of America recommends also using rifampin when dexamethasone is given, but in practice this is not commonly done. If neither of these organisms is found, then dexamethasone should be discontinued. Dexamethasone has been associated with unfavorable outcomes in

L. monocytogenes meningitis, so its use is discouraged. Empiric therapy may include IV acyclovir (dosed 10 mg/kg IV every 8 hours in patients with normal renal function) if there is suspicion for HSV encephalitis. Definitive (targeted) therapy will depend on the patient's clinical response and the results of the CSF studies. Definitive therapy for selected etiologies of acute meningoencephalitis is summarized in Table 54.2.

Failure to improve within a few days (despite seemingly appropriate therapy) should prompt further investigation such as repeating CSF analysis and imaging (if not already done) of the brain and spinal cord to look for parameningeal foci of infection (i.e., epidural abscess).

Now back to our case. The first-line treatment of *Listeria* CNS infection is IV ampicillin (or IV penicillin-G) plus or minus gentamicin for at least 3 weeks (longer duration may be necessary with brain abscesses). The alternative options include trimethoprim/sulfamethoxazole or meropenem. These same medications can be used for *Listeria* bacteremia (without metastatic focus of infection) with duration being 10 to 14 days. *Listeria* gastroenteritis typically goes unnoticed (i.e., never diagnosed), and treatment is not necessary in most cases.

C. neoformans (**option A**) infection can also present as a subacute to chronic meningoencephalitis in an immune-compromised patient such as this one. Cryptococcal meningoencephalitis is typically associated with a mononuclear or lymphocytic pleocytosis, which is not seen in this case. HSV (**option B**) CNS infections include meningitis (HSV-2>HSV-1) and encephalitis (mainly due to HSV-1). HSV CNS infections are typically associated with a lymphocytic pleocytosis and, in the case of HSV-1 encephalitis, temporal lobe (often unilateral) enhancement on CNS imaging. The treatment for HSV encephalitis is IV acyclovir for 14 to 21 days. JC virus (**option C**) infection causes progressive multifocal leukoencephalopathy (PML). PML is a rare infection (often a reactivation of a latent JC virus infection) seen in severely immune-compromised patients such as those with advanced HIV/AIDS (CD4 count <50 cells/uL) or patients on certain immune-suppressing medications (i.e., natalizumab). PML would be highly unlikely to occur in this patient. *B. burgdorferi* (**option E**) is the causative agent of Lyme disease. Neuroborreliosis (CNS Lyme disease) can present as a subacute to chronic meningoencephalitis associated with lymphocytic pleocytosis and cranial neuropathy (classically cranial nerve VII palsy). This case presentation is not consistent with neuroborreliosis.

Table 54.2 – Definitive Therapy in Meningoencephalitis

Organism	First-Line	Alternatives	Duration
Streptococcus pneumoniae (penicillin MIC ≤0.06 ug/mL)	• Penicillin-G or ampicillin	• Third-generation cephalosporin (ceftriaxone)	10–14 days
S. pneumoniae (penicillin MIC >0.12 ug/mL + CFTX MIC <1 ug/mL)	• Third-generation cephalosporin (ceftriaxone)	• Cefepime or meropenem	
S. pneumoniae (penicillin MIC >0.12 ug/mL + CFTX MIC ≥1 ug/mL)	• Vancomycin + third-generation cephalosporin (ceftriaxone)[c]	• Fluroquinolone with streptococcal coverage (moxifloxacin)	
Neisseria meningitidis (penicillin MIC<0.1 ug/mL)	• Penicillin-G or ampicillin	• Third-generation cephalosporin (ceftriaxone)	7 days
N. meningitidis (penicillin MIC 0.1–1 ug/mL)	• Third-generation cephalosporin (ceftriaxone)	• Meropenem or fluoroquinolone	
Haemophilus influenzae (beta-lactamase–negative)	• Ampicillin	• Third-generation cephalosporin (ceftriaxone)	7 days
H. influenzae (beta-lactamase–negative)	• Third-generation cephalosporin (ceftriaxone)	• Cefepime or fluoroquinolone	
Listeria monocytogenes[a]	• Ampicillin or penicillin-G ± aminoglycoside	• Meropenem or TMP/SMX or linezolid	21 days
Aerobic gram-negative rods/ most enterobacteriaceae (i.e., *Escherichia coli*)	• Third-generation cephalosporin (ceftriaxone)	• Meropenem or aztreonam or fluoroquinolone or TMP/SMX	21 days
Pseudomonas spp.	• Cefepime ± aminoglycoside	• Aztreonam, ciprofloxacin, or meropenem ± aminoglycoside	21 days
Acinetobacter spp.	• Meropenem	• Colistin or polymyxin B	21 days
Streptococcus agalactiae (group B streptococcus)	• Ampicillin or penicillin-G ± aminoglycoside	• Third-generation cephalosporin (ceftriaxone)	14–21 days
Methicillin-susceptible *Staphylococcus aureus* (MSSA)[b]	• Nafcillin or oxacillin	• Vancomycin	10–14 days
Methicillin-resistant *S. aureus*[d]	• Vancomycin	• TMP/SMX or linezolid	
Enterococcus	• Penicillin- or ampicillin-susceptible → use ampicillin or penicillin-G + aminoglycoside		10–14 days
	• Penicillin- or ampicillin-resistant → use vancomycin + aminoglycoside		
	• Vancomycin-resistant → use linezolid		

[a]Use of aminoglycosides in *Listeria* meningitis is controversial (data are mixed and not very strong).

[b]Cefazolin cannot be used for MSSA meningoencephalitis due to suboptimal central nervous system penetration.

[c]Addition of rifampicin can be considered if the organism is susceptible, the expected clinical or bacteriological response is delayed, or the cefotaxime/ceftriaxone MIC of the *S. pneumoniae* isolate is >4.0 µg/mL.

[d]Consider addition of rifampin if susceptible (probably most useful in device-associated infections).

CFTX, Ceftriaxone; *MIC*, minimal inhibitory concentration; *TMP/SMX*, trimethoprim/sulfamethoxazole.

KEY LEARNING POINT

Listeria *rhombencephalitis should be suspected in an immune-compromised patient presenting with an acute to subacute meningoencephalitis associated with brainstem or cerebellar signs.*

REFERENCES AND FURTHER READING

- Brower MC, Van de Beek D. Acute and chronic meningitis. In: Cohen J, ed. *Infectious Diseases*. 4th ed. Elsevier; 2017:177–188.
- Johnson JE, Mylonakis E. *Listeria monocytogenes*. In: Bennet JE, Dolin R, Blaser MJ, eds. *Mandell, Douglas, and Bennett's Principles and Practice of Infectious Diseases*. 9th ed. Elsevier; 2020:2543–2549.
- Prod'hom G, Bille J. Aerobic gram-positive bacilli. In: Cohen J, ed. *Infectious Diseases*. 4th ed. Elsevier; 2017: 1537–1552.
- Sotoudeh H, et al. Brainstem encephalitis. The role of imaging in diagnosis. In: *Current Problems in Diagnostic Radiology*. Elsevier; 2020.
- Van de Beek D, Brouwer MC, Thwaites GE, Tunkel AR. Advances in treatment of bacterial meningitis. *Lancet*. 2012;380(9854):1693–1702.

A 55-year-old male presents to the emergency room with a 2-day history of fevers, headache, confusion, and neck discomfort. He has a history of rheumatoid arthritis. Medications include acetaminophen, naproxen, methotrexate, and etanercept. He does not have any medication allergies. Vital signs reveal temperature 102° F, heart rate 95 beats per minute, blood pressure 110/70 mmHg, and respiratory rate 16. On examination, he appears ill, drowsy, and confused. There is nuchal rigidity. Kernig and Brudzinski signs are negative. Cranial nerves are intact. There is no papilledema. Patellar reflexes are 2+ bilaterally. Babinski sign is negative. There is no skin rash. Examination of the hands reveals mild swelling of the metacarpophalangeal and proximal interphalangeal joints bilaterally. The remainder of the examination is unremarkable. Labs reveal white blood cell count 14,000 cells/uL. What is the next best sequence of steps in management?

A. Blood cultures, lumbar puncture, empiric antibiotics, head CT.

B. Blood cultures, empiric antibiotics, head CT, lumbar puncture.

C. Blood cultures, head CT, lumbar puncture, empiric antibiotics.

D. Blood cultures, empiric antibiotics, lumbar puncture, head CT.

E. Head CT, lumbar puncture, blood cultures, empiric antibiotics.

The best next sequence of steps is blood cultures followed by empiric antibiotics followed by head CT and then lumbar puncture (**option B**). This patient's presentation is concerning for acute meningitis. A more appropriate term is meningoencephalitis, as meningitis and encephalitis are not always two distinct entities; rather, they exist on a spectrum. The term meningoencephalitis will be used here.

Acute meningoencephalitis (community-acquired) typically presents with an acute onset of fevers, headache, neck stiffness, and altered mentation. Additional symptoms may include nausea, vomiting, and photophobia. Depending on the etiology, patients may also have rashes, focal neurologic signs, and shock. The most common bacterial cause in adults is *Streptococcus pneumoniae*. Other common etiologies include various viruses, *Neisseria meningitidis* (adolescents and young adults living in close quarters), *Haemophilus influenzae* type B (declining incidence with vaccination), and *Listeria monocytogenes* (elderly, immune-compromised).

The classic triad (fever, neck stiffness, altered mentation) occurs in just under 50% of cases. Interestingly, 95% of patients with culture-proven bacterial meningitis had at least two of the following four symptoms: headache, fever, neck stiffness, and altered mentation. None of the signs or symptoms of meningitis are sensitive enough to exclude the diagnosis. Nuchal rigidity is poorly sensitive and specific. Kernig and Brudzinski signs are fairly specific (95%) but are very insensitive. Jolt accentuation of the headache (i.e., worsening headache when rotating the head horizontally a few times) was once thought to be very sensitive, but recent reviews have established this test is also not sensitive enough to rule out meningitis.

In a patient with suspected acute meningoencephalitis, work-up (at the minimum) should include blood cultures and cerebrospinal fluid (CSF) analysis, ideally before administering antibiotics (note: antibiotic administration mainly affects culture results and potentially the Gram stain, but not the other CSF parameters). Obtaining blood cultures before antibiotics is very important, as this may the only way an organism is identified in some cases (i.e., if CSF analysis delayed). The CSF analysis should include opening pressure, cell count with differential, protein, glucose, and gram stain and culture. Assuming no prior antibiotic exposure, Gram stain is positive in 50% to 90% of cases and CSF culture is positive in 80% of cases. The sensitivity of these tests is not high enough to rule out meningitis. Gram stain is highly specific and is often used to direct targeted therapy.

The CSF profiles of some common forms of meningoencephalitis are shown in Table 55.1.

Table 55.1 – Common Meningoencephalitis Profiles

Type of Meningitis	White Blood Cells (cells/uL)	Protein (mg/dL)	Glucose[a] (mg/dL)	Comments
Normal	0–5	15–45	50–75	• Normal opening pressure is 7–18 cmH$_2$0
Bacterial	↑↑	↑↑	↓	• Neutrophilic pleocytosis
Viral	↑	↑	~Normal	• Neutrophilic pleocytosis acutely but eventually see lymphocytic pleocytosis • May see red blood cells in setting of HSV-1 encephalitis
Tuberculosis and fungal	↑	↑	↓	• Neutrophilic pleocytosis acutely, but eventually see lymphocytic pleocytosis

[a]A glucose ratio (CSF glucose/serum glucose) may be a better estimate. Normal ratio is ~0.65. Less than 0.4 is considered low.

Depending on the results of the CSF analysis and the clinical suspicion, additional testing may be necessary. One common additional test that is performed is the CSF meningitis/encephalitis (M/E) panel (BioFire FilmArray). This panel is a PCR-based panel that tests for common meningitis pathogens, including:

- Bacteria—*S. pneumoniae, N. meningitidis, L. monocytogenes, H. influenzae, Escherichia coli* K1, *Streptococcus agalactiae*

- Viruses—cytomegalovirus, enterovirus, herpes simplex virus 1 and 2, human herpesvirus 6, varicella-zoster virus, human parechovirus

- Fungi/yeast—*Cryptococcus neoformans* and *Cryptococcus gattii*

Additionally, due to suboptimal sensitivity of cryptococcal PCR, a separate CSF cryptococcal antigen test should be done if cryptococcal meningitis is suspected despite negative cryptococcal PCR on the M/E panel. An additional consideration is central nervous system (CNS) imaging to identify space-occupying lesions that could preclude performing a lumbar puncture. Imaging also helps to evaluate for other differential diagnoses such as CNS hemorrhage or parameningeal focus of infection (i.e., CNS abscess). It is important to know the order in which to do these tests (blood cultures, CSF analysis, imaging) relative to administration of antibiotics. This concept is outlined in Fig. 55.1.

Fig. 55.1 explains why **option B** is correct and the remaining options (**options A, C, D, and E**) are incorrect. Given this patient's history of immune compromise and altered level of consciousness, CNS imaging should be performed prior to CSF analysis. When this situation occurs, blood cultures should be obtained immediately, and the patient should be started on

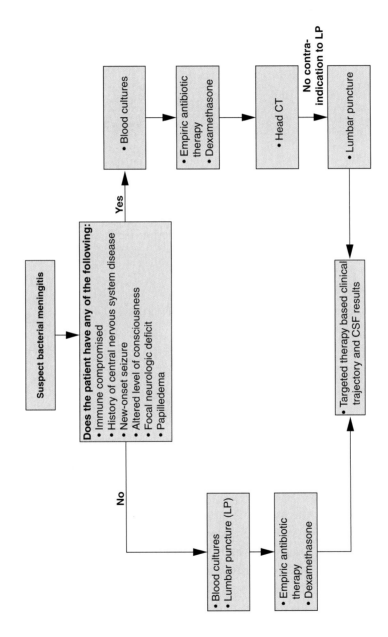

Figure 55.1 – Management of acute bacterial meningitis.
CSF, Cerebrospinal fluid.

appropriate empiric antimicrobial therapy right away. The rationale for this approach lies in the fact that delaying antibiotic administration may result in increased mortality.

Failure to improve within a few days (despite seemingly appropriate therapy) should prompt further investigation, such as repeating CSF analysis and imaging (if not already done) of the brain and spinal cord to look for parameningeal foci of infection (i.e., epidural abscess).

In the case of culture-negative (aseptic) meningoencephalitis, the differential should include (not an exhaustive list) partially-treated bacterial meningoencephalitis (i.e., antibiotics given prior to cultures being obtained), parameningeal focus of infection (i.e., abscess, otitis, sinusitis, etc.), viral meningoencephalitis (i.e., M/E panel viruses [but too early to be detected on PCR], HIV, West Nile virus, arboviruses, etc.), syphilitic meningoencephalitis, neuroborreliosis (Lyme disease), fungal and mycobacterial meningoencephalitis, and noninfectious etiologies such as inflammatory disorders (i.e., sarcoidosis), malignancy (i.e., leptomeningeal carcinomatosis), and various drugs (i.e., nonsteroidal anti-inflammatory drugs, trimethoprim/sulfamethoxazole, etc.). An overview of the approach to common cause of meningoencephalitis is shown in Fig. 55.2 (this is obviously not an exhaustive list).

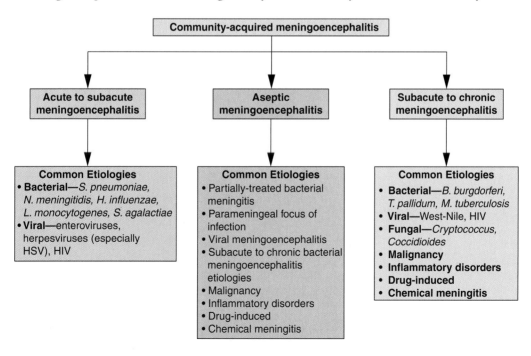

Figure 55.2 – Overview of meningoencephalitis

KEY LEARNING POINT

In certain patients with acute meningoencephalitis (Fig. 55.1), brain imaging should be obtained prior to cerebrospinal fluid analysis. This should not delay antibiotic therapy. After blood cultures are obtained, empiric antibiotic therapy should be started.

REFERENCES AND FURTHER READING

- Brower MC, Van de Beek D. Acute and chronic meningitis. In: Cohen J, et al., eds. *Infectious Diseases*. 4th ed. Elsevier; 2017:177–188.
- Johnson JE, Mylonakis E. *Listeria monocytogenes*. In: Bennet JE, Dolin R, Blaser MJ, eds. *Mandell, Douglas, and Bennett's Principles and Practice of Infectious Diseases*. 9th ed. Elsevier; 2020:2543–2549.
- Prod'hom G, Bille J. Aerobic gram-positive bacilli. In: Cohen J, et al., eds. *Infectious Diseases*. 4th ed. Elsevier; 2017:1537–1552.

A 36-year-old female is admitted to the hospital with a new diagnosis of acute myelogenous leukemia (AML). White blood cell count on admission is 6000 cells/uL (10% neutrophils, 80% myeloblasts). She receives induction chemotherapy with plan for consolidation therapy with stem-cell transplant. On day 7 of hospitalization, she becomes neutropenic with absolute neutrophil count of 100 cells/uL. On the same day, she develops fever and hypotension requiring vasopressor support. Blood cultures are drawn, and she is started on cefepime. The next day, her blood cultures reveal aerobic gram-negative rods. In addition, she develops the lesions shown in Fig. 56.1. These lesions are not painful or pruritic.

Which of the following is the most likely diagnosis?

A. Ecthyma gangrenosum (EG).
B. Acute febrile neutrophilic dermatosis (Sweet syndrome [SS]).
C. Disseminated *Fusarium* infection.
D. Leukemia cutis (LC).
E. Urticarial drug eruption.

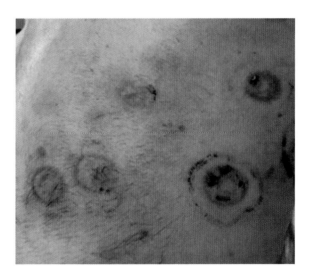

Figure 56.1 – Ecthyma gangrenosum
Saade A, Mirouse A, Zarani L. Ecthyma gangrenosum: an early hint for diagnosis. *Intl J Infect Dis*. 2020;97:19–20.

The most likely diagnosis here is EG (**option A**), likely due to *Pseudomonas aeruginosa* infection. EG is a rare dermatologic manifestation of *P. aeruginosa* infection (although it can be caused by other pathogens) that classically affects neutropenic patients. EG can occur in the setting of *P. aeruginosa* bacteremia (with metastatic seeding of the skin) or, less commonly, as a primary cutaneous lesion with no bacteremia. It is thought that these lesions represent a vasculitis caused by bacterial invasion into vessel walls with resultant ischemic necrosis. EG skin lesions typically start as isolated, red macules (typically not painful) that evolve rapidly into multiple vesiculopustular lesions and finally necrotic ulcerated lesions (with hemorrhage and surrounding erythema). Patients will often be systemically ill (toxic).

Diagnosis is largely clinical, but a definitive diagnosis can be made with skin biopsy showing necrotizing vasculitis and bacterial invasion of vascular walls. Occasionally, a swab from the lesion may demonstrate the causative pathogen. In addition, blood cultures should be obtained to look for associated bacteremia.

Management consists of targeted antimicrobial therapy, typically covering *P. aeruginosa*. Options include cefepime, piperacillin/tazobactam, or meropenem. Transition to oral therapy (fluoroquinolone) to which the isolate is susceptible can be considered once the patient has improved. Duration of therapy is typically 1 to 2 weeks. Resolution of neutropenia is a key prognostic factor. The lesions may take weeks to heal despite appropriate treatment.

Acute febrile neutrophilic dermatosis or SS (**option B**) presents with tender violaceous plaques or nodules. Fever, elevated erythrocyte sedimentation rate, and peripheral neutrophilia may be seen as well (<50%). A characteristic appearance of SS is shown in Fig. 56.2.

Approximately 20% of SS cases are associated with hematologic malignancies, especially AML. There have also been reports of SS being caused by granulocyte colony stimulating factors and various other systemic conditions (i.e., inflammatory bowel disease, pregnancy, etc.). Diagnosis is based on the typical presentation and a skin biopsy showing a neutrophilic dermal infiltrate without leukocytoclastic vasculitis. Treatment involves systemic steroids (tapered over several weeks), which should result in rapid improvement.

Disseminated *Fusarium* infection (**option C**) is a rare invasive fungal (mold) infection (caused by *Fusarium spp.*) that is typically seen in severely immune-compromised patients (i.e., stem-cell transplant patients). Cutaneous lesions occur in three quarters of patients and can occur

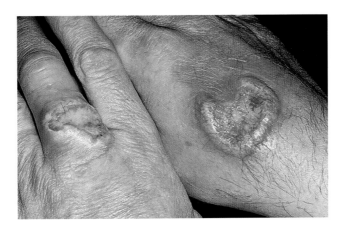

Figure 56.2 – Sweet syndrome
Dinulos JGH. Hypersensitivity syndromes and vasculitis. In: *Habif's Clinical Dermatology*. 7th ed. Elsevier; 2021:713–747.

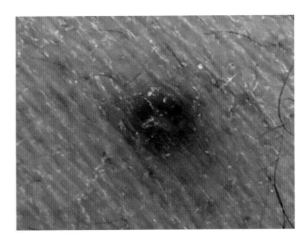

Figure 56.3 – Disseminated mold infection
Bays DJ, Thompson GR 3rd. Fungal infections of the stem cell transplant recipient and hematologic malignancy patients. *Infect Dis Clin North Am*. 2019;33(2):545–566. https://doi.org/10.1016/j.idc.2019.02.006.

as isolated cutaneous lesions or as part of disseminated disease. The typical manifestation is erythematous papules and nodules (often painful) that may or may not have central necrosis (Fig. 56.3).

Fusarium species will grow on routine blood cultures. Skin biopsy should be considered as well to establish the diagnosis. Mortality is very high in disseminated *Fusarium* infections.

The treatment involves amphotericin-B plus or minus voriconazole. Improvement in immunity (i.e., reduction of immune suppression, resolution of neutropenia) is a key factor in management. Surgical debridement may be necessary in severe cases.

LC (**option D**) represents leukemic infiltration of the skin. LC is more common with lymphocytic leukemias (acute and chronic) and chronic myelogenous leukemia than with AML. The most common form of LC presents with multiple violaceous colored papulonodular lesions, as shown in Fig. 56.4.

Management of LC involves managing the underlying malignancy. Unfortunately, LC is associated with a poor prognosis.

Urticarial drug eruptions ("hives," **option E**) typically present soon after exposure to the drug. The classic lesion is a wheal, which is a raised, often very pruritic, erythematous annular-appearing lesion. This patient's presentation is not consistent with this diagnosis.

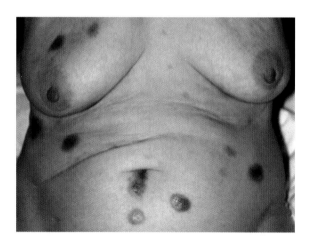

Figure 56.4 – Leukemia cutis
James W, et al. Cutaneous lymphoid hyperplasia, cutaneous T-cell lymphoma, other malignant lymphomas, and allied diseases. In: *Andrew's Diseases of the Skin*. 13th ed. Elsevier; 2020:731–749.

KEY LEARNING POINT

Ecthyma gangrenosum (EG) classically presents as one or more necrotic-appearing lesions in a patient with neutropenia. EG is classically associated with Pseudomonas aeruginosa.

REFERENCES AND FURTHER READING

- Araos R, D'Agata E. *Pseudomonas aeruginosa* and other *Pseudomonas species*. In: Bennet JE, Dolin R, Blaser MJ, eds. *Mandell, Douglas, and Bennett's Principles and Practice of Infectious Disease*. 9th ed. Elsevier; 2020:2686–2699.
- Bays DJ, Thompson GR 3rd. Fungal infections of the stem cell transplant recipient and hematologic malignancy patients. *Infect Dis Clin North Am*. 2019;33(2):545–566. https://doi.org/10.1016/j.idc.2019.02.006.
- Dinulos JGH. Bacterial infections. In: *Habif's Clinical Dermatology*. 7th ed. Elsevier; 2021:331–375.
- Dinulos JGH. Hypersensitivity syndromes and vasculitis. In: *Habif's Clinical Dermatology*. 7th ed. Elsevier; 2021:713–747.
- James W, et al. Cutaneous lymphoid hyperplasia, cutaneous T-cell lymphoma, other malignant lymphomas, and allied diseases. In: *Andrew's Diseases of the Skin*. 13th ed. Elsevier; 2020:731–749.
- Khoo T, Ford F, Lobo Z, Psevdos G. One thing after another: ecthyma gangrenosum. *Am J Med*. 2018;131(5):510–511.
- Saade A, Mirouse A, Zarani L. Ecthyma gangrenosum: an early hint for diagnosis. *Intl J Infect Dis*. 2020;97:19–20.

A 40-year-old male presents to the hospital with a 3-day history of fevers, headache, vomiting, confusion, and general malaise. He returned from a trip to Sudan approximately 2 weeks ago. He did not take any malaria prophylaxis. He is otherwise healthy and does not take any medications routinely. Vital signs reveal temperature 104° F, blood pressure 85/40 mmHg, heart rate 130 beats per minute, respiratory rate 24, and oxygen saturation 90% on room air. On examination, he appears ill and drowsy. There is scleral icterus and conjunctival pallor. Heart exam reveals a regular tachycardia without murmur. Lung exam reveals bibasilar crackles. Abdominal exam reveals hepatosplenomegaly. Pulses are weak, and capillary refill is greater than 3 seconds. Laboratory studies reveal hemoglobin 8 g/dL, platelet count 90,000 cells/uL, white blood cell count 15,000 cells/uL, creatinine 2.5 mg/dL (clearance 20 mL/min), glucose 70 mg/dL, bicarbonate 12 mEq/L, total bilirubin 6 mg/dL, and serum lactate 6 mmol/L. What is the most appropriate next step in diagnosis?

A. Serum PCR.

B. Serologic testing.

C. Rapid antigen testing.

D. Blood smear.

E. Blood cultures.

The most appropriate next step is to obtain a blood smear (**option D**). This patient's presentation is most consistent with severe malaria infection. Malaria is a protozoal infection caused by one of the following *Plasmodium* species: *P. falciparum, P. vivax, P. ovale, P. malariae,* and *P. knowlesi* (Figs. 57.1 and 57.2). Malaria is transmitted by the *Anopheles* mosquito, which is endemic to many tropical and subtropical regions of the world (i.e., Central and South America, sub-Saharan Africa, Middle East, and Southern Asia). *P. falciparum* typically causes the most severe illness. *P. vivax* and *P. ovale* can persist in hepatocytes in a "hypnozoite" form. *P. malariae* causes low-level parasitemia (often not detected on microscopy) and chronic infection. *P. knowlesi* can cause severe infection similar to *P. falciparum* and is typically associated with travel to Southeast Asia (classically Malaysia).

Most malaria infections diagnosed in the United States are related to travel to a malaria-endemic region. After an average incubation of 1 to 4 weeks, patients classically present with fevers, chills (rigors), diaphoresis, headaches, myalgias, arthralgias, and gastrointestinal upset. More severe cases may present with neurologic dysfunction (i.e., depressed consciousness, seizures), respiratory distress, jaundice, and bleeding. Certain fever (and associated rigors) patterns have been associated with certain *Plasmodium* species (although clinically there is substantial variability):

- *P. knowlesi*—every 24 hours
- *P. vivax* and *P. ovale*—every 48 hours (tertian)
- *P. malariae*—every 72 hours (quartan)
- *P. falciparum*—every 48 hours (tertian)

Examination may reveal evidence of shock, altered mentation, icterus, conjunctival pallor, hemoglobinuria, and hepatosplenomegaly. Laboratory studies may reveal leukocytosis, anemia (typically hemolytic with elevated lactate dehydrogenase and decreased haptoglobin), thrombocytopenia, kidney injury (elevated creatinine and/or blood urea nitrogen), hypoglycemia, metabolic acidosis (including lactic acidosis), coagulopathy (i.e., disseminated intravascular coagulopathy), and hyperbilirubinemia. The constellation of symptoms, signs, and laboratory findings in any given malaria patient will depend on the severity of the infection. See Fig. 57.3 for a discussion of "severe malaria" features.

Answer and Explanation

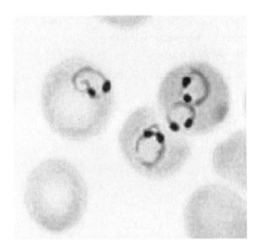

Figure 57.1 – *Plasmodium falciparum*.
From Garcia LS. Malaria. *Clin Lab Med*. 2010;30(1):93–129.

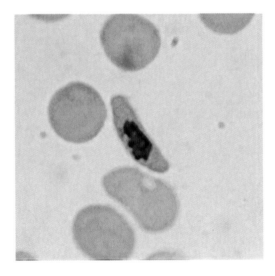

Figure 57.2 – *Plasmodium falciparum*.
From Garcia LS. Malaria. *Clin Lab Med*. 2010;30(1):93–129.

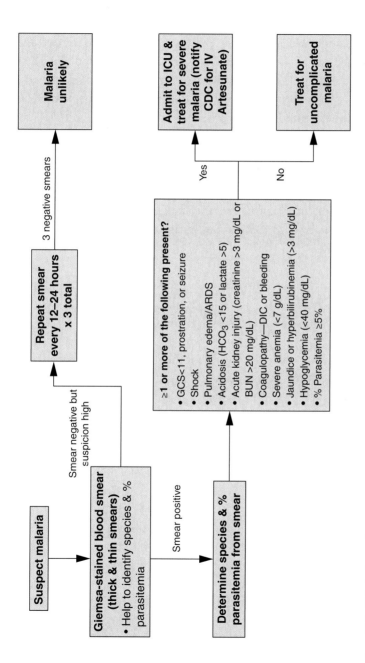

Figure 57.3 – Malaria diagnosis.

ARDS, Acute respiratory distress syndrome; *CDC*, Centers for Disease Control and Prevention; *DIC*, disseminated intravascular coagulopathy; *GCS*, Glasgow coma scale; HCO_3, serum bicarbonate; *ICU*, intensive care unit.

Any traveler returning from a malaria-endemic region with fevers should be evaluated for malaria. The standard method for diagnosis of malaria is light microscopy of Giemsa-stained blood smears (**option D**). If malaria is suspected, the smears should be done and interpreted as quickly as possible. Blood smears can be useful for species identification and calculation of parasite density (i.e., % parasitemia). If the initial smear is negative, then additional smears should be repeated every 12 to 24 hours for a total of at least three smears before considering malaria to be ruled out. Some common smears are shown later.

If microscopy is not available, another diagnostic option is the rapid detection test (RDT; **option C**), which detects malaria antigens. This is more commonly used in resource-limited areas, but one platform (BinaxNOW) is available in the United States. RDTs provide rapid results, but they cannot provide information on parasite density (% parasitemia). In addition, RDTs are less sensitive than microscopy. Consequently, positive and negative RDT results must be confirmed with microscopy.

PCR (**option A**) testing is actually more sensitive and specific than microscopy, but its use is limited by lack of widespread availability and slower turnaround time (i.e., time to get results). PCR can be used to confirm the species and assess for drug resistance.

Serologic testing (**option B**) is not commonly used for the diagnosis of malaria, because antibodies may remain positive for years after malaria infection. Blood cultures (**option E**) should be obtained in any patient presenting with a sepsis syndrome (such as this one), but diagnosing malaria infection actually takes precedence in this patient with likely severe malaria infection.

The approach to malaria diagnosis is shown in Fig. 57.3. HIV screening should always be considered as well.

If malaria is ruled out, then differential diagnosis may include (not an exhaustive list) routine infections that are seen in nontravelers (i.e., viral respiratory infection, bacteremia/septic shock, etc.), enteric (typhoid) fever, dengue fever, meningococcemia, yellow fever, acute schistosomiasis (Katayama fever), leptospirosis, rickettsial disease, East African trypanosomiasis (sleeping sickness), and viral hemorrhagic fever (i.e., Ebola virus). Most of these infections present like malaria (at least initially) and can be acquired in similar regions. Distinguishing features of some these infections are summarized in Table 57.1.

Table 57.1 – Selected Causes of Fever in the Returning Traveler

Infection	Tip-offs/Clues
Malaria (*Plasmodium spp.*)	• Onset 1–4 weeks after travel to an endemic region. Some cases have occurred up to 3 months after travel. • Lack of chemoprophylaxis prior to travel (although chemoprophylaxis does not eliminate the risk).
Enteric (typhoid) fever (*Salmonella typhi* or *S. paratyphi*)	• Incubation 1–3 weeks. Consumption of unsanitary food or water. • Lack of vaccination prior to travel (although vaccination does not eliminate risk, as it is 80% effective at best). • Salmon-colored rose spots (typically on the abdomen/trunk) and relative bradycardia.
Dengue fever (dengue virus)	• Incubation ~1 week. Mosquito-borne (*Aedes* mosquito). • Severe myalgias and arthralgias ("break-bone fever"), retro-orbital headache, maculopapular rash ("islands of white macules on a sea of red"), thrombocytopenia, bleeding, hemoconcentration, positive Tourniquet sign (petechiae after blood pressure cuff inflation). • Recurrent infection associated with more severe illness.
Meningococcemia (*Neisseria meningitidis*)	• Rapid onset (incubation—few days) with meningeal symptoms/signs, shock, and petechial or purpuric rash. • Travel to Mecca (Hajj) or African meningitis belt. • Asplenia or on terminal complement inhibitor (i.e., eculizumab).
Yellow fever (YF, yellow fever virus)	• Incubation 3–6 days. Mosquito-borne (*Aedes* and *Haemogogus*). • Travel to South America and sub-Saharan Africa. • Prior YF vaccination (prior 10 years) makes YF very unlikely. • Conjunctival suffusion. Severe illness associated with hemorrhage, liver failure, and renal failure (similar to dengue and leptospirosis).
Acute schistosomiasis (Katayama fever)	• Incubation 1–2 months. Exposure to freshwater. • Represents a hypersensitivity reaction with urticaria, pruritic rash at site of cercarial penetration (usually legs), and eosinophilia.
Leptospirosis (*Leptospira spp.*)	• Incubation 1–2 weeks. Exposure to freshwater, rodents, or dogs. • Conjunctival suffusion. Severe illness (Weil disease) characterized by hemorrhage, renal failure, and liver failure (striking hyperbilirubinemia).
Rickettsial disease (many types)	• African tick-bite fever (*Rickettsia africae*)—travel to South Africa, eschar skin lesions. • Boutonneuse (Mediterranean spotted) fever (*Rickettsia connorii*)—travel to Mediterranean, rash or eschar.
Oroya fever (*Bartonella bacilliformis*)	• Transmitted by sand fly bite. Travel to Peru, Colombia, or Ecuador (higher elevations). • Acutely, causes a hemolytic anemia.
African trypanosomiasis (*Trypanosoma brucei*)	• Sleeping sickness—eastern (Rhodesian) form is more acute (incubation <1 month) than western (Gambian) form. Acquired from tsetse fly bite. • Red chancre at the bite site, lymphadenopathy, and meningoencephalitis.
Viral hemorrhagic fever	• Travel to areas (often sub-Saharan Africa) with outbreaks of certain viruses (i.e., Lassa fever, Ebola, Marburg). • Hemorrhagic manifestations more common with certain viruses (i.e., Marburg).

KEY LEARNING POINT

Microscopy of Giemsa-stained blood smears is the best initial test to perform in the diagnosis of suspected malaria.

REFERENCES AND FURTHER READING

- Bennet JE, Dolin R, Blaser MJ, eds. *Mandell, Douglas, and Bennett's Principles and Practice of Infectious Diseases*. 9th ed. Elsevier; 2020.
- Boggild AK, Liles WC Travel-acquired illnesses associated with fever. In: Sanford CA, Pottinger PS, Jong EC, eds. *Travel and Tropical Medicine Manuel*. Elsevier; 2017:271–299. 5th ed.
- Centers for Disease Control and Prevention. Treatment of malaria: guidelines for clinicians (United States). https://www.clinicalkey.com/#!/content/practice_guide_summary/31-s2.0-EPG-f1e39c17-bfa3-4713-83f3-2a7134d52f49. Last reviewed May 29, 2020. Accessed on November 8, 2021.

A 40-year-old African American female presents to the hospital with a 3-day history of fevers, headache, vomiting, confusion, and general malaise. She returned from a trip to Sudan approximately 2 weeks ago. She did not take any malaria prophylaxis. She is 22 weeks pregnant. Medications include prenatal vitamin and folic acid. Vital signs reveal temperature 104° F, blood pressure 95/60 mmHg, heart rate 110 beats per minute, respiratory rate 22, and oxygen saturation 90% on room air. On examination, she appears ill and drowsy. There is scleral icterus and conjunctival pallor. Heart exam reveals a regular tachycardia without murmur. Lung exam reveals bibasilar crackles. Abdominal exam is limited by a gravid uterus. Pulses are weak. Laboratory studies reveal hemoglobin 8 g/dL, platelet count 90,000 cells/uL, white blood cell count 15,000 cells/uL, creatinine 2.5 mg/dL (clearance 20 mL/min), glucose 80 mg/dL, bicarbonate 12 mEq/L, total bilirubin 6 mg/dL, and serum lactate 6 mmol/L. Blood smear is shown in Fig. 58.1. The patient is admitted to the ICU. What is the best treatment for this patient?

A. Artesunate.

B. Artemether-lumefantrine.

C. Atovaquone-proguanil.

D. Quinine plus clindamycin.

E. Mefloquine.

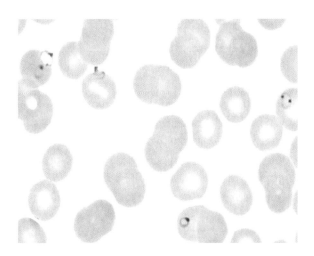

Figure 58.1 – Blood Smear
Courtesy DPDx - Laboratory Identification of Parasites of Public Health Concern [the CDC's website for parasitology identification] at https://www.cdc.gov/dpdx/index.html.

Table 58.1 – Features of Severe Malaria

One or more of the following:
• GCS <11, prostration, or seizure
• Shock
• Pulmonary edema/ARDS
• Acidosis (bicarbonate <15 or lactate >5)
• Acute kidney injury (creatinine >3 mg/dL or blood urea nitrogen >20 mg/dL)
• Coagulopathy—DIC or bleeding
• Severe anemia (<7 g/dL)
• Jaundice or hyperbilirubinemia (>3 mg/dL)
• Hypoglycemia (<40 mg/dL)
• % Parasitemia ≥5%

ARDS, Acute respiratory distress syndrome; *DIC*, disseminated intravascular coagulation; *GCS*, Glasgow coma scale.

The best treatment for this patient is intravenous artesunate (**option A**). This patient is presenting with severe malaria infection in the setting of pregnancy (second trimester). Based on the smear, the most likely causative organism is *Plasmodium falciparum*. This is not surprising, because *P. falciparum* is the most common etiology of severe malaria. Features of severe malaria are shown in Table 58.1.

Several factors need to be considered when treating malaria infections. These include the infecting species, the patient's clinical status (i.e., severe/complicated infection vs. uncomplicated infection), potential for resistant species (i.e., location where infection was acquired), and prior antimalarial exposure (i.e., should avoid using the prior agent as part of the treatment regimen). In general, malaria treatment should not be initiated until the diagnosis has been established definitively. If severe malaria is suspected but a timely laboratory diagnosis cannot be made, appropriate diagnostic testing should be obtained, and parenteral antimalarial drugs should be started empirically. Patients with any manifestations of severe malaria should be treated promptly and aggressively with IV antimalarial therapy, regardless of the species of malaria seen on the blood smear. The management of malaria in nonpregnant patients (Centers for Disease Control and Prevention algorithm) is summarized in Fig. 58.2.

After initiation of treatment, the patient's clinical and parasitological status should be monitored. If the infection is severe or due to *P. falciparum*, *Plasmodium knowlesi*, or suspected chloroquine-resistant *Plasmodium vivax*, blood smears should be checked every 12 to 24 hours

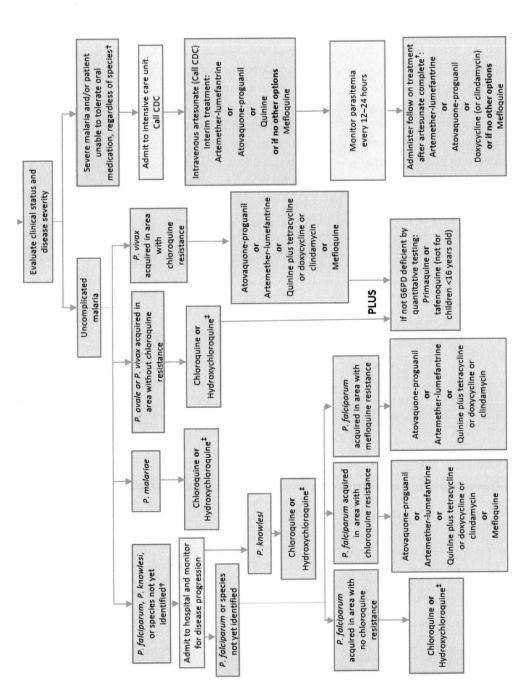

Figure 58.2 – Management of malaria in nonpregnant individuals

†If species later identified as *Plasmodium vivax* or *Plasmodium ovale*, add primaquine or tafenoquine if not glucose-6-phosphate dehydrogenase–deficient by quantitative testing; ‡Drug options for chloroquine-resistant *Plasmodium falciparum* may be used. The "areas without chloroquine-resistance" (i.e., chloroquine-sensitive areas) include:

- *Plasmodium falciparum*—Central America west of the Panama Canal, Haiti, and the Dominican Republic
- *Plasmodium vivax*—Papua New Guinea or Indonesia

CDC, Centers for Disease Control and Prevention.

to monitor treatment response. Documentation of a negative malaria smear after treatment is recommended. All persons treated for severe malaria with IV artesunate should be monitored weekly for up to 4 weeks after treatment initiation for evidence of hemolytic anemia. Exchange transfusion no longer recommended for severe malaria.

Malaria infection during pregnancy is associated with significant mortality and can lead to miscarriage, premature delivery, low birth weight, congenital infection, and/or perinatal death. In general, doxycycline and atovaquone/proguanil should be avoided in pregnant patients, unless there are no alternative options. Treatment for malaria in pregnancy is summarized in Fig. 58.3.

In this pregnant patient with severe malaria infection, the best therapy is IV artesunate. While awaiting IV artesunate to be obtained, interim treatment with artemether-lumefantrine

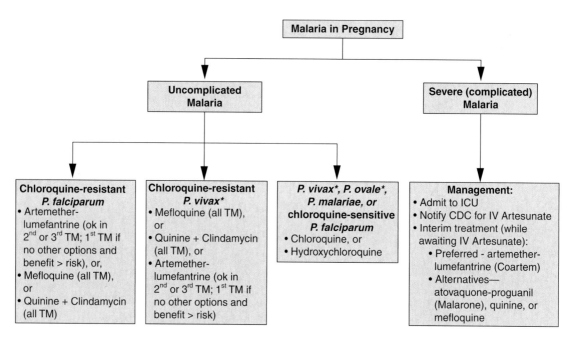

Figure 58.3 – Management of malaria in pregnancy
*For hypnozoite forms (*Plasmodium vivax* and *Plasmodium ovale*), primaquine and tafenoquine cannot be used during pregnancy. Recommendation is to continue chloroquine prophylactically during pregnancy. Postpartum, if glucose-6-phosphate dehydrogenase (G6PD) level is normal, can treat with primaquine (baby must be G6PD-normal if using) or tafenoquine (cannot use if breastfeeding). If unable to use either drug, then continue chloroquine prophylaxis for 1 year.
CDC, Centers for Disease Control and Prevention; *ICU*, intensive care unit; *TM*, Trimester.

(**option B**) can be considered. Alternative options for interim treatment include atovaquone/proguanil (**option C**), quinine with or without clindamycin (**option D**), and mefloquine (**option E**).

KEY LEARNING POINT

The best (most effective) therapy for patients with severe malaria is IV artesunate, even in pregnancy.

REFERENCES AND FURTHER READING

- Centers for Disease Control and Prevention. Treatment of malaria: guidelines for clinicians (United States). https://www.clinicalkey.com/#!/content/practice_guide_summary/31-s2.0-EPG-f1e39c17-bfa3-4713-83f3-2a7134d52f49. Last reviewed May 29, 2020. Accessed November 8, 2021.

A 50-year-old male is admitted to the hospital with a 2-week history of fevers, anorexia, night sweats, and cough. He has a history of chronic obstructive pulmonary disease. Medications include albuterol as needed and inhaled budesonide/formoterol. He has no medication allergies. He lives alone. He was born in Vietnam and moved to the United States 10 years ago. He frequently travels back to visit family in Vietnam. He smokes one pack of cigarettes a day. He denies alcohol and illicit drug use. Vital signs reveal temperature 101° F, heart rate 90 beats per minute, blood pressure 110/75 mmHg, respiratory rate 24, and oxygen saturation 94% on 2 L/min oxygen by nasal cannula. On examination, he is thin and appears ill. He exhibits pursed-lip breathing. Heart sounds are difficult to hear. He has diffuse wheezing and amphoric breath sounds in the right upper lobe posteriorly. There is no cyanosis or clubbing. The remainder of the examination is within normal limits. Anteroposterior chest x-ray shows hyperinflation. Chest CT is shown in Fig. 59.1. What is the next best step in management?

A. HIV screening.

B. Airborne isolation.

C. Sputum acid-fast bacillus (AFB) smear.

D. Bronchoscopy.

E. Multidrug therapy for *Mycobacterium tuberculosis*.

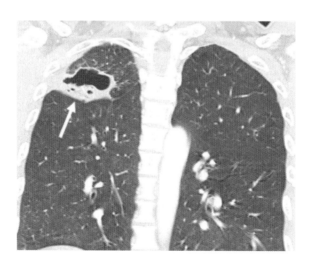

Figure 59.1 – CT chest
Santiago Restrepo C, Katre R, Mumbower A. Imaging manifestations of thoracic tuberculosis. *Radiol Clin North Am*. 2016;54(3):453–473.

The best next step in management is to place the patient on airborne isolation (**option B**). This patient's presentation is highly concerning for cavitary pulmonary tuberculosis (TB). TB is caused by an AFB called *M. tuberculosis* complex (consists of *M. tuberculosis*, *Mycobacterium bovis*, and others), but *M. tuberculosis* is the most relevant. TB is acquired by inhalation of aerosolized droplet nuclei containing *M. tuberculosis*. The natural history is summarized in Fig. 59.2.

Pulmonary TB should be suspected in patients with TB risk factors (i.e., exposure to endemic area, exposure to a person with TB, congregate setting exposure [homelessness, incarceration, etc.], healthcare exposure, or immune suppression—especially HIV) who present with constitutional symptoms (i.e., fevers, night sweats, weight loss, etc.) and a pneumonia-like illness. Importantly, the presentation can be highly variable; so having a high index of suspicion is paramount. If pulmonary (or laryngeal) TB is suspected, airborne isolation should be instituted immediately. The factors associated with high infectivity include symptomatic pulmonary disease, laryngeal disease, smear positivity, culture positivity, aerosolization procedures, and cavitary disease.

Diagnosis of pulmonary TB can be challenging. TB is one of the great imitators and can present in various different ways (i.e., it can almost always be on the differential diagnosis). In addition, there is not a single test that can rule out TB completely. With this in mind, we will discuss the tests that can be used in the diagnosis of pulmonary TB. Fig. 59.3 summarizes the approach to the diagnosis of pulmonary TB. Table 59.1 summarizes the major diagnostic tests that can be used to diagnose pulmonary TB.

In patients with suspected (but not confirmed/proven) pulmonary TB, airborne isolation can be discontinued if the likelihood of TB is very low and there is either a better, alternative explanation for the illness or three sputum AFB smears are negative (+/- at least one negative NAAT). In patients with proven pulmonary TB who are on treatment, airborne isolation can be discontinued once effective treatment has been given for at least 2 weeks, the patient has clinically improved, and three sputum AFB smears are negative.

HIV screening (**option A**) and sputum AFB smear (**option C**) should be done, but airborne isolation takes precedence. Bronchoscopy (**option D**) can be done if sputum cannot be obtained, but airborne isolation takes precedence. Multidrug TB therapy (**option E**) will likely be necessary, but in this otherwise reasonably stable patient, diagnostic work-up can be obtained prior to starting therapy in order to avoid false-negative culture results.

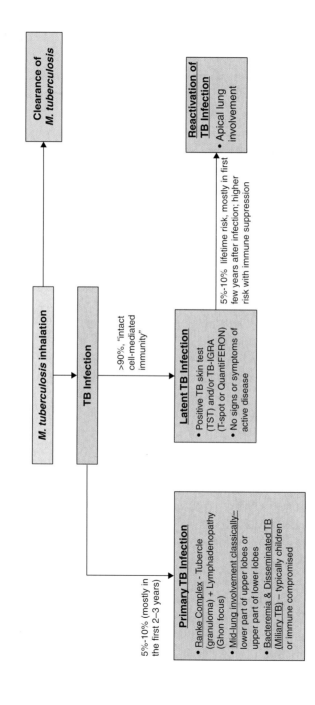

Figure 59.2 – Natural history of tuberculosis
IGRA, Interferon-gamma release assay; *TB,* tuberculosis; *TST,* tuberculin skin test.

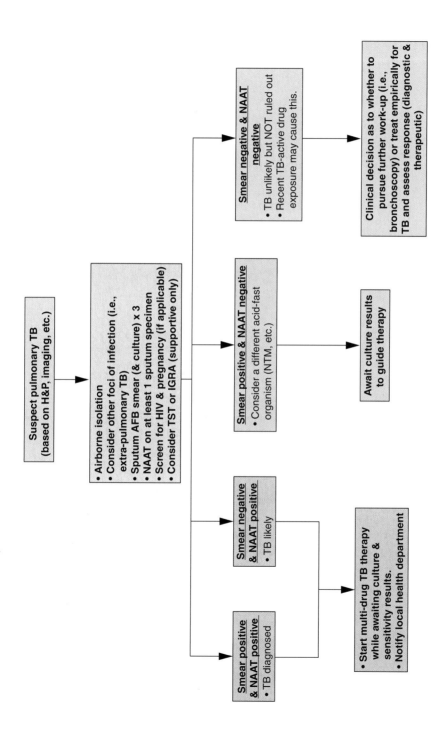

Figure 59.3 – Approach to pulmonary tuberculosis diagnosis

AFB, Acid-fast bacillus; *HIV*, human immunodeficiency virus; *H&P*, history and physical exam; *IGRA*, interferon-gamma release assay; *NAAT*, nucleic acid amplification testing; *NTM*, nontuberculous mycobacteria; *TST*, tuberculin skin test.

Table 59.1 – Tests Used to Diagnose Pulmonary Tuberculosis (TB)

Test	Description
Chest imaging	• Chest x-ray (CXR) is typically the first-line imaging test. In immune-compromised patients (i.e., those with HIV), chest imaging may appear "atypical" (i.e., not the classic TB appearance), and cavities may be absent.
	• CXR can be normal despite having active TB disease. CT is more sensitive and can be used if suspicion is high despite negative CXR.
Sputum AFB smear (microscopy)	• Should obtain at least three sputum specimens (separated by 8 hours, with one being an early morning specimen) for AFB smear/culture. Studies show that the yield of the third specimen is minimal, and only two specimens are probably needed in most cases.
	• Sputum can be expectorated or induced (need at least 3 mL, but ideally 5–10 mL). Induced sputum has similar yield to bronchoscopy but is considered safer.
	• AFB smear—Se 45%–80% and PPV 50%–80%. ↑ Sensitivity with concentration of the specimen, organism load, and number of specimens. ↓ Sensitivity with lower organism burden (i.e., HIV).
Nucleic acid amplification testing (NAAT, or TB PCR)	• NAAT should be done on at least one of the sputum samples.
	• NAAT is more Se than smear but less Se than culture. Highly Sp though.
	• If AFB smear-positive, then NAAT 95% Se and 98% Sp.
	• If AFB smear-negative, then NAAT 75%–88% Se and 95% Sp.
	• Relatively rapid turn-around time.
	• Detects live and dead organisms, so cannot be used for monitoring response to treatment.
	• Most common test in the United States is the Xpert MTB/RIF, which can actually detect rifampin (RIF) resistance (*RPOB* gene presence). RIF resistance can be used as a proxy for isoniazid (INH) resistance, as most RIF-resistant TB is also resistant to INH, but isolate should still be sent for formal resistance testing.
Sputum AFB culture	• Considered the gold standard—Se 80% and Sp 98%.
	• Can take weeks (up to 8 weeks in some formats) to result but will provide species identification and sensitivity data.
Bronchoscopy	• Often not necessary unless unable to obtain sputum, sputum studies negative but suspicion for TB still high, needing tissue diagnosis (biopsy), or indicated to evaluate for alternative diagnoses.
	• Biopsy may show granulomatous (typically caseous) inflammation.
Tuberculin skin test	• Only considered a supportive test, as cannot differentiate between active TB infection and prior exposure/latent TB infection.
	• False positive may be seen in setting of previous BCG vaccination, NTM infection, or booster effect.
	• False negative can occur with immune suppression.
Interferon-gamma release assay	• Only considered a supportive test, as cannot differentiate between active TB infection and prior exposure/latent TB infection.
	• Examples include T-spot and QuantiFERON Gold.
	• Unaffected by prior BCG vaccination.
	• False positives with certain NTMs—*Mycobacterium szulgai*, *Mycobacterium marinum*, and *Mycobacterium kansasii*.
Urinary LAM test	• Point-of-care test that detects a mycobacterial cell wall antigen. This test is most useful in patients with HIV who are seriously ill or who have a CD4 count of 100 cells/uL or lower.

AFB, Acid-fast bacillus; *BCG*, Bacillus-Calmette-Guerin; *LAM*, lipoarabinomannan; *NTM*, nontuberculous mycobacteria; *PPV*, positive predictive value; *Se*, sensitivity; *Sp*, specificity.

KEY LEARNING POINT

In a patient with suspected pulmonary tuberculosis, airborne isolation should be instituted immediately, even before initiating diagnosis and treatment.

REFERENCES AND FURTHER READING

- Bernardo J, et al. Diagnosis of pulmonary tuberculosis in adults. In: C Fordham von Reyn, ed. *UpToDate*. Waltham: UpToDate; 2020.
- Santiago Restrepo C, Katre R, Mumbower A. Imaging manifestations of thoracic tuberculosis. *Radiol Clin North Am.* 2016;54(3):453–473.
- Forbes BA, Hall GS, Miller MB, et al. Practice guidelines for clinical microbiology laboratories: mycobacteria. *Clin Microbiol Rev.* 2018;31(2):e00038-17. https://doi.org/10.1128/CMR.00038-17.
- Lee RW, et al. Tuberculosis: natural history, microbiology, and pathogenesis. In: C Fordham von Reyn, ed. Waltham: UpToDate; 2020.
- Punjabi CD, Perloff SR, Zuckerman JM. Preventing transmission of *Mycobacterium tuberculosis* in health care settings. *Infect Dis Clin North Am.* 2016;30(4):1013–1022. https://doi.org/10.1016/j.idc.2016.07.003.

A 40-year-old male is admitted to the hospital with a 2-week history of fevers, malaise, headaches, blurry vision, and more recently, confusion and vomiting. He has a history of chronic HIV infection. He does not take his antiretroviral therapy. He has no medication allergies and does not take any other medications routinely. He was born in Sudan and moved to the United States 10 years ago. He does not smoke or use drugs. He drinks a bottle of wine daily. Vital signs reveal temperature 102° F, heart rate 95 beats per minute, blood pressure 100/65 mmHg, respiratory rate 20, and oxygen saturation 94% on room air. On examination, he is somnolent. There is no icterus or conjunctival injection. Ears, nose, and throat are normal. He cannot abduct his eyes bilaterally. Cranial nerves are intact otherwise. Nuchal rigidity is present. He cannot cooperate with the remainder of the neurologic examination. Heart is tachycardic and regular. There is no murmur. Abdomen is soft and nontender. There is no rash, palpable lymphadenopathy, or joint swelling. Laboratory studies reveal sodium 128 mEq/L, glucose 120 mg/dL, creatinine 1.2 mg/dL, white blood cell (WBC) count 12,000 cells/uL, hemoglobin 9 g/dL, platelet count 450,000 cells/uL, alanine aminotransferase 60 U/L, aspartate aminotransferase 130 U/L, total bilirubin 2.0 mg/dL, and normal alkaline phosphatase. CD4 count 6 months prior was 140 cells/uL (10%). Chest x-ray is normal. Blood cultures are drawn. Head CT is unremarkable. Cerebrospinal fluid (CSF) analysis reveals opening pressure 20 cmH$_2$O (normal 7–18 cmH$_2$O), WBC count 120 cells/uL (60% lymphocytes, 30% polymorphonuclear cells), protein 125 mg/dL, and glucose 40 mg/dL. Routine bacterial gram stain is negative. CSF film array (meningitis/encephalitis) panel and CSF cryptococcal antigen are negative. What is the most appropriate next step in management?

A. Obtain MRI of the brain with and without contrast.

B. Restart antiretroviral therapy.

C. Start vancomycin, cefepime, ampicillin, and dexamethasone.

D. Start rifampin, isoniazid, pyrazinamide, and ethambutol.

E. Start rifampin, isoniazid, pyrazinamide, ethambutol, and dexamethasone.

The most appropriate next step in management is to start rifampin, isoniazid, pyrazinamide, ethambutol, and dexamethasone (**option E**). This patient's presentation is highly concerning for tuberculous (TB) meningitis. TB meningitis is a rare manifestation of tuberculosis seen more commonly in immune-compromised individuals (especially those HIV) and in children in the developing world (vs. adults in the developed world). TB meningitis is more commonly caused by the rupture of a subependymal tubercle into the subarachnoid space (as opposed to hematogenous spread). The meningitis typically involves the base of the brain ("basilar meningitis"). The associated inflammation may result in fibrosis and vasculitis, which can lead to infarction, aneurysm formation, thrombosis, and encasement of local structures (i.e., cranial nerves).

The presentation is typically subacute to chronic in nature. Symptoms include constitutional symptoms (i.e., fevers, malaise, weight loss, etc.), headaches, confusion, neck stiffness, nausea, vomiting, seizures, and even focal neurologic deficits. Examination may reveal nuchal rigidity and focal neurologic deficits (i.e., cranial neuropathy [abducens nerve palsy], as seen in this patient). Laboratory studies may reveal anemia of chronic disease and hyponatremia (related to syndrome of inappropriate antidiuretic hormone secretion). In many cases, the WBC count is normal or only mildly elevated. Erythrocyte sedimentation rate and C-reactive protein may be elevated. Of note, the liver function abnormality in this patient is likely related to his underlying alcohol use. CSF analysis typically shows mildly elevated opening pressure, often mild lymphocytic pleocytosis (may be neutrophilic early on in the disease), mild protein elevation, and, characteristically, low glucose (hypoglycorrhachia). Given the paucibacillary nature of TB meningitis, isolation of the organism is often difficult. To optimize the yield, larger volumes of CSF should be sent (may need to be done on serial lumbar punctures). None of the available tests (i.e., acid-fast bacillus [AFB] smear, nucleic acid amplification testing [NAAT], culture) can rule out TB meningitis completely. NAAT is the typical standard diagnostic test, but all of the aforementioned tests should be obtained in order to increase the chance of making the diagnosis. Chest imaging will show concomitant pulmonary TB in a good majority of cases, but a normal chest x-ray can also be seen, especially in advanced HIV patients. Chest CT is often a more sensitive test in these cases. Central nervous system (CNS) imaging (CT or MRI) may reveal tuberculomas, basilar arachnoiditis, stroke, hydrocephalus, or spinal cord involvement (i.e., myelitis, tuberculomas, etc.). Lastly, additional testing considerations should include HIV screening, pregnancy testing (if applicable), and evaluation for tuberculosis at other sites (i.e., sputum analysis, AFB blood culture, dedicated imaging, etc.).

Due to the high morbidity and mortality associated with TB meningitis, appropriate treatment should be initiated as soon as possible in suspected cases (such as this case). Appropriate therapy consists of four-drug tuberculosis therapy (rifampin, isoniazid, ethambutol, and pyrazinamide) and corticosteroids. Some experts advocate for higher doses of rifampin in TB meningitis. Corticosteroids have been shown to have a mortality benefit in TB meningitis. Typical options include dexamethasone and prednisolone. Steroids are typically given for a prolonged period of time with slow taper. The overall duration of antimicrobial therapy is 9 to 12 months. In addition, adjunctive aspirin may reduce mortality and risk of stroke in TB meningitis. Lastly, complications of the infection (i.e., hydrocephalus, intracranial pressure, seizures, etc.) should be managed accordingly. The general approach to the management of drug-susceptible TB in HIV-negative patients is outlined in Fig. 60.1.

Obtaining an MRI (**option A**) may be considered, but it should not take precedence over starting the appropriate therapy, which should include four-drug tuberculosis therapy (**option D**) and steroids. The decision to start or restart antiretroviral therapy (ART; **option B**) in the setting of HIV and tuberculosis coinfection deserves some mention. Early initiation of ART (in patients not already on ART) in HIV/tuberculosis coinfected patients is associated with reduced mortality. Consequently, for patients not on ART (or those with poor adherence to ART), the appropriate timing of ART initiation depends on the CD4 count and whether TB meningitis is present:

- **Any CD4 count in setting of suspected TB meningitis**—delay starting ART for at least 8 weeks after initiation of tuberculosis treatment (due to risk of severe consequences with immune reconstitution inflammatory syndrome in the CNS).
- **CD4 <50 cells/uL (no TB meningitis)**—start ART within 2 weeks after initiation of tuberculosis treatment.
- **CD4 ≥50 cells/uL (no TB meningitis)**—start ART within 8 to 12 weeks after initiation of tuberculosis treatment.

ART should be continued in patients who were already on ART. In addition, drug-drug interactions should be considered anytime tuberculosis treatment is started and particularly when treating HIV/tuberculosis coinfected patients. Rifabutin can be used instead of rifampin, because it has fewer drug-drug interactions. A typical regimen would include tenofovir DF and emtricitabine (Truvada), plus a third drug that depends on which rifamycin is used:

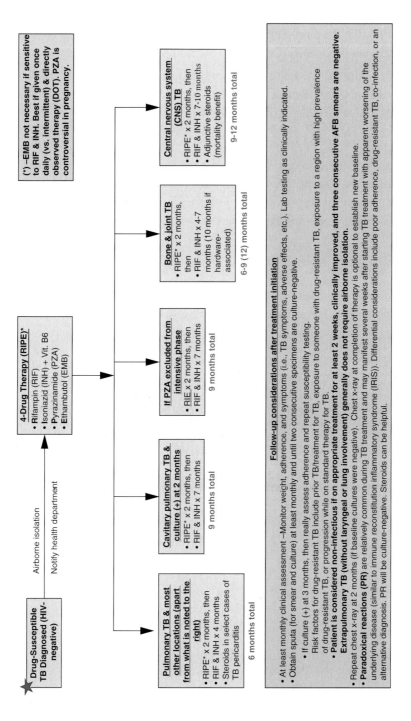

Figure 60.1 – Treatment of drug-susceptible tuberculosis (TB) (in HIV-negative patients).

- If using rifampin, the third drug can be efavirenz (Atripla combination), higher-dose dolutegravir (50 mg twice daily) or higher-dose raltegravir (800 mg twice daily).
- If using rifabutin, the third drug can be efavirenz (Atripla combination), regular-dose dolutegravir (50 mg daily), regular-dose raltegravir (400 mg twice daily), or boosted protease inhibitor (but have to reduce rifabutin dose to 150 mg daily).

Starting vancomycin, cefepime, ampicillin, and dexamethasone (**option C**) would be appropriate for suspected community-acquired bacterial meningitis in an immune-compromised patient. This patient's presentation is not consistent with acute bacterial meningitis, so this option is not the best choice.

KEY LEARNING POINT

In a patient with suspected tuberculous meningitis, appropriate therapy (four-drug tuberculosis therapy and steroids) should be instituted as soon as possible.

REFERENCES AND FURTHER READING

- Donovan J, Figaji A, Imran D, Phu NH, Rohlwink U, Thwaites GE. The neurocritical care of tuberculous meningitis. *Lancet Neurol.* 2019;18(8):771–783. https://doi.org/10.1016/S1474-4422(19)30154-1.
- Fitzgerald DW, et al. *Mycobacterium tuberculosis.* In: Bennet JE, Dolin R, Blaser MJ, eds. *Mandell, Douglas, and Bennett's Principles and Practice of Infectious Diseases.* 9th ed. Elsevier; 2020:2985–3021.
- Griffith DE, et al. Antimycobacterial agents. In: Bennet JE, Dolin R, Blaser MJ, eds. *Mandell, Douglas, and Bennett's Principles and Practice of Infectious Diseases.* 9th ed. Elsevier; 2020:477–496.
- Zha BS, Nahid P. Treatment of drug-susceptible tuberculosis. *Clin Chest Med.* 2019;40(4):763–774. https://doi.org/10.1016/j.ccm.2019.07.006.

A 20-year-old male is admitted to the hospital with bloody diarrhea and abdominal pain. His symptoms started 3 days ago with watery diarrhea and abdominal pain. He took some leftover azithromycin that he had at home. The bloody diarrhea developed today, and he was not able to keep up with oral intake, so he decided to come to the hospital. He is otherwise healthy and does not take any medications routinely. Vital signs reveal temperature 100° F, heart rate 120 beats per minute, blood pressure 95/60 mmHg, respiratory rate 16, and oxygen saturation 98% on room air. On examination, he appears ill and uncomfortable. There is mild scleral icterus present. He has diffuse abdominal tenderness with hypoactive bowel sounds, and no rebound tenderness. Rectal examination reveals blood-tinged liquid stool. Laboratory studies reveal white blood cell count 15,000 cells/uL, hemoglobin 8 g/dL, platelet count 75,000 cells/uL, creatinine 2.0 mg/dL (creatinine clearance 30 mL/min), ALT 60 U/L, and total bilirubin 5.0 mg/dL (indirect bilirubin 4.0 mg/dL). Which of the following organisms is the most likely cause of this patient's presentation?

A. *Shigella dysenteriae.*

B. *Escherichia coli O157:H7.*

C. *Campylobacter jejuni.*

D. *Salmonella spp.* (nontyphoidal).

E. *Yersinia enterocolitica.*

The most likely cause is *E. coli* O157:H7 (**option B**). This patient's presentation is most consistent with hemolytic uremic syndrome (HUS), a type of thrombotic microangiopathy. HUS is typically caused by Shiga-toxin producing *E. coli* (STEC; also known as enterohemorrhagic *E. coli* [EHEC]). The most common serotype causing HUS is *E. coli* O157:H7, but other species of STEC and *S. dysenteriae* (**option A**) can also cause HUS. Antibiotic treatment of STEC (EHEC) diarrhea increases the risk of developing HUS. The *E. coli* infection is classically acquired by ingestion of raw or undercooked beef. A few days after ingestion, patients develop watery diarrhea that frequently becomes bloody. Abdominal pain and cramping are common, but fever is not very common. Approximately 15% of patients with bloody diarrhea go on to develop HUS (typically approximately 1 week after symptom onset). Patients classically present with microangiopathic hemolytic anemia (anemia, elevated lactate dehydrogenase, decreased haptoglobin, indirect hyperbilirubinemia, and presence of schistocytes on peripheral blood smear), thrombocytopenia, and acute kidney injury. The diagnosis is largely clinical, but the toxins can be assayed for (not commonly done). The management of HUS is supportive. This includes volume repletion, avoidance of antibiotics and antimotility agents, and if necessary, renal replacement therapy. There is no role for steroids or plasmapheresis.

The most common *Shigella* species (**option A**) that infect humans are *S. dysenteriae, S. flexneri, S. sonnei*, and *S. boydii*. Humans are the natural host. *Shigella* has a very low infectious dose. Infection can be foodborne (fecal-contaminated food or water) or spread person-to-person (especially in the men who have sex with men [MSM] population). Raw vegetables are a classic association. The incubation period is a few days. After incubation, patients develop a gastroenteritis that can be bloody and rarely (mostly with *S. dysenteriae*) associated with HUS. Fever is also more common with *Shigella* infection. In most people, the infection is self-limited. Treatment is highly recommended for patients with severe illness and immune compromise. Treatment may shorten the duration of illness, but this comes at the risk of developing resistance and prolonging shedding. First-line treatment options include azithromycin, ciprofloxacin (if minimum inhibitory concentration <0.12 ug/mL), or ceftriaxone.

C. jejuni (**option C**) is a curved, microaerophilic, gram-negative rod that is acquired by ingestion of undercooked poultry or exposure to certain animals (i.e., puppies, kittens, reptiles, etc.). The typical presentation is fever, vomiting, and often bloody diarrhea. *C. jejuni* has been associated with Guillain–Barre syndrome and reactive arthritis. Treatment may shorten the duration of illness and should be given in cases that are prolonged or severe. First-line treatment is azithromycin.

Nontyphoidal *Salmonella* (NTS) species (**option D**) are a common cause of infectious diarrhea. NTS can be acquired via the foodborne route (commonly raw or undercooked eggs or chicken) or exposure to certain animals (especially reptiles, amphibians, and poultry). Visiting petting zoos is a risk factor. Symptoms typically start within 72 hours of exposure. Patients present with a febrile gastroenteritis. The diarrhea is initially watery but may become bloody. Most cases resolve on their own without the need for antibiotic treatment. In fact, antibiotics do nothing to shorten the duration of the illness, but they may prolong fecal carriage of NTS. Certain patients (particularly the immune-suppressed, elderly [>50 years old], and patients with cardiovascular disease or joint disease including prostheses) are at risk for more invasive *Salmonella* infections (i.e., bacteremia, etc.). Treatment is reserved for high-risk patients or those with invasive infection. Options include ceftriaxone, fluoroquinolone, trimethoprim/sulfamethoxazole (TMP/SMX), or an aminopenicillin.

Y. enterocolitica (**option E**) infections are classically seen in patients with iron overload states (i.e., hemochromatosis, cirrhosis). The infection can be acquired via ingestion of unpasteurized dairy or undercooked pork (especially pork chitlins [intestines]). The incubation period is 4 to 6 days. Patients typically present with a gastroenteritis associated with "pseudoappendicitis" and pharyngitis. Bacteremia may occur with iron-overload diseases. First-line treatment (reserved for severe disease or at-risk host) is TMP/SMX.

An overview of infectious diarrhea is shown in Fig. 61.1 and common associations in gastroenteritis in Table 61.1.

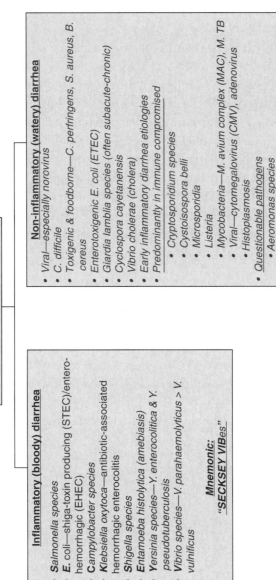

Infectious Diarrhea/Gastroenteritis

Inflammatory (bloody) diarrhea
- *Salmonella species*
- *E. coli*—shiga-toxin producing (STEC)/entero-hemorrhagic (EHEC)
- *Campylobacter species*
- *Klebsiella oxytoca*—antibiotic-associated hemorrhagic enterocolitis
- *Shigella species*
- *Entamoeba histolytica (amebiasis)*
- *Yersinia species—Y. enterocolitica & Y. pseudotuberculosis*
- *Vibrio species—V. parahaemolyticus > V. vulnificus*

Mnemonic:
"SECKSEY VIBes"

Non-inflammatory (watery) diarrhea
- *Viral*—especially norovirus
- *C. difficile*
- *Toxigenic & foodborne—C. perfringens, S. aureus, B. cereus*
- *Enterotoxigenic E. coli (ETEC)*
- *Giardia lamblia species (often subacute-chronic)*
- *Cyclospora cayetanensis*
- *Vibrio cholerae (cholera)*
- *Early inflammatory diarrhea etiologies*
- Predominantly in immune compromised
  - *Cryptosporidium species*
  - *Cystoisospora belli*
  - *Microsporidia*
  - *Listeria*
  - *Mycobacteria—M. avium complex (MAC), M. TB*
  - *Viral—cytomegalovirus (CMV), adenovirus*
  - *Histoplasmosis*
- Questionable pathogens
  - *Aeromonas species*
  - *Plesiomonas species*
  - *Blastocystis hominis*

Figure 61.1 – An overview of infectious diarrhea

Table 61.1 – Common Associations in Gastroenteritis

- Raw seafood—*Vibrio spp., Plesiomonas shigelloides*
- Raw eggs—*Salmonella spp.*
- Undercooked meat (i.e., beef, pork, poultry)—*Salmonella spp., Campylobacter spp., Clostridium perfringens, E. coli, Yersinia spp.* (undercooked pork)
- Unpasteurized dairy—*Salmonella spp., Campylobacter spp., Yersinia spp., Brucella spp.*, and rarely *Listeria monocytogenes*
- Raw hot dogs or deli meats—*L. monocytogenes*
- Imported raspberries or herbs—*Cyclospora*
- Reheated rice—*Bacillus cereus*
- Liver disease—*Vibrio spp., Yersinia spp.*
- Reactive arthritis—*Salmonella spp., Shigella spp., Yersinia spp., Campylobacter spp.*, and rarely *Clostridioides difficile*
- Antibiotic exposure—*C. difficile, Klebsiella oxytoca*
- Healthcare-associated—*C. difficile*, Norovirus
- Swimming pools or hiking—*Giardia lamblia, Cryptosporidium parvum*
- Brackish water exposure—*Vibrio spp., Aeromonas spp.*
- Daycare/young child exposure—*G. lamblia, C. parvum*, Norovirus, *Shigella spp.*
- Cruise ship—Norovirus
- Animal exposure—*Salmonella spp., Campylobacter spp., Balantidium coli* (pig feces)
- MSM population—*Shigella spp., Entamoeba histolytica*
- HIV/AIDS—*C. parvum, Cyclospora, Cystoisospora, Microsporidia, Mycobacterium avium complex*, cytomegalovirus, *Histoplasma*
- Vomiting-predominant, short incubation—Norovirus, preformed toxin (*Staphylococcus aureus, B. cereus*)
- Pseudoappendicitis +/- pharyngitis—*Y. enterocolitica*
- Ekiri syndrome (encephalopathy and seizures)—*Shigella spp.*

KEY LEARNING POINT

Escherichia coli O157:H7 is the most common cause of infection-associated hemolytic uremic syndrome.

REFERENCES AND FURTHER READING

- Shane AL, Mody RK, Crump JA, et al. 2017 Infectious Diseases Society of America Clinical Practice Guidelines for the diagnosis and management of infectious diarrhea. *Clin Infect Dis.* 2017;65(12):e45–e80. https://doi.org/10.1093/cid/cix669.
- Fleckenstein J, Kuhlmann FM, Sheikh A. Acute bacterial gastroenteritis. *Gastroenterol Clin North Am.* 2021;50(2):283–304. https://doi.org/10.1016/j.gtc.2021.02.002.
- LaRocque R, Harris JB. Causes of acute infectious diarrhea and other foodborne illnesses in resource-rich settings. In: Post TW, ed. *UpToDate*. Waltham: UpToDate; 2020.
- Orenstein R. Select gastrointestinal and hepatobiliary infections. In: *A Rational Approach to Clinical Infectious Diseases*. Elsevier; 2022:132–145.

A 40-year-old male presents to the emergency room with a 3-day history of fever, nausea, watery diarrhea, and right lower quadrant abdominal pain. He also has a sore throat, which he relates to vomiting. He has history of cirrhosis related to hereditary hemochromatosis. He had a liver transplant 2 years ago. Medications includes tacrolimus, mycophenolate, and low-dose prednisone. He has no medication allergies. He does not drink alcohol, use drugs, smoke, or vape. He denies any recent travel. He does not have any pets or animal exposures. He does not consume undercooked food or seafood. He does not know of anyone else with similar symptoms. Vital signs show temperature 101° F, heart rate 105 beats per minute, blood pressure 85/50 mmHg, and respiratory rate 18. There is no conjunctival injection or scleral icterus. There is pharyngeal erythema and mild tonsillar enlargement. Oral mucosa is very dry. Heart is regular in terms of rate and rhythm, and there is no murmur. Lungs are clear. Abdominal exam reveals tenderness in the right lower quadrant but no rebound tenderness. The reminder of the exam is unremarkable. Laboratory studies reveal white blood cell count 14,000 cells/uL and creatinine 1.5 mg/dL (creatinine clearance 40 mL/min). Abdominal x-ray is unremarkable. Lipase is normal. Blood cultures are obtained. What is the next best step in the management of this patient?

A. Symptom control (i.e., antiemetics, antimotility agents).

B. Obtain CT of the abdomen with contrast.

C. Obtain a stool sample for PCR testing (i.e., Film-Array).

D. Consult a general surgeon.

E. Start ceftriaxone and doxycycline.

The next best step in management is to start ceftriaxone and doxycycline (**option E**). This patient's presentation is most consistent with *Yersinia enterocolitica* infection. *Y. enterocolitica* infections are classically seen in patients with iron overload states (i.e., hemochromatosis [as in this patient], cirrhosis, contaminated blood products, etc.). The infection can be acquired via ingestion of unpasteurized dairy or undercooked pork. After an incubation period of 4 to 6 days, patients typically present with a febrile gastroenteritis (diarrhea may be bloody) associated with "pseudoappendicitis" and pharyngitis. Invasive infections (i.e., bacteremia) may be seen more commonly with iron-overload diseases. Rarely, *Yersinia* may cause aortitis/ mycotic aneurysm and osteomyelitis (similar to *Salmonella spp.*). Other classic associations (postinfectious sequelae) include erythema nodosum and reactive arthritis. Diagnosis can be made by stool PCR (i.e., Film-Array) or stool culture. Blood and pharyngeal (throat) cultures should be considered as well. Treatment is reserved for immune-compromised individuals and those with severe disease. First line-regimen is trimethoprim/sulfamethoxazole. Alternatives include fluoroquinolones (i.e., ciprofloxacin), doxycycline, or third-generation cephalosporin (ceftriaxone). In this patient, the other organism to potentially worry about would be *Vibrio parahaemolyticus*. Therefore, the combination of ceftriaxone and doxycycline would provide ideal coverage for both organisms.

Symptom control (i.e., antiemetics, antimotility agents; **option A**) may be necessary, but this should not take precedence over starting appropriate empiric antimicrobial therapy. Antimotility agents should generally be avoided in patients with suspected enterohemorrhagic *Escherischia coli* infection and *Clostridioides difficile* infection. Obtaining CT of the abdomen with contrast (**option B**) may be considered as well to rule out complicated disease (i.e., aortitis, etc.) or other etiologies (i.e., appendicitis, occult perforation), but this should not delay starting appropriate antimicrobial therapy. In the setting of renal dysfunction, contrast can be used if it is deemed that the benefit of obtaining a contrasted image outweighs the risk of contrast-induced kidney injury. Obtaining a stool sample for PCR testing (i.e., Film-Array, **option C**) should be considered because the patient is significantly ill and immune-compromised. The results of stool studies likely will not be affected by antimicrobial therapy in most cases, so there is no need to delay antimicrobial therapy to obtain this work-up. The typical gastrointestinal pathogen panel (i.e., Film-Array or PCR panel) is highly sensitive and specific, and it tests for the following pathogens:

- **Bacteria**—*Campylobacter spp., C. difficile, Plesiomonas shigelloides, Salmonella spp., Y. enterocolitica, Vibrio spp., E. coli, Shigella spp.*

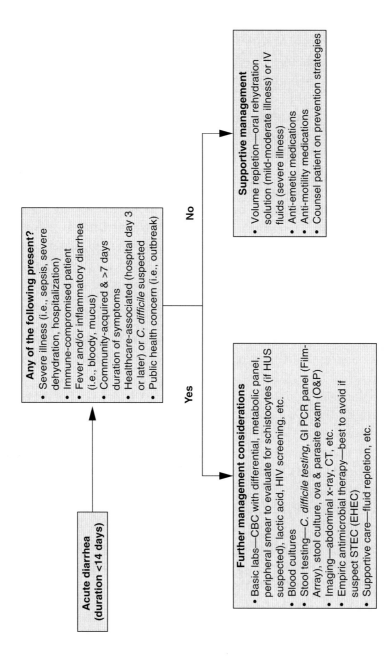

Figure 62.1 – Approach to the management of acute diarrhea
CBC, Complete blood count; *EHEC*, enterohemorrhagic E. coli; *GI*, gastrointestinal; *HUS*, hemolytic uremic syndrome; *PCR*, polymerase chain reaction; *STEC*, Shiga-toxin producing *Escherichia coli.*

- **Viruses**—Adenovirus, Astrovirus, Norovirus, Rotavirus, Sapovirus
- **Parasites**—*Crytposporidium, Cyclospora cayetanensis, Entamoeba histolytica, Giardia lamblia*

Because the gastrointestinal pathogen panel is PCR-based, one caveat to be aware of is that it will detect viable and dead organisms, and, due to the sensitivity, it may pick up pathogens that are just being shed in small amounts and not actually causing disease. Therefore, clinical correlation is always advised.

Consulting a general surgeon (**option D**) may be necessary if a surgical problem is discovered (i.e., appendicitis, perforated viscus, etc.).

A general approach to the management of acute diarrheal illness is shown in Fig. 62.1.

Table 62.1 summarizes the diagnosis and treatment of common infectious diarrheal pathogens.

Table 62.1 – Diagnosis and Treatment of Selected Diarrheal Pathogens

Pathogen	Diagnosis	First-Line Treatment	Alternative Treatment
Campylobacter spp.[a]	• NAAT (PCR) • Stool culture	• Azithromycin	• Ciprofloxacin
Nontyphoidal *Salmonella* spp.	• NAAT (PCR) • Stool culture	• Only treat if high-risk for severe disease • Ceftriaxone	• Ciprofloxacin or • TMP/SMX or • Aminopenicillin
Typhoid fever (*S. enteric* subspecies *typhi* and *paratyphi*)	• Culture of stool, blood, or bone marrow (may be the best source)	• Ceftriaxone or • Ciprofloxacin	• TMP/SMX or • Aminopenicillin
Shigella spp.[a]	• NAAT (PCR) • Stool culture	• Azithromycin, or • Ciprofloxacin (if MIC <0.12)	• TMP/SMX or • Ceftriaxone or • Aminopenicillin
Vibrio cholerae[a]	• NAAT (PCR)	• Primary treatment is rehydration • Doxycycline	• Ciprofloxacin or • Azithromycin or • Ceftriaxone

(Continued)

Table 62.1 – Diagnosis and Treatment of Selected Diarrheal Pathogens *(Cont'd)*

Pathogen	Diagnosis	First-Line Treatment	Alternative Treatment
Other *Vibrio spp.* (*V. parahaemolyticus, V. vulnificus*)[a]	• NAAT (PCR)	• Ceftriaxone + doxycycline	• TMP/SMX + aminoglycoside
Yersinia enterocolitica[a]	• NAAT (PCR) • Culture of stool, blood, or pharynx (throat)	• TMP/SMX	• Ciprofloxacin or • Third-generation cephalosporin (ceftriaxone)
Cryptosporidium	• NAAT (PCR) • Ova and parasite stool exam	• Nitazoxanide (and antiretroviral therapy if advanced HIV)	• N/A
Cyclospora cayetanensis	• NAAT (PCR) • Ova and parasite stool exam (modified acid-fast stain)	• TMP/SMX	• Nitazoxanide
Cystoisospora belli	• Ova and parasite stool exam (modified acid-fast stain)	• TMP/SMX	• Pyrimethamine
Giardia lamblia	• NAAT (PCR) • Stool antigen • Ova and parasite stool exam	• Tinidazole	• Metronidazole
Entamoeba histolytica	• NAAT (PCR) • Stool microscopy • Stool antigen	• Metronidazole + paromomycin	• Tinidazole + iodoquinol

[a]Treatment only if severe disease or at-risk host (i.e., immune-compromised).

MIC, Minimum inhibitory concentration; *NAAT*, nucleic-acid amplification testing; *PCR*, polymerase chain reaction; *TMP/SMX*, trimethoprim/sulfamethoxazole.

KEY LEARNING POINT

*For patients presenting with acute diarrhea and certain alarm features (**Fig. 62.1**), additional work-up and treatment should be pursued.*

REFERENCES AND FURTHER READING

- Shane AL, Mody RK, Crump JA, et al. 2017 Infectious Diseases Society of America Clinical Practice Guidelines for the Diagnosis and Management of Infectious Diarrhea. *Clin Infect Dis.* 2017;65(12):e45–e80. https://doi.org/10.1093/cid/cix669.
- Barr W, Smith A. Acute diarrhea. *Am Fam Physician.* 2014;89(3):180–189.
- Fleckenstein J, Kuhlmann FM, Sheikh A. Acute bacterial gastroenteritis. *Gastroenterol Clin North Am.* 2021;50(2):283–304. https://doi.org/10.1016/j.gtc.2021.02.002.

- Kotloff KL, Riddle MS, Platts-Mills JA, Pavlinac P, Zaidi AKM Shigellosis. *Lancet*. 2018;391(10122):801–812. https://doi.org/10.1016/S0140-6736(17)33296-8.
- LaRocque R, Harris JB. Causes of acute infectious diarrhea and other foodborne illnesses in resource-rich settings. In: Post TW, ed. *UpToDate*. Waltham: UpToDate; 2020.
- Orenstein R. Select gastrointestinal and hepatobiliary infections. In: *A Rational Approach to Clinical Infectious Diseases*. Elsevier; 2022:132–145.

A 35-year-old male presents to the emergency room with a 3-day history of fevers, chills, headaches, myalgias, vomiting, and back pain. Approximately 1 week ago, he returned from a trip to Hawaii. He was there for approximately 1 week and, while there, he swam in freshwater. He does not recall any mosquito bites and used mosquito repellant obsessively. He is otherwise healthy and does not take any medications routinely. Vital signs show temperature 101.5° F, heart rate 105 beats per minute, blood pressure 110/80 mmHg, respiratory rate 18, and oxygen saturation 96% on room air. On examination, he appears ill. There is mild scleral icterus and conjunctival injection with suffusion. Heart exam shows a regular tachycardia with no murmurs. Lungs are clear. Abdomen is soft and nontender. A liver edge is palpable below the right costal margin. There is no skin rash or joint swelling. Laboratory studies reveal white blood cell (WBC) count 4,000 cells/uL, hemoglobin 13 g/dL, platelet count 100,000 cells/uL, creatinine 1.5 mg/dL (creatinine clearance 45 mL/min), total bilirubin 3.5 mg/dL, and alanine aminotransferase level of 150 U/L. What is the most likely diagnosis?

A. Dengue virus infection.

B. Zika virus infection.

C. Chikungunya virus infection.

D. Leptospirosis.

E. Malaria.

The most likely diagnosis is leptospirosis (**option D**). Leptospirosis is caused by a spirochete called *Leptospira*. The infection is acquired by exposure to the bodily fluids (especially urine) of infected animals (i.e., rodents, dogs, etc.) or exposure to environment that has been contaminated by such animals (the organisms can survive for long periods of time in the soil). The organisms enter the human via skin abrasions or mucosal surfaces. Individuals in certain occupations that involve work with animals (i.e., veterinarians, farmers, etc.) are at risk for infection. A classic board exam favorite is the whitewater rafter who recently returned from Hawaii, the area with the highest incidence of leptospirosis in the United States. Leptospirosis is typically found in more tropical environments.

The median incubation period is 10 days (can be up to 1 month in some cases). Infection can be mild and subclinical. Patients initially experience an abrupt onset of influenza-like illness (i.e., fever, rigors, myalgias, gastrointestinal upset, etc.). Highly suggestive features of leptospirosis are lumbosacral and calf pain, muscle tenderness (with palpation), and conjunctival suffusion (Fig. 63.1). The initial phase (septicemic phase) lasts approximately 1 week. After that, most patients become asymptomatic, but some go on to have a second phase of illness (the immune phase) that is variable in nature. The onset of the immune phase is associated with clearance of the spirochetes from the blood, tissues, and cerebrospinal fluid (CSF) with a rise in antibody titer. Interestingly, spirochetes can be found in the urine during the second phase of illness. A hallmark of the second stage of illness is aseptic meningitis. Late sequelae include anterior uveitis. A more severe form of illness called icterohemorrhagic fever (Weil disease) occurs in some individuals in the second week of the illness (~10% of cases). Weil disease carries a high rate of mortality and is characterized by jaundice (but there is no

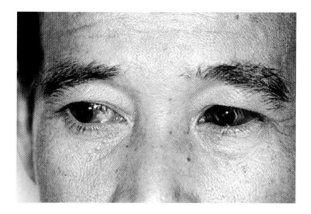

Figure 63.1 – Conjunctival suffusions
Vinetz JM, Watt G. Leptospirosis. In: *Hunter's Tropical Medicine and Emerging Infectious Diseases*. 10th ed. Elsevier; 2020:636–640.

pathologic liver damage), hemorrhage, renal failure, and shock. Death can occur via severe pulmonary hemorrhage syndrome, cardiovascular arrythmia/collapse, complications of renal failure, or other hemorrhage.

Diagnosis requires a high index of suspicion. Laboratory studies may show normal WBC count or leukocytosis (often neutrophilia-predominant), mild thrombocytopenia, transaminase elevation, hyperbilirubinemia (strikingly high bilirubin levels, out of proportion to degree of transaminase elevation), kidney injury, active urinary sediment, and elevated creatine kinase. CSF analysis may reveal lymphocytic pleocytosis, normal glucose, and mildly elevated protein. Chest imaging may show various patterns including effusions, focal opacities, or acute respiratory distress syndrome pattern (bilateral and diffuse infiltrates). *Leptospira* can be recovered (i.e., culture) from the blood or CSF in the initial phase of illness, as well as from the urine during the second phase of illness. Serology is the most commonly used method of diagnosis. The gold standard is the microscopic agglutination test, which requires demonstration of at least a four-fold rise in titer between acute and convalescent samples. Delayed seroconversion and crossreactivity with other infections may limit the usefulness. PCR may be used in early infection, but it is not widely available.

Treatment is probably most effective when given early on in the illness (i.e., during the initial phase of illness). Doxycycline is the treatment of choice for milder forms of leptospirosis. Intravenous penicillin-G is the treatment of choice for severe disease. An alternative choice in either severity of illness is ceftriaxone. Treatment duration is typically 1 week. Jarisch–Herxheimer reactions have been reported with penicillin treatment. Supportive care may be necessary for the complications of the disease (i.e., dialysis for renal failure, mechanical ventilation, etc.).

Options A, B, and C are compared in Table 63.1. Zika and Chikungunya have not been reported in Hawaii. Dengue is rarely reported in Hawaii, but this presentation and exposure history is not consistent with Dengue fever.

Table 63.1 – Zika Versus Dengue Versus Chikungunya

Category	Zika Virus	Dengue Fever (DF)	Chikungunya
Pathogen	• Zika virus	• Dengue virus	• Chikungunya virus
Vector and transmission	• *Aedes* mosquito • Vertical transmission (mother to fetus) • Sexual transmission • Blood product transfusion and organ transplantation • Accidental lab exposures	• *Aedes* mosquito	• *Aedes* mosquito
Epidemiology	• Americas, including Florida and Texas; Central and South America, Africa, Southeast Asia	• Central and South America, Southern Africa, Southeast Asia, Northeast Australia, Southern United States and Hawaii	• Nearly global—North America (including United States), Central and South America, Europe, tropical Africa, Southeast Asia
Incubation period	• 3–12 days	• 4–10 days	• 3–7 days (can be up to 12 days)
Distinguishing clinical manifestations[a]	• Conjunctivitis (Fig. 63.2) • Maculopapular rash (see Fig. 63.2) • Peripheral edema (see Fig. 63.2) • Rare cases Guillain–Barre syndrome, meningoencephalitis, myelitis • Congenital malformations in pregnancy (↓ risk with ↑ trimester)	• **Classic DF** – myalgias and arthralgias ("breakbone fever"), retro-orbital pain, Herman's rash ("white islands in a sea of red"—Fig. 63.3) • **Dengue hemorrhagic fever (severe Dengue)**—↑ risk after reinfection with different serotype; ↑ vascular permeability (as viremia clears and patient defervesces) → hemoconcentration, effusions, shock, hemorrhage, thrombocytopenia	• Severe polyarthralgia or polyarthritis—symmetric, small joints, can become chronic (similar to rheumatoid arthritis) • Maculopapular rash • "Saddle-back" fever curve—bimodal fever pattern
Diagnosis[c]	• Clinical • If <14 days since symptom onset (<12 weeks in pregnant women) → RT-PCR on serum and urine (note: if negative, cannot rule out) • If RT-PCR negative (but suspicion high) or >14 days of symptoms → serology (IgM and confirmatory plaque reduction neutralization test)	• Clinical • Positive tourniquet test (petechiae after using blood pressure cuff or tourniquet) • First week of illness → RT-PCR or NS1 antigen • >1 week of illness → serology (paired acute and convalescent)	• Clinical • First week of illness → RT-PCR • >1 weeks of illness → serology (paired acute and convalescent)—can persist up to 3 months

(Continued)

Table 63.1 – Zika Versus Dengue Versus Chikungunya *(Cont'd)*

Category	Zika Virus	Dengue Fever (DF)	Chikungunya
Management	• Supportive • Abstain from sex (or use barrier precautions) for 2 months (females) or 3 months (males) after exposure or illness onset	• Supportive • Monitor very closely if signs of severe Dengue[b] • Avoid aspirin and NSAIDs	• Supportive

[a]All three of these infections can be asymptomatic infections or present as a nonspecific viral syndrome ("flu-like illness"). Leukopenia, thrombocytopenia, and transaminase elevations can be seen in Dengue and Chikungunya.

[b]**Warning signs of severe Dengue**—abdominal pain or tenderness, persistent vomiting, clinical fluid accumulation, mucosal bleeding, lethargy or restlessness, hepatomegaly >2 cm, increase in hematocrit concurrent with a rapid decline in platelet count.

[c]There is crossreactivity between these viruses when using serologic testing. For paired serology, need to demonstrate at least a four-fold rise between acute and convalescent samples.

NSAIDs, nonsteroidal anti-inflammatory drugs; *RT-PCR*, Reverse transcriptase polymerase chain reaction.

Malaria (**option E**) is not endemic to Hawaii, so this patient is not at risk for malaria.

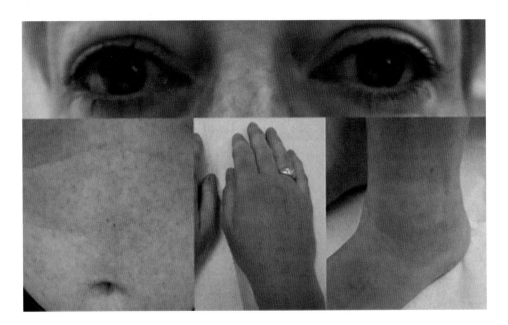

Figure 63.2 – Zika virus infection: conjunctivitis, rash, and peripheral edema
Neumayr A, et al. A 51-year-old female traveler returning from Central America with conjunctivitis, rash, and peripheral edema. In: *Clinical Cases in Tropical Medicine*. 2nd ed. Elsevier; 2022:214–216.

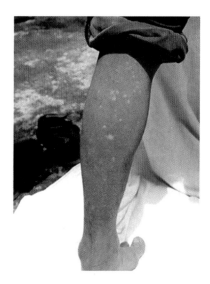

Figure 63.3 – Dengue fever rash
Simmons CP, et al. Dengue and chikungunya. In: Cohen J, ed. *Infectious Diseases*. 4th ed. Elsevier; 2017:1119–1122.

KEY LEARNING POINT

The diagnosis of leptospirosis requires a high index of suspicion. It should be suspected in a patient who has traveled to an area with high incidence (i.e., tropical areas such as Hawaii, etc.) and had exposure to certain animals or potentially contaminated soil/water.

REFERENCES AND FURTHER READING

- Endy T. Viral febrile illnesses and emerging pathogens. In: *Hunter's Tropical Medicine and Emerging Infectious Diseases*. 10th ed. Elsevier; 2020:325–350.
- Haake, DA, Levett PN. *Leptospira* species (Leptospirosis). In: Bennet JE, Dolin R, Blaser MJ, eds. *Mandell, Douglas, and Bennett's Principles and Practice of Infectious Diseases*. 9th ed. Elsevier; 2020:2898–2905.
- Neumayr A, et al. A 51-year-old female traveler returning from Central America with conjunctivitis, rash, and peripheral edema. In: *Clinical Cases in Tropical Medicine*. 2nd ed. Elsevier; 2022:214–216.
- Sayres L, Hughes BL. Contemporary understanding of Ebola and Zika virus in pregnancy. *Clin Perinatol.* 2020;47(4):835–846. https://doi.org/10.1016/j.clp.2020.08.005.
- Simmons CP, et al. Dengue and chikungunya. In: Cohen J, ed. *Infectious Diseases*. 4th ed. Elsevier; 2017: 1119–1122.
- Vinetz JM, Watt G. Leptospirosis. In: *Hunter's Tropical Medicine and Emerging Infectious Diseases*. 10th ed. Elsevier; 2020:636–640.

A 50-year-old male is admitted to the hospital with a 1-week history of fevers, cough, pleuritic chest pain, and shortness of breath. He had a deceased-donor kidney transplant 5 months ago for end-stage renal disease related to diabetic nephropathy. Medications include insulin, rosuvastatin, tacrolimus, mycophenolate, and low-dose prednisone. He lives in Nebraska with his wife. He enjoys gardening. He does not have any pets and denies any large animal exposures. He denies any recent travel. Vital signs reveal temperature 100.4° F, heart rate 95 beats per minute, blood pressure 110/75 mmHg, respiratory rate 24, and oxygen saturation 90% on room air. On examination, he appears drowsy. There are no oral mucosal lesions. Heart is regular in terms of rate and rhythm. Lung exam reveals rales in the right upper lobe posteriorly. There are no skin lesions. The remainder of the examination is unremarkable. Laboratory studies reveal white blood cell count 11,000 cells/uL, creatinine 1.4 mg/dL (creatinine clearance 55 mL/min), and normal liver function testing. Noncontrast CT of the chest shows a 2-cm irregular-appearing mass in the peripheral right upper lung. Percutaneous biopsy of the lesion is performed; a representative stain is shown in Fig. 64.1. Histopathology shows neutrophilic infiltration, but no granulomas.

What is the next best step in the management of this patient?

A. Liposomal amphotericin-B.

B. Itraconazole.

C. Levofloxacin and rifampin.

D. Isoniazid, rifampin, pyrazinamide, and ethambutol.

E. MRI of the brain with contrast.

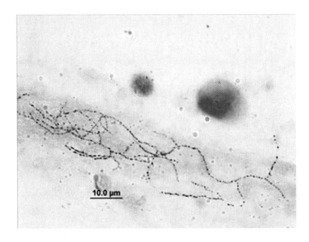

Figure 64.1 – Percutaneous biopsy
Cabada M, Nishi SP, Lea AS, et al. Concomitant pulmonary infection with *Nocardia transvalensis and Aspergillus ustus* in lung transplantation. *J Heart Lung Transplant*. 2010;29(8):900–903. https://doi.org/10.1016/j.healun.2010.04.016.

The next best step in management is to obtain an MRI of the brain with contrast (**option E**). This patient's presentation is most consistent with *Nocardia* infection. *Nocardia* is an environmental organism found in soil and water. Various species of *Nocardia* can infect humans. Most infections occur in patients who are significantly immune-compromised (i.e., solid-organ transplant recipients >1 month posttransplant) or who have chronic lung disease (i.e., cystic fibrosis, bronchiectasis, etc.). *Nocardia* is often described as an aerobic, beaded, branching, filamentous gram-positive rod that is weakly acid-fast (see Fig. 64.1). Even in the setting of trimethoprim/sulfamethoxazole (TMP/SMX) prophylaxis (i.e., for *Pneumocystis*), breakthrough *Nocardia* infections may occur.

Infection is acquired by inhalation or direct inoculation. Manifestations of *Nocardia* infection include pneumonia (often nodular or cavitary), cutaneous infection (often sporotrichoid in appearance and can occur in immune-competent individuals), and disseminated disease. Dissemination to the central nervous system (CNS) is not uncommon and manifests as a brain abscess. When a *Nocardia* infection is diagnosed in a non-CNS location (i.e., pneumonia), CNS infection needs to be ruled out, as in this case. The rationale behind this recommendation is that *Nocardia* has a propensity for causing CNS infection (especially *N. farcinica*), and CNS infection may not always be clinically evident (overtly symptomatic). Asymptomatic colonization has been described, but in general isolation of *Nocardia* should not be dismissed, especially in immune-compromised individuals.

Diagnosis often requires isolating the organism from the area of involvement. This may involve bronchoscopy for bronchoalveolar lavage or lesion biopsy. The tissue should be sent for microbiologic analysis (including aerobic, anaerobic, fungal, and acid-fast stain and culture) and histopathology. Differential diagnosis includes the usual pathogens (pathogens that affect immune-competent hosts), fungal infection, and mycobacterial infection. Additional work-up may include blood cultures (potentially including acid-fast bacillus [AFB] and fungal blood cultures), sputum gram stain and cultures (potentially including AFB and fungal sputum stain and cultures), *Legionella* urine antigen, respiratory viral panel (PCR-based Film-Array), HIV screening, and fungal antigens.

If patients are severely ill, and empiric therapy is required, three drugs may be necessary. Options include TMP/SMX plus carbapenem plus amikacin, ceftriaxone, or linezolid. Definitive treatment (choice and duration) will depend on the subspecies (and associated susceptibility profile), the site of the infection, and the severity of the infection. The drug of choice for most subspecies is TMP/SMX, but some subspecies may be resistant. In most cases (especially in the case of severe illness or an immune-compromised host), a second agent is required. Options include linezolid, carbapenems, ceftriaxone, and amikacin. Reduction of immune suppression should be considered. Surgical drainage or debridement may be necessary as well. Treatment is often prolonged (on the order of 6–12 months).

Liposomal amphotericin-B (**option A**) and itraconazole (**option B**) are used for the treatment of fungal infections (i.e., endemic mycoses). Fungal pneumonias can present in a similar fashion, but the stain in this case is not consistent with fungal infection.

The combination of levofloxacin and rifampin (**option C**) is a regimen that can be used to treat *Rhodococcus* infections. Rhodococci are aerobic gram-positive coccobacilli that cause infections (typically a pneumonia) in patients with defective cell-mediated immunity (classically patients with advanced HIV). A characteristic microbiologic feature of *Rhodococcus* is the formation of "salmon pink–colored" colonies. Occasionally, it may stain partially acid-fast as well. Treatment typically involves at least two to three drugs, with options being macrolides, fluoroquinolones, vancomycin, carbapenems, aminoglycosides, and rifampin.

Isoniazid, rifampin, pyrazinamide, and ethambutol (**option D**) are used to treat most infections caused by *Mycobacterium tuberculosis* (TB). TB is less likely in this patient based on the exposure history and the available stain.

AN APPROACH TO INFECTIONS IN SOLID-ORGAN TRANSPLANT RECIPIENTS

Solid-organ transplant (SOT) patients are at risk for various infectious and noninfectious conditions. The infections they are at risk for are a product of their "net state of immune suppression," their exposures, and how far out from the transplant they are. The timeline below is a general guideline and may be altered by the patient's immune suppression regimen, use of additional immune suppression (i.e., to treat rejection), and use of prophylactic antimicrobials. Table 64.1 shows the general timeline of infection and rationale for each time frame (note—there is some overlap here).

These patients can also get the usual infections that nonimmune-compromised patients get, so it is important not to overlook these. Moreover, they often have more than one (often unrelated) infection at any given time. In addition, they may have less obvious symptoms and clinical findings. Consequently, infections are often advanced/disseminated at the time

Table 64.1 – Infections in Solid-Organ Transplant Patients

Timing	Differential

0–1 months posttransplant	• **Rationale**—effects of immune suppression (IS) are not yet evident unless the patient received immune suppression prior to transplant or has a pre-existing immune deficiency
	• **Infectious complications of surgery and hospitalization**—some are unique, such as superinfection of ischemic or injured graft tissues (anastomotic suture lines) or fluid collections (urinomas, lymphoceles, etc.)
	• **Pre-existing infection (either from donor or recipient)**—patients may even have pre-existing colonization with resistant pathogens
	• **Donor-derived infections:**
	  • **Viral**—herpes viruses (CMV, EBV, HSV, VZV, HHV), LCMV and other arenaviruses (Lassa, hemorrhagic fever viruses, etc.), WNV, HTLV, HIV, hepatitis viruses, rabies
	  • **Bacterial**—mycobacterial, meningococcus, syphilis, bacteremia at time of donation (some pathogens can stick to anastomotic sites), antimicrobial-resistant organisms (colonization or infection)
	  • **Fungal**—*Candida spp., Aspergillus spp., Cryptococcus*, endemic mycoses
	  • **Parasitic**—*Toxoplasma, Trypanosoma cruzi*, malaria, *Babesia, Strongyloides, Ballimuthia*

1–6 months posttransplant	• **Rationale**—effect of IS is maximal, so now patients are at risk for **opportunistic infections**. Prophylaxis does not completely eliminate the risk of infection, and delayed infections occur after stopping prophylaxis • **Bacterial**—*Mycobacteria, Listeria, Nocardia* • **Viral**—herpes (CMV, EBV, HHV, VZV, HSV), hepatitis B/C (HBV and HCV), polyoma (BK virus, JC virus), respiratory viruses, HIV, parvovirus, norovirus, papillomavirus, and rarely, WNV, rabies, HTLV, and LCMV • **Fungal**—*Pneumocystis, Cryptococcus*, endemic mycoses, molds • **Parasitic**—*Toxoplasma, Strongyloides, Leishmania, T. cruzi, Echinococcus*, gastrointestinal pathogens (*Cryptosporidium, Microsporidium*, etc.)
>6 months posttransplant	• **Rationale**—IS is now at a stable, usually reduced, level • **Community-acquired infections including typical and atypical pathogens** • **Late-onset viral infections**—delayed-onset CMV, HBV, HCV, HSV, JC virus, EBV (PTLD), etc.

CMV, Cytomegalovirus; *EBV*, Epstein–Barr virus; *HHV*, human herpes virus; *HIV*, human immunodeficiency virus; *HSV*, herpes simplex virus; *HTLV*, human T-cell leukemia virus; *LCMV*, lymphocytic choriomeningitis virus; *PTLD*, posttransplant lymphoproliferative disease; *VZV*, varicella zoster virus; *WNV*, West Nile virus.

of presentation. Serologic testing is not as useful for diagnosis of acute infections because seroconversion is either delayed or does not occur. In general, we tend to be more aggressive in evaluating and managing these patients (i.e., obtaining bronchoscopy to get deep sample/tissue sent for pathology and microbiology). Lastly, various noninfectious conditions can mimic infection, including malignancy, organ rejection, and drug adverse effects/reactions. Treatments for infections in SOT patients can be complex. One should always consider drug-drug interactions when prescribing therapy. Reduction of the overall immune suppression should always be considered, as many of these infections (>1 month posttransplant) are either reactivations of latent infections or infections caused by opportunistic pathogens.

In either case, successful management may require better immunity. Lastly, obtaining source control should always be considered (i.e., draining a fluid collection).

KEY LEARNING POINT

*Patients diagnosed with **Nocardia** infection in a non–central nervous system (CNS) site (i.e., pneumonia) should have CNS imaging (typically MRI) done to evaluate for CNS **Nocardia** infection (i.e., brain abscess).*

REFERENCES AND FURTHER READING

- Cabada M, Nishi SP, Lea AS, et al. Concomitant pulmonary infection with *Nocardia transvalensis* and *Aspergillus ustus* in lung transplantation. *J Heart Lung Transplant*. 2010;29(8):900–903. https://doi.org/10.1016/j.healun.2010.04.016.
- Chen S, et al. *Nocardia* species. In: Bennet JE, Dolin R, Blaser MJ, eds. *Mandell, Douglas, and Bennett's Principles and Practice of Infectious Disease*. 9th ed. Elsevier; 2020:3059–3070.
- Fishman JA. Infection in the solid-organ transplant recipient. In: Blumberg EA, Bond S, eds. *UpToDate*. Waltham: UpToDate; 2020.
- Kim R, Reboli AC. Other coryneform bacteria, *Arcanobacterium haemolyticum*, and rhodococci. In: Bennet JE, Dolin R, Blaser MJ, eds. *Mandell, Douglas, and Bennett's Principles and Practice of Infectious Diseases*. 9th ed. Elsevier; 2020:2532–2542.
- Kumar R, Ison MG. Opportunistic infections in transplant patients. *Infect Dis Clin North Am*. 2019;33(4):1143–1157. https://doi.org/10.1016/j.idc.2019.05.008.

A 26-year-old female presents with a 2-day history of low-grade fever, malaise, myalgias, and a skin rash. One week ago, she returned from a trip to Connecticut to visit family. She notes she spent a lot of time outdoors while there. She is currently 22 weeks pregnant. She has no medication allergies. Her current medications include a multivitamin and folic acid supplement. Vital signs are within normal limits, and she is afebrile. Physical examination reveals a healthy-appearing woman with a gravid uterus on abdominal examination. Skin examination is shown in Fig. 65.1. The remainder of the examination is within normal limits.

What is the next best step in the management of this patient?

A. Treat empirically with doxycycline.

B. Treat empirically with amoxicillin.

C. Serologic testing.

D. Skin biopsy with PCR testing.

E. Observe without any further diagnostic or therapeutic intervention.

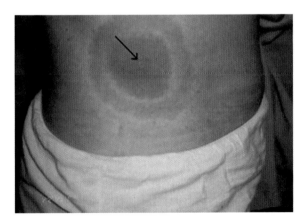

Figure 65.1 – Skin examination
Nadelman R. Erythema migrans. *Infect Dis Clin North Am*. 2015;29(2):211–239. https://doi.org/10.1016/j.idc.2015.02.001.

The next best step in management is empiric treatment with amoxicillin (**option B**). This patient's presentation is most consistent with early localized Lyme disease. Lyme disease is tickborne illness (*Ixodes scapularis* tick) caused by a spirochete called *Borrelia burgdorferi*. The presentation, diagnosis, and management of Lyme disease is summarized in Table 65.1. As shown in the table, the diagnosis of early localized Lyme disease is largely clinical (i.e., no further testing is necessary), and empiric treatment is recommended. Options for pregnant women include amoxicillin or cefuroxime.

A few additional points are worth mentioning with regards to Lyme disease:

- If a tick is removed, it should be sent for species identification, but not for *B. burgdorferi* testing.
- Lyme-endemic regions include Northeast United States, upper Midwest United States (Wisconsin, MN), and Northern California.
- *Borrelia afzelii* infection (typically acquired in Europe) has been associated with the following cutaneous manifestations:
  - Borrelial lymphocytoma (BL)—BL is an inflammatory skin lesion (blue-purple papule, nodule, or plaque) that occurs weeks to months after exposure. Classic location is the earlobe or breast.
  - Acrodermatitis chronica atrophicans (ACA)—ACA is an atrophic dermatitis that classically affects the extensor surfaces (i.e., hands) and occurs months to years after exposure.
- Asymptomatic patients should not be tested for Lyme disease. Testing should only be done on symptomatic patients with high pretest probability of Lyme disease.
- The most commonly used diagnostic test is the two-tier serologic test. This test starts with a screening enzyme immunoassay or immunofluorescence assay. The screening test is highly sensitive for those with more than a 1-month duration of symptoms. A negative screen makes Lyme disease unlikely, but if it is early in infection (<1 month) and ongoing suspicion exists, then consider repeating testing in several weeks (convalescent sample). A positive screen is sent for confirmatory western blot (IgG and IgM immunoblot). The presence of two out of three IgM bands (if illness duration <1 month) or five out of ten IgG bands is considered positive. IgM antibody should not be considered if symptoms have been going on for more than 1 month. The antibodies may persist for a long time, but they are not protective, so repeat infections can occur. Lyme disease diagnosis is summarized in Fig. 65.2.

Table 65.1 – Manifestations and Diagnosis of Lyme Disease

Category	Early Localized	Early Disseminated	Late or Chronic
Manifestations	• Days to weeks (within first month of exposure) • Influenza-like symptoms • Erythema migrans rash (see Fig. 65.1) at site of tick bite in 80% of patients	• Weeks to months after exposure • Multiple erythema migrans (EM) lesions • Cardiac—AV block, myopericarditis • Neurologic—cranial neuropathy (classically facial nerve), meningoencephalitis (lymphocytic/aseptic), radiculitis • Musculoskeletal pain • Ocular manifestations—conjunctivitis is most common	• Months to years after exposure • Arthritis—typically monoarthritis involving the knee • Neurologic—encephalomyelitis, neuropathy
Diagnosis	• Clinical diagnosis in most cases • If presentation atypical, then can perform skin biopsy (lesion margin) with PCR, OR serology (may need paired acute and convalescent samples if initial test is negative)	• Clinical diagnosis if isolated presentation of multiple EM lesions • Serology otherwise	• Serology preferred • Joint disease—can do PCR of synovial fluid or tissue • CNS—elevated CSF Lyme index (CSF to serum ratio) is highly specific for neuroborreliosis but is not sensitive enough to exclude the diagnosis

Treatment[a]	**First-line options**
	• Doxycycline (10 days) or
	• Amoxicillin (14 days) or
	• Cefuroxime (14 days)
	Second-line treatment
	• Azithromycin (7 days, less efficacious)
		• **Cardiac disease**
		  • Hospitalize if high-risk for cardiac complications—PR interval >300 ms, arrhythmia, or myopericarditis
		  • Temporary pacing should be used for refractory bradycardia. The rule is that permanent pacing is often not necessary
		  • Treat with IV ceftriaxone initially; can change to PO (as for early localized Lyme) once improved. Duration 14–21 days
		• **CNS disease and no parenchymal involvement (i.e., meningitis, radiculo-neuropathy, cranial neuropathy)**—IV ceftriaxone, IV penicillin-G, or PO doxycycline for 14–21 days
		• **CNS disease + parenchymal involvement (based on MRI or focal neurologic findings)**—IV therapy preferred
		• **Lyme arthritis**—PO therapy for 28 days; if no or minimal response, then trial of IV ceftriaxone for 2–4 weeks
		• **Borrelial lymphocytoma**—PO therapy for 14 days
		• **Acrodermatitis chronica atrophicans**—PO therapy for 21–28 days	

[a]Preferred PO therapy is doxycycline, amoxicillin, or cefuroxime. Preferred IV therapy is ceftriaxone (alternative is IV penicillin-G).

AV, Atrioventricular; *CNS*, central nervous system; *CSF*, cerebrospinal fluid; *IV*, intravenous; *PCR*, polymerase chain reaction; *PO*, oral therapy.

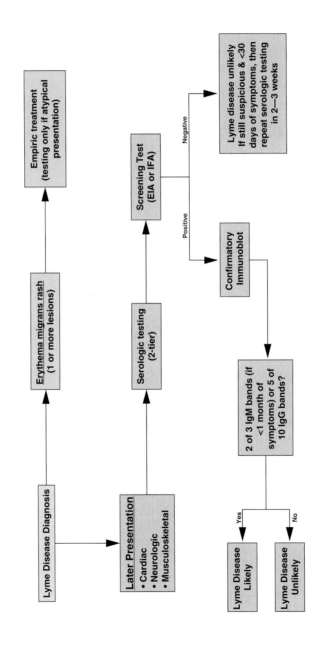

Figure 65.2 – Diagnosis of Lyme disease

EIA, Enzyme immunoassay; *IFA,* immunofluorescence assay.

- Treatment may be complicated by Jarisch–Herxheimer reactions. These reactions are managed supportively.

- Failure to respond to treatment should prompt consideration of coinfections. The most common coinfections are *Babesia* and *Anaplasma*. Less common coinfections include *Borrelia miyamotoi, Borrelia mayonii, Ehrlichia muris eauclairensis* (formerly *Ehrlichia muris-like agent*) and Powassan virus (deer tick virus). The likely coinfection will depend on the treatment used and other available clinical data.

- Prophylaxis (doxycycline 200 mg PO once) for Lyme disease after a tick bite can be given if all of the following criteria are met:
  - Tick was removed within the last 72 hours
  - Tick is identified as *Ixodes* tick
  - The tick bite occurred in a highly endemic area for Lyme
  - Tick was attached for at least 36 hours

Empiric treatment with doxycycline (**option A**) is not the best choice during pregnancy due to the teratogenic potential (i.e., dental discoloration and skeletal growth impairment). Serologic testing (**option C**) is unlikely to be helpful in early localized Lyme disease. In a clear-cut case of early Lyme disease, the best step in most cases is empiric treatment. Skin biopsy with PCR testing (**option D**) can be done, but it is not very common. In addition, a biopsy would put the patient through an unnecessary procedure to verify a diagnosis that can be made clinically. Observing without any further diagnostic or therapeutic intervention (**option E**) would not be appropriate, as the later stages of Lyme disease carry significant morbidity and potentially mortality.

KEY LEARNING POINT

If a patient presents with classic erythema migrans lesion(s), empiric treatment for Lyme disease is warranted. Testing is not necessary.

REFERENCES AND FURTHER READING

- Nadelman R. Erythema migrans. *Infect Dis Clin North Am.* 2015;29(2):211–239. https://doi.org/10.1016/j.idc.2015.02.001.
- Lantos PM, Rumbaugh J, Bockenstedt LK, et al. Clinical Practice Guidelines by the Infectious Diseases Society of America (IDSA), American Academy of Neurology (AAN), and American College of Rheumatology (ACR): 2020 Guidelines for the Prevention, Diagnosis and Treatment of Lyme Disease. *Clin Infect Dis.* 2012;72(1):e1–e48. https://doi.org/10.1093/cid/ciaa1215.
- Steere AC. Lyme disease (Lyme borreliosis) due to *Borrelia burgdorferi.* In: Bennet JE, Dolin R, Blaser MJ, eds. *Mandell, Douglas, and Bennett's Principles and Practice of Infectious Diseases.* 9th ed. Elsevier; 2020:2911–2922.

A 40-year-old male presents to the emergency room with a 3-day history of fevers, headache, confusion, and vomiting. While in the ambulance on the way to the hospital, he suffered a seizure event. Medical history is unremarkable. Vitals reveal temperature 101 ° F, heart rate 95 beats per minute, blood pressure 110/75 mmHg, respiratory rate 18, and oxygen saturation 98% on 1 to 2 L/min oxygen by nasal cannula. On examination, he is confused, and his speech is aphasic. He does not cooperate with the neurological exam. There is no conjunctival injection or sinus tenderness. External ear canals and tympanic membranes appear normal. He has several dental caries, but no oral mucosal lesions. Heart exam shows a regular rate and rhythm with no heart murmur. Lung exam reveals decreased breath sounds over the right lower lobe. The remainder of the examination is unremarkable. The white blood cell count is 15,000 cells/uL (85% neutrophils). Noncontrast head CT is unremarkable. Contrast MRI of the brain is shown in Fig. 66.1.

HIV screen is negative. Blood cultures are drawn. What is the best next step in management?

A. Hold antibiotics while obtaining biopsy for gram stain and culture.

B. Start empiric therapy with vancomycin, ceftriaxone, and metronidazole.

C. Start empiric therapy with ceftriaxone and metronidazole.

D. Lumbar puncture.

E. Transthoracic echo.

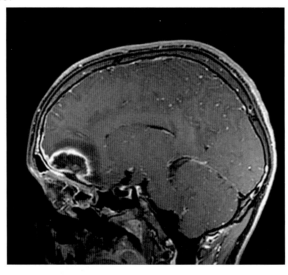

Figure 66.1 – Magnetic resonance image of the brain
From Swaiman KF et al. *Swaiman's Pediatric Neurology, Principles and Practice.* 6th ed. Philadelphia: Elsevier; 2017.

The best next step in management is to start empiric therapy with ceftriaxone and metronidazole (**option C**). This patient's presentation is most consistent with a brain abscess. Based on the location of the abscess (frontal lobe) and history of dental caries, the most likely source of infection is an odontogenic source.

Most bacterial brain abscesses (~50%) are caused by contiguous spread from a nearby infection (i.e., otitis, mastoiditis, sinusitis, odontogenic infection, trauma, surgery, etc.). Hematogenous spread from a distant area (i.e., infective endocarditis, lung abscess, congenital heart disease, etc.) accounts for approximately 30% of cases. The remaining 20% are idiopathic (cryptogenic) in nature. Aside from bacteria, brain abscess may be caused by fungal and parasitic organisms. The microbiology of brain abscesses is summarized in Table 66.1.

The presentation may include fevers, headache, confusion, vomiting, and focal neurologic deficits. The presentation will depend on the causative organism, the mode of acquisition, and the abscess location. The history and physical examination should focus on identifying the most likely etiology. Patients should be asked about prior medical and surgical issues (i.e., repaired heart valve, recent neurosurgical procedure), alcohol use, intravenous drug use, and epidemiologic exposures (i.e., animal exposure, travel, tuberculosis risk factors, sexual history and HIV status). Examination should involve a detailed neurologic exam, close examination of the ears, sinuses, and teeth, and a good general medical examination look for distant sources of infection.

Laboratory studies may reveal leukocytosis, hyponatremia (related to syndrome of inappropriate antidiuretic hormone), elevated inflammatory markers, and findings specific to the source of infection (i.e., murmur in endocarditis). HIV screening should always be considered. In certain cases, testing for unusual pathogens (i.e., *Toxoplasma*) may be warranted. At least two sets of blood cultures (before antibiotics) should be obtained. CT and MRI with contrast are the imaging tests of choice for the diagnosis of brain abscess. As for bacterial meningitis (which is often in the differential), imaging (prior to even considering lumbar puncture) should be performed in patients with depressed consciousness, history of central nervous system (CNS) disease, new-onset seizure, immune compromise, papilledema, or focal neurologic deficit. MRI is more sensitive than CT, and imaging may show cerebritis (early finding), a ring-enhancing lesion (or lesions) with diffusion restriction, ventriculitis (when abscess ruptures into ventricular system), and evidence of cerebral edema. Certain sources of infection have a predilection for particular areas of the brain—otitis (temporal lobe or cerebellum), sinusitis or odontogenic (frontal lobe), or hematogenous (typically multifocal CNS lesions).

Table 66.1 – Microbiology of Brain Abscesses

Source of Infection	Microbial Causes[a]	Empiric Treatment
Otitis and mastoiditis	• Streptococci, *Prevotella* spp., *Bacteroides* spp., Enterobacteriaceae	• Ceftriaxone (CNS dose – 2 grams IV q12h) + metronidazole 500 mg PO/IV every 8 hours • Penicillin-G can be used instead of ceftriaxone in odontogenic infections
Sinusitis	• Similar to otitis/mastoiditis + *Staphylococcus aureus* and *Haemophilus influenzae*	
Odontogenic	• Streptococci, *Prevotella* spp., *Bacteroides* spp., *Fusobacterium* spp., *Actinomyces* spp.	

Penetrating trauma, neurosurgical, or hospital-acquired (HA)	• *S. aureus* (including MRSA in postneurosurgery)
	 • Enterobacteriaceae, *Clostridium* spp.
	 • Coagulase-negative staphylococci and *Pseudomonas* spp. (postsurgery)
		• Penetrating trauma:
		  • Ceftriaxone (CNS dosing) + metronidazole
		 • Postneurosurgical or HA:
		  • Vancomycin + cefepime
		  • Alternative to vancomycin—linezolid
		  • Alternative to cefepime—meropenem

Pulmonary—empyema, abscess, etc.	• Streptococci, *Prevotella* spp., *Bacteroides* spp., *Nocardia* spp., *Actinomyces* spp., *Fusobacterium* spp.	• Ceftriaxone (CNS dosing) + metronidazole
Infective endocarditis	• *S. aureus* and streptococci	• Vancomycin + ceftriaxone (CNS dosing)
Immune compromise	• *Listeria monocytogenes* • *Salmonella* spp. • *Cryptococcus* spp. • *Nocardia* spp. • *Toxoplasma gondii* • Mycobacteria • Fungal—*Candida* spp., endemic mycoses, invasive molds—*Aspergillus* spp., Mucorales, etc.	• Variable—depends on suspicion and clinical context
Immigrant	• Neurocysticercosis • *Echinococcus* spp. • *Mycobacterium tuberculosis*	• Variable—depends on suspicion and clinical context

[a]The most common cause overall is streptococci. Polymicrobial infections are very common to see as well.

CNS, Central nervous system; *MRSA*, methicillin-resistant *Staphylococcus aureus*.

Lumbar puncture (cerebrospinal fluid analysis) in the setting of a brain abscess is relatively contraindicated due to risk of cerebral herniation. If a brain abscess is suspected, then neurosurgical consultation should be requested in order to obtain a stereotactic biopsy of the lesion and potentially perform surgical evacuation and decompression (in select patients). If biopsy is obtained, it should be sent for routine aerobic and anaerobic gram stain and culture, and, if indicated, fungal staining and culture and acid-fast bacillus staining and culture. If possible, some tissue should be sent for histopathologic analysis (and/or held for more sophisticated testing such as broad-range PCR testing in the event of no organism being recovered). Differential diagnosis includes malignancy, inflammatory lesions (i.e., neurosarcoidosis, CNS vasculitis), mycotic aneurysm, and septic emboli (i.e., infective endocarditis).

The approach to management is summarized in Fig. 66.2.

Management should be multidisciplinary and include specialists in neurology, neurosurgery, and infectious disease. If a patient is neurologically and hemodynamically stable, then antibiotics can be withheld until culture data is obtained. Otherwise, empiric therapy should be started as soon as possible. Empiric therapy depends on suspected organism(s), source of infection, and patient stability (see Table 66.1 for antimicrobial selection). If the organism and source are unknown (and/or patient is unstable) and there are no concerns for odd organisms (i.e., mycobacteria, nocardia, fungi, etc.), a reasonable empiric regimen could be vancomycin plus metronidazole plus either a third- or fourth-generation cephalosporin (i.e., ceftriaxone or cefepime). Targeted therapy is based on the results of gram stain and culture, suspected source of infection, and patient's clinical response. As with bacterial meningitis, it is important to consider the appropriate CNS dosing and CNS penetration of the chosen agents. In addition, anaerobes may need to be covered in many situations, as they are often difficult to isolate, and polymicrobial infection is common. Table 66-2 covers the targeted (definitive) therapy for brain abscesses.

Surgical management should always be considered. Most lesions greater than 1 cm in size are amenable to stereotactic aspiration. Aspiration is both diagnostic and therapeutic (reduces burden of infection and compression). Surgical decompression and debridement should be pursued if there is concern for impending herniation or rupture into ventricular system (i.e., abscess near ventricular system), if the patient is failing to respond to adequate therapy, or if the abscess is large (>2.5–3 cm). Duration of therapy needs to be individualized and will depend on the effectiveness of source control (i.e., optimal drainage/debridement vs.

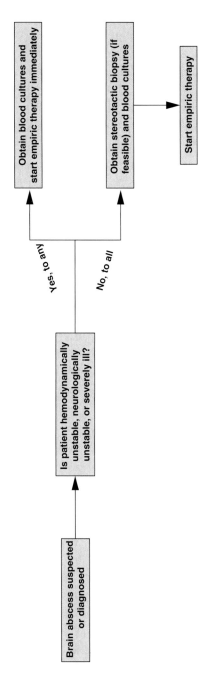

Figure 66.2 – Overview of brain abscess management

Table 66.2 – Definitive Therapy for Select Causes of Brain Abscesses

Organism	First-Line Treatment[a]	Alternative Treatment[a]
Streptococci	• Penicillin-G or ceftriaxone (CNS dosing)—choice depends on species and susceptibility profile	• Vancomycin
Anaerobes (i.e., *Fusobacterium, Prevotella, Bacteroides*, etc.)	• Metronidazole	• Meropenem
Methicillin-susceptible staphylococci (MSSA)	• Nafcillin or oxacillin	• Vancomycin • NOTE: Cefazolin does not have reliable CNS penetration, so best to avoid
Methicillin-resistant staphylococci (MRSA)	• Vancomycin	• TMP/SMX or linezolid
Pseudomonas spp.	• Cefepime	• Meropenem or aztreonam or fluoroquinolone
Most gram-negatives (i.e., *Enterobacteriaceae*)	• Ceftriaxone or cefepime	• Meropenem or aztreonam or fluoroquinolone
Actinomyces spp.	• Penicillin-G	• Ceftriaxone
Listeria monocytogenes	• Penicillin-G or ampicillin +/- aminoglycoside	• TMP/SMX or meropenem
Candida spp.	• Liposomal amphotericin-B + flucytosine	• Fluconazole

[a]The choice of agent will depend on the susceptibility profile of the organism. Many infections will be polymicrobial (anaerobes may not always be recovered), so coverage may need to broader than what is listed (i.e., adding metronidazole for anaerobic coverage).

CNS, Central nervous system; *TMP/SMX*, trimethoprim-sulfamethoxazole.

suboptimal) and clinical response. Most patients will get at least 6 weeks of targeted (often intravenous) therapy with repeat imaging toward the end of therapy (or sooner if warranted) to determine if further therapy is necessary or not. If further therapy is needed based on clinical evaluation, then oral therapy with good CNS penetration should be considered. Lastly, management of complications (i.e., seizures, cerebral edema, etc.) may be necessary as well.

Holding antibiotics while obtaining cultures (**option A**) can be considered in patients who are hemodynamically and neurologically stable and are not septic. Given this patient's seizure and early sepsis presentation, he should be provided appropriate antibiotic therapy as soon as possible. Starting empiric therapy with vancomycin, ceftriaxone and metronidazole (**option B**) could be considered if there is concern for resistant gram-positive organisms (i.e., methicillin-resistant *Staphylococcus aureus* [MRSA]). Situations in which this should be considered include history of MRSA infection, hospital-acquired infection (i.e., postneurosurgical), or a patient with severe illness (i.e., septic shock) with no room for error. Lumbar puncture (**option D**) is relatively contraindicated in the setting of a space-occupying CNS lesion. Transthoracic echo (**option E**) would be useful to evaluate for a hematogenous source such as infective endocarditis. This patient's presentation is most consistent with an odontogenic source.

KEY LEARNING POINT

Antibiotic therapy can be withheld (while working to obtain appropriate culture data) in patients with brain abscesses who are hemodynamically and neurologically stable.

REFERENCES AND FURTHER READING

- Gea-Banacloche JC, Tunkel AR. Brain abscess. In: Bennet JE, Dolin R, Blaser MJ, eds. *Mandell, Douglas, and Bennett's Principles and Practice of Infectious Disease*. 9th ed. Elsevier; 2020:1248–1261.
- Hardy E. Brain abscess. In: *Ferri's Clinical Advisor 2022*. Elsevier; 2022:269–270.
- Tunkel A, et al. Brain abscess. In: Youmans and Winn Neurological Surgery. 7th ed. 2017:e187–e204.

A 55-year-old male is admitted to the hospital with a 2-day history of fevers, rigors, headaches, blurry vision, and sinus pain and congestion. He has a history of hereditary hemochromatosis complicated by diabetes mellitus and chronic heart failure. Medications include metformin, insulin, atorvastatin, metoprolol, lisinopril, and furosemide. He has no medication allergies. Vital signs reveal temperature 102.5° F, heart rate 120 beats per minute, blood pressure 85/50 mmHg, respiratory rate 22, and oxygen saturation 92% on room air. Examination reveals an ill-appearing man. He is somnolent. There is proptosis and periorbital edema around the right eye. He is unable to move the right eye. Oral mucosa is dry, and there are no lesions. His breath smells fruity. Heart exam reveals a regular tachycardia without murmur. He has increased work of breathing, but the lungs sound clear. Abdomen is mildly tender, but there is no rebound tenderness. Skin is tan, but there are no skin lesions. The remainder of the examination is unremarkable. Laboratory studies reveal white blood cell count 20,000 cells/uL (95% neutrophils), creatinine 1.5 mg/dL (creatinine clearance 45 mL/min), glucose 600 mg/dL, sodium 125 mEq/L, potassium 4.8 mEq/L, bicarbonate 10 mEq/L, chloride 90 mEq/L, ALT 60 U/L, AST 70 U/L, and lactate 5 mmol/L. Urinalysis reveals ketonuria. Blood cultures are obtained. Noncontrast head CT reveals right maxillary sinus mucosal thickening with an air-fluid level, right-sided periorbital edema, and thickening of the extraorbital muscles in the right eye. The patient is started on intravenous fluids and intravenous insulin.

In addition to surgical consultation, what is the next best step in management?

A. Amphotericin-B.
B. Isavuconazole.
C. Posaconazole.
D. Voriconazole.
E. Fluconazole.

The next best step in management is to start Amphotericin-B (**option A**). This patient's presentation is highly concerning for rhinocerebral mucormycosis (RM). Mucormycosis (previously known as zygomycosis) is an invasive mold infection (IMI) caused by *Mucorales* species (*Rhizopus, Mucor, Rhizomucor, Lichtheimia* [formerly *Absidia*], *Cunninghamella, Apophysomyces, Saksenaea,* etc.). These molds are found in the environment in decaying organic matter. Risk factors for *Mucorales* infections include hyperglycemia (i.e., corticosteroids or diabetes with ketoacidosis [DKA], as in this patient), prolonged neutropenia, as seen in hematologic malignancy and hematopoietic stem cell transplantation (HSCT), iron-overload states (such as hemochromatosis seen in this patient), HIV infection, use of iron-chelating agents (i.e., deferoxamine), and prolonged voriconazole use (voriconazole does not cover *Mucorales* and may select for *Mucorales* growth). Interestingly, patients with diabetes are more likely to present with RM, whereas patients with hematologic malignancies (or HSCT) are more likely to present with pulmonary or disseminated infection. Fungal spores can be ingested, inhaled, or directly inoculated (often traumatic in nature). The mode of acquisition defines the presentation.

RM presents like most acute sinus infections. As the infection progresses, it will spread to invade local structures such as the eyes, palate, and brain, resulting in vision loss, proptosis, periorbital edema, cranial neuropathies, and central nervous system infection (i.e., brain abscess). A characteristic clinical finding is an eschar involving the palate or nasal mucosa. The absence of an eschar obviously does not rule this infection out. This is especially true for early infections, because the eschar takes time to develop. In terms of imaging, head CT (especially if done with contrast) may show sinus mucosal thickening, fluid-filled sinuses, and invasion into neighboring structures. CT is particularly good at demonstrating bony destruction, which is typically seen later in the disease. MRI of the brain should also be done to evaluate extent of infection and associated complications (i.e., dural venous sinus thrombosis, etc.).

Pulmonary mucormycosis (PM) classically presents as a severe acute pneumonia that can be complicated by hemorrhage (due to angioinvasion) and extension to neighboring structures (i.e., mediastinitis). A classic sign of PM is the "reverse-halo" sign (Fig. 67.1), which is an area of ground-glass opacification surrounded by consolidation. In addition, the presence of multiple pulmonary nodules, a pleural effusion, and sinusitis in an immune-compromised host may be suggestive of *Mucorales* as opposed to other fungi.

Cutaneous mucormycosis (CM) can be seen in immune-competent and immune-compromised individuals. It is typically acquired by traumatic inoculation. CM can be an

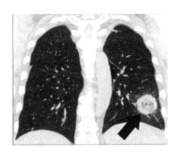

Figure 67.1 – Reverse halo sign depicted by red arrow
Steinbrink JM, Miceli MH. Mucormycosis. *Infect Dis Clin North Am*. 2021;35(2):435–452. https://doi.org/10.1016/j.idc.2021.03.009.

isolated syndrome or a manifestation of systemic infection; thus, systemic infection needs to always be considered. The skin lesions are initially erythematous, painful, and indurated, but over time they become necrotic. Less common forms of infection include gastrointestinal mucormycosis (related to spore ingestion; may see ulceration, bleeding, or perforation), renal mucormycosis, and disseminated infection.

Early recognition and diagnosis are key to successful treatment and good outcome. If mucormycosis is suspected, a tissue diagnosis should be obtained. In general, proving a diagnosis of IMIs requires demonstrating hyphal forms on histopathology, cytopathology, or direct microscopic evaluation from a sterile site obtained via needle aspiration or biopsy. Furthermore, a positive culture for a mold from a normally sterile site obtained via a sterile procedure (excluding bronchoalveolar lavage) is considered a "proven IMI." A diagnosis of "probable IMI" is characterized by the presence of a host risk factor (i.e., neutropenia, HSCT, etc.), a clinical factor (i.e., suggestive presentation or imaging findings), and a microbiologic factor (i.e., nonsterile culture growing mold, positive fungal antigen, etc.). In terms of mucomycosis, a proven diagnosis would be demonstration of broad, ribbon-like, nonseptate hyphae (often with irregular right-angle branching) invading tissue on histopathology, along with culture growth from the involved site. These characteristics can be seen in Fig. 67.2.

Effort should be made to identify the specific subspecies and, if possible, sensitivity testing should be performed (minimum inhibitory concentration values). In addition, additional sites of *Mucorales* involvement should be considered. The serum galactomannan and 1,3-beta-D-glucan (Fungitell) tests are characteristically negative in *Mucorales* infections. Blood cultures very rarely grow *Mucorales*. Assessment for an underlying predisposition (i.e., HIV screening, iron overload, etc.) should be done. Depending on the presentation, testing for other infections (i.e., endemic mycoses, *Cryptococcus, Nocardia*, mycobacteria, etc.) may be indicated.

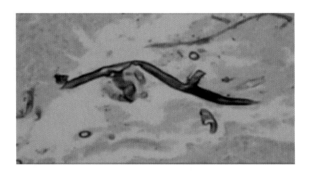

Figure 67.2 – *Mucorales* in tissue biopsy

Management is multifactorial, including antifungal therapy, surgical debridement (very important, as surgery improves survival), correction of the underlying cause (i.e., treat DKA), and reduction of immune suppression (if applicable). Treatment should be started as soon as possible, as delays in treatment are associated with worse outcomes. First-line antifungal therapy is amphotericin-B (Amp-B). Some experts recommend higher doses (i.e., up to 10 mg/kg) of Amp-B, despite lack of evidence showing improved outcomes. In fact, higher doses of Amp-B have been shown to cause more toxicity. Case reports have shown some efficacy for combination therapy with Amp-B and posaconazole. Options for salvage therapy or oral step-down include posaconazole (**option C**) and isavuconazole (**option B**). Breakthrough infections can occur with these agents. Voriconazole (**option D**), fluconazole (**option E**), and itraconazole are not active against *Mucorales*. Echinocandins are not active either. Therapy duration is typically long and continued until all clinical and radiographic signs of infection have resolved. If the underlying risk factor cannot be reversed (i.e., ongoing neutropenia), then secondary prophylaxis may be considered. Despite all this, morbidity and mortality are high.

KEY LEARNING POINT

The first-line therapy for infections due to Mucorales *species is amphotericin-B and surgical debridement. Antifungal options for salvage therapy or oral step-down therapy are posaconazole or isavuconazole.*

REFERENCES AND FURTHER READING

- Bays DJ, Thompson GR 3rd. Fungal infections of the stem cell transplant recipient and hematologic malignancy patients. *Infect Dis Clin North Am.* 2019;33(2):545–566. https://doi.org/10.1016/j.idc.2019.02.006.
- Nathan CL, Emmet BE, Nelson E, Berger JR. CNS fungal infections: a review. *J Neurol Sci.* 2021:422. https://doi.org/10.1016/j.jns.2021.117325.
- Steinbrink JM, Miceli MH. Mucormycosis. *Infect Dis Clin North Am.* 2021;35(2):435–452. https://doi.org/10.1016/j.idc.2021.03.009.

A 40-year-old male is admitted to the hospital with several days of fevers, fatigue, night sweats, anorexia, and diarrhea. He has a history of rheumatoid arthritis. Current medications include etanercept, methotrexate, and folic acid. He is a farmer in rural Iowa. He owns cattle, horses, and chickens. He has never traveled abroad. Vital signs reveal temperature 102° F, heart rate 95 beats per minute, blood pressure 100/60 mmHg, respiratory rate 20, and oxygen saturation 94% on room air. On examination, he appears ill. There is mild scleral icterus. Examination of the oral mucosa reveals mucosal ulceration. Heart has regular rate and rhythm, and there is no murmur. Lungs are clear. There is hepatosplenomegaly. The remainder of the examination is unremarkable. Laboratory studies reveal white blood cell count 2,500 cells/uL, hemoglobin 8 g/dL, platelet count 90,000 cells/uL, creatinine 1.4 mg/dL (creatinine clearance 50 mL/min), AST 70 U/L, ALT 75 U/L, alkaline phosphatase 350 U/L, and total bilirubin 3.5 mg/dL. Prior to starting etanercept, he had documented negative HIV antigen/antibody, hepatitis B and C serology, and tuberculosis interferon-gamma release assay. Chest x-ray reveals mediastinal calcification but is otherwise normal. A peripheral blood smear sample stained with Wright–Giemsa stain is shown in Fig. 68.1.

What is the best initial therapy for this patient?

A. Liposomal amphotericin-B.

B. Itraconazole.

C. Voriconazole.

D. Azithromycin, ethambutol, and rifampin.

E. Miltefosine.

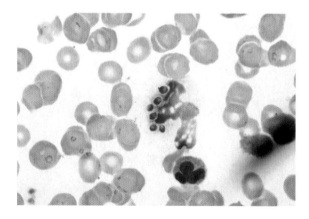

Figure 68.1 – Wright–Giemsa stain
Deepe G. *Histoplasma capsulatum* (histoplasmosis). In: Bennet JE, Dolin R, Blaser MJ, eds. *Mandell, Douglas, and Bennett's Principles and Practice of Infectious Disease.* 9th ed. Elsevier; 2020:3162–3176.

The best initial therapy is liposomal amphotericin-B (**option A**). This patient's presentation is most consistent with disseminated histoplasmosis (DH).

Histoplasmosis is an endemic mycosis caused by the dimorphic fungus *Histoplasma capsulatum*. The two most common species are *H. capsulatum var capsulatum* (global distribution) and *H. capsulatum var duboisii* (West Africa). In the United States, *Histoplasma* is commonly associated with the Ohio and Mississippi river valleys. As a dimorph, it can exist in two forms: a yeast form (at body temperature) and a mold form (in the environment). In the environment, it is found in the soil, especially soil contaminated with bird or bat droppings (i.e., bat guano in caves or chicken coops). Consequently, certain people are at increased risk of infection including farmers, construction workers, and spelunkers (cave explorers).

The presentation of histoplasmosis depends on the host's immune status and the type and degree of exposure. The infection is acquired either by inhalation (most commonly) or direct inoculation. More severe disease occurs in those with large inoculum of exposure or with immune deficiency (i.e., HIV, TNF-alpha antagonists, etc.). Once inhaled, macrophages phagocytose the organism. Inside macrophages, the fungus converts to the yeast form, replicates, and disseminates via the reticuloendothelial system. If cell-mediated immunity (CMI) is impaired, then the infection often disseminates and causes severe illness. If CMI is intact, the infection is contained after a few weeks. This containment may result in necrotizing granuloma formation. If CMI becomes impaired, then the infection may reactivate to cause more severe illness.

Incubation period is 1 to 3 weeks. Most cases of acute infection are either asymptomatic or mild and self-limited (especially if immune-competent). Acute pulmonary histoplasmosis may present like any community-acquired pneumonia and may be associated with mediastinal or hilar lymphadenopathy. Chronic (cavitary) pulmonary histoplasmosis occurs in individuals with pre-existing lung disease and can resemble reactivation tuberculosis with cavitary lesions. In addition, pulmonary nodules may be seen, which can represent calcified granulomas or histoplasmomas. Several mediastinal manifestations are described, and these are more commonly seen with acute infections. Mediastinal lymphadenitis often appears as a subcarinal necrotic lymph node that may cause local compression (bronchial or esophageal), hemoptysis, and broncholithiasis (via erosion into airways). Mediastinal granuloma represents multiple enlarged lymph nodes that coalesce to form a mass that can behave like mediastinal lymphadenitis and even cause fistula formation. Lastly, mediastinal fibrosis (fibrosing mediastinitis) is a rare late complication that is seen in young adults who acquired the infection at a younger age. This complication is caused by a chronic fibrosing response to mediastinal lymph node infection and may envelope mediastinal structures (i.e., superior vena cava syndrome, etc.).

Fibrosing mediastinitis is pauciorganismal, so recovering viable organisms is very unlikely. DH can occur as a new infection or as a result of reactivation of a latent infection (as is the likely case in this patient). DH may present with constitutional symptoms, respiratory symptoms, gastrointestinal upset, oral ulceration, skin lesions, hepatosplenomegaly, and even adrenal insufficiency. Labs may show pancytopenia, coagulopathy, liver function abnormalities (especially elevated bilirubin and alkaline phosphatase), elevated lactate dehydrogenase, elevated ferritin, and hypercalcemia. Less common manifestations of histoplasmosis include central nervous system histoplasmosis, ocular histoplasmosis, endovascular infection, and various inflammatory phenomena (i.e., erythema nodosum, arthralgias, pericarditis, etc.).

Diagnosis of histoplasmosis may involve serology, antigenic testing, culture, and/or histopathology. Serologic testing is typically used to diagnose the chronic forms of infection. Because it takes time to develop antibody responses (i.e., 4–8 weeks), serology may be negative early in infection (or with immune suppression). Therefore, repeat serologic testing may be necessary. The two types of serologic testing are complement fixation (CF) and immunodiffusion (ID). A CF titer of 1:32 or greater is highly suggestive of infection, and a four-fold rise in titer is diagnostic. CF titer can be present at low level for years after the resolution of the infection. ID is more specific than CF. With ID, the M band becomes positive sooner and lasts longer than the H band. The H band is rarely seen and is associated with acute and more severe infections. Antigenic testing can be done on various tissues, including serum, urine, cerebrospinal fluid, or bronchoalveolar lavage fluid. The serum and urine antigens are the most commonly done antigenic tests. They are most useful in immune-compromised patients or patients with severe pulmonary disease. The urine antigen is considered more sensitive than the serum antigen, and the combination (serum and urine antigens) is more sensitive than either alone. The antigen can be used to follow disease activity, and the same antigen is used for the diagnosis of *Blastomyces* infection (so there is often no need to order antigen tests for *Blastomyces* as well). Culture is considered the gold standard, but it can take up to 6 weeks to identify the organism. Histopathology can be very useful. The most useful stain is the Grocott–Gomori methenamine silver, and the organism can be found in peripheral blood smears using Wright–Giemsa staining (see Fig. 68.1). The organism typically appears as small, oval yeast forms in tissues or within phagocytic cells. Additional testing should include HIV screening, and, depending on the presentation, evaluation for other differential diagnoses (i.e., other endemic mycoses and fungi, mycobacterial infections, etc.) should be considered.

Management is summarized in Table 68.1. In general, management depends on the presentation/severity of infection and the host's immune status. Asymptomatic,

Table 68.1 – Management of Histoplasmosis

Presentation	Mild Infection[a]	Severe Infection or Immune Compromise[a]
Acute pulmonary histoplasmosis	• If immune competent and symptoms <1-month duration → no treatment • If symptoms >1 month or immune compromised → itraconazole for 6–12 weeks	• Amp-B for 1–2 weeks then itraconazole for 3 months (1 year if immune suppressed) • Steroids can be used in the first couple weeks of treatment in those with severe pulmonary involvement and those who develop pulmonary complications
Chronic pulmonary histoplasmosis	• Itraconazole for at least 1 year	• Same as above, but itraconazole should be continued for at least 1 year
Disseminated histoplasmosis	• Itraconazole for at least 1 year	• Same as for chronic pulmonary histoplasmosis
Inflammatory phenomena (i.e., pericarditis)	• Nonsteroidal anti-inflammatory drugs	• Pericardiocentesis • Itraconazole for 6–12 weeks • Steroid taper
Mediastinal lymphadenitis	• If symptomatic (>1 month) or causing obstruction/compression, then itraconazole and steroids as for inflammatory phenomena	
Mediastinal granuloma	• If symptomatic (>1 month), consider itraconazole for up to 12 weeks or longer, depending on clinical response. Steroids are not recommended	
Fibrosing mediastinitis	• Antifungals not indicated unless cannot differentiate between fibrosis and mediastinal granuloma. If this is the case, then treat like mediastinal granuloma. • Management of complications (i.e., stenting) may be necessary.	
Central nervous system histoplasmosis	• Liposomal Amp-B 5 mg/kg/day for a total of 175 mg/kg over 4–6 weeks followed by itraconazole 200 mg PO BID to TID for at least 1 year and until CSF abnormalities, including histoplasma antigenemia, resolve	
Endovascular infection	• Amp-B and surgery (valve replacement), then treatment as for disseminated infection	
Pregnancy	• Amp-B is the drug of choice and is typically given for 4–6 weeks • Azole therapy can be considered after the first trimester.	
Primary prophylaxis in HIV	• HIV patients living in endemic area and having a CD4 count <150 cells/uL can consider taking itraconazole 200 mg PO daily until CD4 recovers to >150 cells/uL and is maintained for at least 6 months in the setting of ART/virologic control	

[a]**Itraconazole**—Typical dosing is 200 mg by mouth three times daily for 3 days, then 200 mg by mouth twice daily (unless noted otherwise). Compared with the capsule formulation, the solution formulation is better absorbed and less likely to be affected by antacid medications. The solution form should be taken on an empty stomach, while the capsule form needs to be taken with food and an acidic beverage. Therapeutic drug monitoring is often necessary and is typically obtained ~2 weeks after starting therapy with itraconazole. Goal drug level (itraconazole level + hydroxyitraconazole level) is >1 ug/mL.

Amp-B, Amphotericin-B; *ART,* antiretroviral therapy; *CSF,* cerebrospinal fluid.

immune-competent patients do not need to be treated. Amphotericin-B (Amp-B) is used as the initial therapy in severe infections. The liposomal Amp-B formulation is preferred in most cases due to reduced toxicity compared with conventional Amp-B. Itraconazole (**option B**) is the preferred agent in mild-moderate infections.

Salvage treatment options for histoplasmosis include posaconazole (first-line salvage), voriconazole (second-line salvage, **option C**), isavuconazole (active *in vitro*, but clinical experience limited), and fluconazole (last-line, as shown to be inferior to itraconazole, and there is a risk of developing resistance with treatment). During treatment, *Histoplasma* antigen (if elevated to begin with) should be monitored. The antigen should decline within a few weeks of starting therapy. Repeat imaging may be necessary to monitor treatment response. Prolonged or life-long therapy may be warranted in those with ongoing immune suppression (that cannot be reversed) or with relapsed disease.

Azithromycin, ethambutol, and rifampin (**option D**) is the treatment for disseminated *Mycobacterium avium* complex (MAC) infection. Disseminated MAC is typically seen in advanced HIV and actually presents very similarly to DH. The peripheral smear finding in this case makes histoplasmosis the more likely diagnosis. Miltefosine (**option E**) is a drug used to treat visceral leishmaniasis (visceral LM; Kala-azar). Interestingly, liposomal Amp-B can also be used to treat visceral LM. Visceral LM can present similarly to histoplasmosis, but the lack of travel abroad and peripheral smear finding make visceral LM unlikely.

KEY LEARNING POINT

Severe histoplasmosis should initially be treated with amphotericin-B. Mild-moderate histoplasmosis is initially treated with itraconazole.

REFERENCES AND FURTHER READING

- Araúz AB, Papineni P. Histoplasmosis. *Infect Dis Clin North Am.* 2021;35(2):471–491. https://doi.org/10.1016/j.idc.2021.03.011.
- Deepe G. *Histoplasma capsulatum* (histoplasmosis). In: Bennet JE, Dolin R, Blaser MJ, eds. *Mandell, Douglas, and Bennett's Principles and Practice of Infectious Disease.* 9th ed. Elsevier; 2020:3162–3176.

A 35-year-old male presents to the hospital with fevers, night sweats, anorexia, and a new skin lesion. He has a history of psoriatic arthritis. Medications include naproxen, methotrexate, and etanercept. He has no medication allergies. He lives in Wisconsin by himself. He works in construction. He denies any travel abroad. He denies any substance abuse. Vital signs reveal temperature 100.6° F, heart rate 85 beats per minute, blood pressure 110/70 mmHg, and respiratory rate 18. He appears fairly well. He is diaphoretic. There are no oral ulcerations. The skin lesion is shown in Fig. 69.1. He has no evidence of active psoriasis or arthritis in the extremities. The remainder of the physical examination is unremarkable. A biopsy of the lesion is performed. A representative Grocott–Gomori methenamine silver (GMS) stain is shown in Fig. 69.2.

What is the next best step in the management of this patient?

A. Liposomal amphotericin-B (Amp-B).
B. Wide excision by a dermatologist.
C. Itraconazole.
D. Rifampin, isoniazid, pyrazinamide, and ethambutol.
E. Topical corticosteroid.

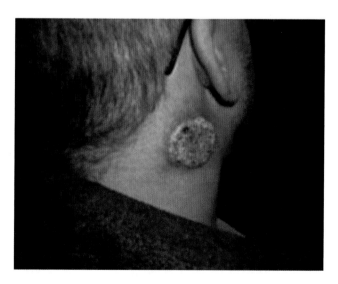

Figure 69.1 – Skin lesion
Mazi PB, Rauseo AM, Spec A. Blastomycosis. *Infect Dis Clin North Am.* 2021;35(2):515–530. https://doi.org/10.1016/j.idc.2021.03.013.

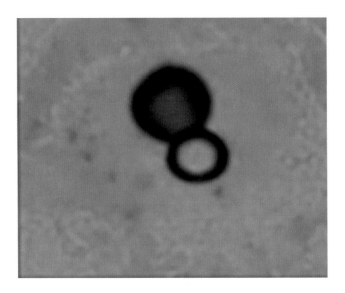

Figure 69.2 – Grocott–Gomori methenamine silver stain
Thompson GR 3rd, Le T, Chindamporn A, et al. Global guideline for the diagnosis and management of the endemic mycoses: an initiative of the European Confederation of Medical Mycology in cooperation with the International Society for Human and Animal Mycology. *Lancet Infect Dis*. 2021;21(12):e364–e374. https://doi.org/10.1016/S1473-3099(21)00191-2. Courtesy of Dr Carol Kauffman.

The next best step is to start Amp-B (**option A**), as the most likely diagnosis is cutaneous blastomycosis in an immune-suppressed patient.

Blastomycosis is an endemic mycosis caused by the dimorphic fungus *Blastomyces*. There are several subspecies of *Blastomyces*. The most common subspecies in North America is *Blastomyces dermatitidis*. This species infects immune-competent and immune-compromised individuals. As a dimorph, it exists as a mold in the environment and a yeast at body temperature. In the environment, *Blastomyces spp.* are classically found in moist soil and near decomposing matter (i.e., rotting wood). The distribution is similar to that of *Histoplasma capsulatum*, including the Ohio and Mississippi river valleys and Midwest states surrounding the Great Lakes (Wisconsin may have a disproportionately high number of reported cases). Certain occupations are at risk, including construction work and forest work. The presence of blastomycosis in a pet dog may be an important diagnostic clue.

Infection is acquired by inhalation of spores or direct inoculation. Incubation period is 1 to 3 months (longer than *H. capsulatum*, which has an incubation period <1 month). Many acute infections are either asymptomatic or mild and self-limited, especially in immune-competent individuals. In patients with immune compromise or high inoculum exposure the disease can be more severe/disseminated. Symptomatic acute pulmonary blastomycosis presents as a protracted community-acquired pneumonia (similar to histoplasmosis). Chronic pulmonary blastomycosis can present with cavitary or mass-like lesions resembling tuberculosis (TB) or malignancy. More severe cases can present with acute respiratory distress syndrome, which carries a high rate of mortality. Disseminated blastomycosis can be seen in immune-compromised individuals and, in rare cases, in immune-competent individuals. Most extrapulmonary blastomycosis actually represents disseminated infection, so disseminated disease always needs to be ruled out. The most common extrapulmonary site of infection is the skin (as seen in this patient). The classic lesion is an ulcerated, verrucous lesion with irregular heaped-up borders (Fig. 69.1). Additional sites of disseminated include bones/joints (septic arthritis, osteomyelitis; may appear as lytic lesions in bone), genitourinary organs (prostatitis, epididymo-orchitis, tubo-ovarian abscess, etc.), and the central nervous system (meningoencephalitis and abscesses).

The gold standard for diagnosis is culture from the involved site, but culture can take several weeks to identify the organism. Histopathology (e.g., fungal staining with GMS) will show the classic broad-based budding yeast with a thick, double-refractile wall (Fig. 69.2). Serology is not useful for blastomycosis. The same antigenic test used to diagnose histoplasmosis can be used for the diagnosis of blastomycosis. Although it can be done on various bodily fluids, it is most commonly checked on serum and urine. The urinary antigen test may be more sensitive, but the combination of serum and urine is more sensitive than either alone. The antigen is more likely to be positive in disseminated or more severe infections. In addition, the antigen can be followed to assess response to therapy. Interestingly, the 1,3-beta-D-glucan test (Fungitell) is typically negative in blastomycosis (similar to *Cryptococcus* and *Mucorales*). Additional testing should include HIV screening, and, depending on the presentation, evaluation for other differential diagnoses (i.e., other endemic mycoses and fungi, mycobacterial infections, etc.) should be considered.

Management is largely similar to that for histoplasmosis. All symptomatic patients need to be treated. The selection of an antifungal regimen and its duration should be based on the site and severity of infection, the immune status of the host, and the toxicities associated with each antifungal agent. Amp-B is used as the initial therapy in severe infections or infections in immune-suppressed individuals (such as the patient in this case). The liposomal Amp-B formulation is preferred in most cases due to reduced toxicity compared with conventional Amp-B. Itraconazole (**option C**) is the preferred agent in mild-moderate infections. The other azole antifungals also have activity and may be used as salvage therapy. The management of the various forms of blastomycosis is summarized in Table 69.1.

During treatment, *Blastomyces* antigen (if elevated to begin with) should be monitored to assess treatment response. Repeat imaging may be necessary to monitor response as well. Prolonged or life-long therapy may be warranted in those with ongoing immune suppression (that cannot be reversed) or with relapsed disease. Surgical intervention can be considered in certain situations (i.e., draining an abscess).

Wide excision by a dermatologist (**option B**) would be useful for a squamous cell carcinoma (SCC). SCC can have this type of verrucous appearance, but the presentation and biopsy findings are not consistent with SCC. Rifampin, isoniazid, pyrazinamide, and ethambutol (**option D**) would be indicated to treat TB. Cutaneous TB (tuberculosis verrucose cutis) can present similar to this, but the biopsy in this case is most consistent with blastomycosis. Topical corticosteroids (**option E**) could be used to treat psoriasis or localized pyoderma gangrenosum. These could be considered in the differential, but both are unlikely given the otherwise well-controlled psoriasis, the atypical appearance for either condition, and the biopsy finding.

Table 69.1 – Management of Blastomycosis

Presentation	Management[a]
Mild-moderate blastomycosis (pulmonary and non-CNS extrapulmonary)	• Itraconazole for 6–12 months. • 12-month duration preferred in bone/joint disease.
Severe blastomycosis	• Amphotericin-B (Amp-B) for 1–2 weeks or until improvement is noted. • In severely ill patients, Amp-B can be given concurrently with itraconazole. • Adjunctive steroids may be helpful in severe pulmonary presentations (esp. ARDS). • Provide step-down therapy with itraconazole for 6–12 months for pulmonary disease and 12 months for extrapulmonary (non-CNS) disease.
CNS blastomycosis	• Amp-B for 4–6 weeks followed by step-down therapy with a triazole antifungal such as fluconazole, itraconazole, or voriconazole for 6–12 months or more (often at least 12 months). Voriconazole and fluconazole have better CNS penetration and may be preferred.
Pregnancy	• Amp-B is preferred as azoles are teratogenic (esp. in the first trimester)
Immune suppression	• Amp-B is preferred initially and can be followed up by oral step-down to itraconazole for 12 months (at least).

[a]Itraconazole—Typical dosing is 200 mg by mouth three times daily for 3 days, then 200 mg by mouth twice daily (unless noted otherwise). Compared with the capsule formulation, the solution formulation is better absorbed and less likely to be affected by antacid medications. The solution form should be taken on an empty stomach, while the capsule form needs to be taken with food and an acidic beverage. Therapeutic drug monitoring is often necessary and is typically obtained ~2 weeks after starting therapy with itraconazole. Goal drug level (itraconazole level + hydroxyitraconazole level) is >1 ug/mL.

ARDS, Acute respiratory distress syndrome; *CNS*, central nervous system.

KEY LEARNING POINT

The best initial therapy for blastomycosis in an immune-suppressed patient (regardless of severity) is amphotericin-B.

The B's of blastomycosis:

- *Broad-based budding*
- *Affects breath (lungs), brain, bones, body-covering (skin), baby-makers (genitourinary organs)*

REFERENCES AND FURTHER READING

- Gauthier GM, Klein BS. Blastomycosis. In: Bennet JE, Dolin R, Blaser MJ, eds. *Mandell, Douglas, and Bennett's Principles and Practice of Infectious Diseases*. 9th ed. Elsevier; 2020:3177–3189.

- Mazi PB, Rauseo AM, Spec A. Blastomycosis. *Infect Dis Clin North Am.* 2021;35(2):515–530. https://doi.org/10.1016/j.idc.2021.03.013.
- Thompson GR 3rd, Le T, Chindamporn A, et al. Global guideline for the diagnosis and management of the endemic mycoses: an initiative of the European Confederation of Medical Mycology in cooperation with the International Society for Human and Animal Mycology. *Lancet Infect Dis.* 2021;21(12):e364–e374. https://doi.org/10.1016/S1473-3099(21)00191-2.

A 35-year-old male presents to the emergency room (ER) in June with a 1-week history of fevers, malaise, headache, myalgias, and a mild cough. These symptoms started abruptly, and he was able to manage them at home until he developed shortness of breath, which prompted his presentation to the ER. He is otherwise healthy and does not take any medications. He has no medication allergies. He does not smoke, drink alcohol, or use illicit drugs. He owns a dog and a parrot. He lives alone in rural Iowa. He denies any recent travel. He works as an accountant. Vital signs reveal temperature 100.6° F, heart rate 90 beats per minute, blood pressure 110/75 mmHg, respiratory rate 24, and oxygen saturation 96% on 2 L/min oxygen by nasal cannula. On examination, he is diaphoretic. Head, eyes, ears, nose, and throat examination is within normal limits. Heart exam is normal. Lung exam reveals decreased breath sounds over the right lower lobe posteriorly. The remainder of the exam is within normal limits. Laboratory studies reveal white blood cell count 8,000 cells/uL (12% band forms), AST 125 U/L, creatinine 1.2 mg/dL (creatinine clearance 50 mL/min), and sodium level 135 mEq/L. *Legionella* urine antigen testing is negative. Chest x-ray shows a hazy opacity over the right lower lobe. Which of the following agents is the most likely cause of this patient's illness?

A. *Chlamydophila psittaci.*

B. *Legionella pneumophila.*

C. *Cryptococcus gattii.*

D. *Coccidioides immitis.*

E. Influenza virus.

The most likely cause is *C. psittaci* (**option A**). This patient likely has psittacosis (also known as parrot fever or ornithosis). Psittacosis is a zoonotic infection caused by a gram-negative, intracellular aerobe called *C. psittaci*. A major risk factor for infection is exposure to birds, but this is not always found, and it is not necessary for the diagnosis. Infection is acquired by inhalation of aerosolized organisms, contact with respiratory secretions of infected birds, or direct contact with birds. Consequently, certain individuals are at risk, including bird owners, veterinarians, pet shop employees, and poultry-processing employees.

The spectrum of illness ranges from a mild, subclinical infection to severe illness with multiorgan failure. After an incubation period of 1 to 3 weeks, most patients present with an influenza-like illness. Headache is a prominent feature, and patients may have meningoencephalitis. Eventually, patients may develop pneumonia-like symptoms (i.e., cough, shortness of breath, etc.). Additional findings include relative bradycardia, a pale macular rash (Horder spots), and hepatosplenomegaly. There have been reports of seizures, ataxia, brainstem encephalitis with cranial nerve deficits, and Guillain–Barre syndrome. Fulminant psittacosis classically presents as severe acute respiratory failure (i.e., acute respiratory distress syndrome) with multiorgan failure in a previously healthy individual. Cardiac psittacosis may present with culture-negative endocarditis (often associated with glomerulonephritis) and myopericarditis. Gestational psittacosis presents with multiorgan failure (especially coagulopathy, hepatic, and pulmonary), placentitis, and fetal compromise. A variant called chronic follicular conjunctivitis is often unilateral and characterized by preauricular lymphadenopathy and punctate epithelial keratitis. Lastly, psittacosis has been associated with ocular mucosa-associated lymphoid tissue lymphoma (this is controversial).

Laboratory studies may reveal toxic granulation with left shift (but no frank neutrophilia), liver enzyme disturbances, and elevated inflammatory markers. Chest x-ray is abnormal in 80% of patients and often shows a lobar consolidation. A normal chest x-ray does not rule out psittacosis. Additional findings will depend on the manifestation (i.e., glomerulonephritis, etc.). Routine blood cultures are unlikely to grow the organism. Culture is not commonly done, as it is difficult to perform, and *C. psittaci* is a laboratory biohazard. Serology is the most common method of diagnosis. Microimmunofluorescence (MIF) is more sensitive and specific than complement fixation. The major drawback to serology is the issue with crossreactivity with other species. Nucleic acid amplification testing (NAAT) allows more rapid and species-specific diagnosis. Unfortunately, most commercial respiratory NAAT panels (i.e., Film-Array panel) do not test for *C. psittaci*. Based on the Centers for Disease Control and Prevention case definition, the diagnosis is typically established in patients presenting with a compatible illness and at least one of the following:

- Isolation of *C. psittaci* from respiratory secretions.
- Positive serology—a four-fold or greater rise in antibody titer between acute and convalescent serum samples (2 weeks apart) to a titer 1:32 or higher. Alternatively, a single IgM titer of 1:16 or greater by MIF may be used.

Additional testing to evaluate the differential diagnosis may include *Legionella* urine antigen, sputum culture, respiratory pathogen panel (i.e., Film-Array), and, as with most cases, screening for HIV and, if applicable, pregnancy.

The treatment of choice is doxycycline for 14 days. An alternative therapy is a macrolide (i.e., azithromycin), especially in pregnant women or children. Clinical improvement is typically seen within 48 hours. Surgery is often necessary for endocarditis, and concurrent treatment should include doxycycline as well (duration is unknown). Because psittacosis is not spread from person to person, only standard precautions are needed when caring for these patients. Treatment of the offending bird (if known) should be considered as well.

The general approach to the management of community-acquired pneumonia is summarized in Fig. 70.1.

L. pneumophila (**option B**) can have a very similar presentation, but the lack of water exposure, the normal *Legionella* urine antigen test, and normal sodium level makes *Legionella* an unlikely cause. In addition, *Legionella* is more commonly seen in older patients who smoke, and the response to treatment of *Legionella* is much slower than that seen with psittacosis. *C. gattii* (**option C**) infection can present with a pneumonia initially and may affect immune-competent hosts. It is less likely to be the cause here, as *C. gattii* infection is typically acquired in the Pacific Northwest United States (to which the patient has not traveled). *C. immitis* (**option D**) can also cause an acute pneumonia and may be associated with meningoencephalitis in certain populations. This infection is typically acquired in the Southwest United States (i.e., Arizona, New Mexico, etc.). The lack of travel to this area makes this infection unlikely in this patient. Influenza virus (**option E**) infection presents very similar to psittacosis. Because the infection in this case occurred in June, influenza would be very unlikely.

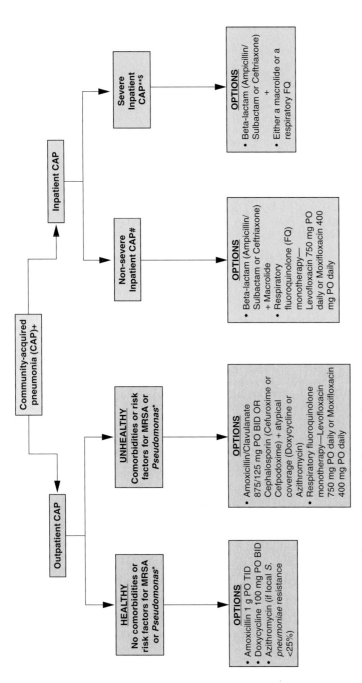

Figure 70.1 – Management of community-acquired pneumonia

MRSA, Methicillin-resistant *Staphylococcus aureus.*

(+) – Typical duration of treatment is 5–7 days (at least 7 days for *Pseudomonas* and MRSA). Anaerobic coverage is only necessary if there is evidence of lung abscess or empyema. Routine anaerobic coverage for aspiration events is not necessary. Steroids should only be used in steroid-responsive situations (i.e., refractory shock, COPD exacerbation, etc.).

(*) – Prior isolation of *methicillin-resistant staphylococcus aureus* (MRSA) or *Pseudomonas,* or hospitalization and receipt of IV antibiotics in the preceding 90 days.

(**) – **Severe CAP requires one or more major criteria or three or more minor criteria**
- Major criteria – septic shock requiring vasopressor or respiratory failure requiring mechanical ventilation
- Minor criteria – respiratory rate >30, PaO2/FiO2 ratio <250, multi-lobar infiltrates, confusion, uremia (BUN>20), leukopenia (WBC count <4K), thrombocytopenia (platelet count <100K), hypothermia (<36 degrees C), hypotension

(#) **Therapy modifications in non-severe inpatient CAP**
- If prior respiratory isolation of MRSA → add MRSA coverage (i.e., Vancomycin or Linezolid) and obtain MRSA nasal PCR and cultures to allow de-escalation
- If prior respiratory isolation of *Pseudomonas* → add *Pseudomonas* coverage (i.e., Piperacillin/Tazobactam, Cefepime) and obtain cultures to allow de-escalation
- If recent hospitalization and IV antibiotics and locally validated risk factors for MRSA → withhold MRSA coverage, obtain cultures and MRSA PCR to guide necessity for coverage (i.e., if PCR negative, withhold coverage; if PCR positive, start coverage and await cultures)
- If recent hospitalization and IV antibiotics and locally validated risk factors for *Pseudomonas* → withhold *Pseudomonas* coverage unless cultures become positive

($) **Therapy modifications in severe inpatient CAP**
- If prior respiratory isolation of MRSA → add MRSA coverage (i.e., Vancomycin or Linezolid) and obtain MRSA nasal PCR and cultures to allow de-escalation
- If prior respiratory isolation of *Pseudomonas* → add *Pseudomonas* coverage (i.e., Piperacillin/Tazobactam, Cefepime) and obtain cultures to allow de-escalation
- If recent hospitalization and IV antibiotics and locally validated risk factors for MRSA → add MRSA coverage (i.e., Vancomycin or Linezolid), obtain cultures and MRSA PCR to guide necessity for coverage
- If recent hospitalization and IV antibiotics and locally validated risk factors for *Pseudomonas* → add *Pseudomonas* coverage and obtain cultures to guide therapy necessity

Community-acquired pneumonia (CAP)+

Outpatient CAP

HEALTHY
No comorbidities or risk factors for MRSA or *Pseudomonas**

OPTIONS
- Amoxicillin 1 g PO TID
- Doxycycline 100 mg PO BID
- Azithromycin (if local *S. pneumoniae* resistance <25%)

UNHEALTHY
Comorbidities or risk factors for MRSA or *Pseudomonas**

OPTIONS
- Amoxicillin/Clavulanate 875/125 mg PO BID OR Cephalosporin (Cefuroxime or Cefpodoxime) + atypical coverage (Doxycycline or Azithromycin)
- Respiratory fluoroquinolone monotherapy—Levofloxacin 750 mg PO daily or Moxifloxacin 400 mg PO daily

Inpatient CAP

Non-severe Inpatient CAP#

OPTIONS
- Beta-lactam (Ampicillin/Sulbactam or Ceftriaxone) + Macrolide
- Respiratory fluoroquinolone (FQ) monotherapy—Levofloxacin 750 mg PO daily or Moxifloxacin 400 mg PO daily

Severe Inpatient CAP$**

OPTIONS
- Beta-lactam (Ampicillin/Sulbactam or Ceftriaxone) + Either a macrolide or a respiratory FQ

KEY LEARNING POINT

Psittacosis should be suspected in a patient presenting with a community-acquired pneumonia and exposure to birds.

REFERENCES AND FURTHER READING

- Dockrell DH, et al. Community-acquired pneumonia. In: *Murray & Nadel's Textbook of Respiratory Medicine*. 7th ed. Elsevier; 2022:600–619.
- Metlay JP, Waterer GW, Long AC, et al. Diagnosis and treatment of adults with community-acquired pneumonia. An official clinical practice guideline of the American Thoracic Society and Infectious Diseases Society of America. *Am J Respir Crit Care Med*. 2019;200(7):e45–e67. https://doi.org/10.1164/rccm.201908-1581ST.
- Stewardson AJ, Grayson ML. Psittacosis. *Infect Dis Clin North Am*. 2010;24(1):7–25. https://doi.org/10.1016/j.idc.2009.10.003.

While doing medical work abroad in Thailand, you see a 50-year-old male who is hospitalized with pneumonia. He initially presented a few days prior with high-grade fevers, cough, pleuritic chest pain, and shortness of breath. He has a history of chronic hepatitis B virus infection complicated by cirrhosis. He does not seek medical care routinely and does not take any medications. He works as a rice farmer. He smokes one pack of cigarettes daily and drinks a "fifth of rum" every few days. He denies any animal exposures. Vital signs reveal temperature 102° F, heart rate 115 beats per minute, blood pressure 90/65 mmHg, respiratory rate 24, and oxygen saturation 94% on 4 L/min oxygen by nasal cannula. On examination, he appears ill. Heart exam reveals regular tachycardia with no murmur. Lung exam shows decreased breath sounds and rales over the right upper lung fields. Abdomen is distended with ascites. A skin lesion is noted over the right forearm (Fig. 71.1). The remainder of the examination is unremarkable. Gram stain of expectorated sputum shows gram-negative bacilli that are oxidase-positive. A chest x-ray is performed (Fig. 71.2).

Which of the following entities is the most likely cause of this patient's presentation?

A. *Mycobacterium tuberculosis.*

B. *Burkholderia pseudomallei.*

C. *Burkholderia mallei.*

D. *Talaromyces marneffei.*

E. Primary lung malignancy.

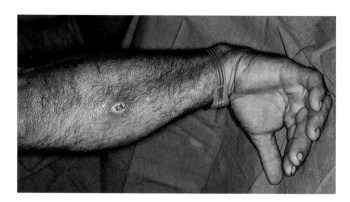

Figure 71.1 – Skin lesion
Bart JC, eds. *Mandell, Douglas, and Bennett's Principles and Practice of Infectious Diseases.* 9th ed. Elsevier; 2020.

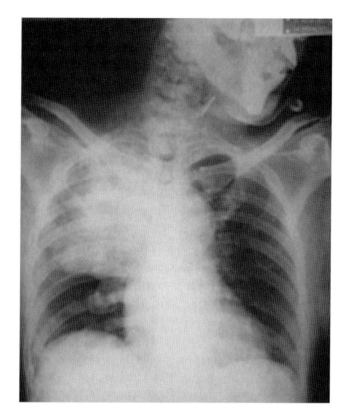

Figure 71.2 – Chest x-ray
Courtesy Sharon J. Peacock and Direk Limmathurotsakul. From Peacock JS, Limmathurotsakul D. Chapter 125 Melioidosis. In: Cohen J, Powderly WG, Opal SM, eds. *Infectious Diseases*. 4th ed. Elsevier; 2017. Figure 125-2A.

The most likely cause is *B. pseudomallei* (**option B**). *B. pseudomallei* is a gram-negative, oxidase-positive, aerobic bacillus that causes an infection known as melioidosis. This organism is endemic to Southeast Asia and Northern Australia. Infections are most likely to occur during rainy seasons and after natural disasters (i.e., tsunamis) because the organism is a water- and soil-dwelling organism. A classic association is with rice paddies and rice farmers. Infection is acquired by inhalation, ingestion, or inoculation of the organism. Certain populations are at risk, including those with chronic comorbidities (i.e., diabetes mellitus, alcoholism, chronic liver disease, chronic lung disease, immunosuppression, thalassemia, etc.).

The incubation period is highly variable and depends on the inoculum, the mode of acquisition, and the type of host. More severe infections occur in those with the aforementioned risk factors ("populations at risk"). Most cases of *B. pseudomallei* infection are asymptomatic. Symptomatic infections present as an acute infection (85% of cases), chronic infection (~10%), or reactivation of latent infection (rare, may occur years later if patients develop risk factors). Acute presentation may include bacteremia with septic shock, pneumonia, and/or lung abscess. Abscesses can form in virtually any organ, including genitourinary organs, hepatosplenic areas, and kidneys. Some patients may have meningoencephalitis and/or focal suppurative central nervous system (CNS) complications. Other manifestations include skin and soft-tissue infections, mycotic aneurysms, and bone/joint infections. Chronic infection (symptoms for >2 months) often presents very similarly to tuberculosis (based on symptoms and imaging). Because of this, melioidosis has been referred to as the "Vietnamese tuberculosis" or the "Vietnamese time-bomb."

The gold standard for diagnosis is microbiologic culture and identification of *B. pseudomallei* from any involved site (i.e., blood, urine, sputum, pus, etc.). If melioidosis is suspected, the microbiology lab should be notified to avoid issues with misidentification and to alert the lab, because *B. pseudomallei* is a biohazard concern. Ashdown's medium is a colistin-containing medium that can be selective for *B. pseudomallei*. Given the disseminated nature of the organism, investigation for additional sites of involvement should be done (i.e., imaging, cultures). Blood cultures will readily grow the organism. PCR can be done, but it is not widely available. Serology is not useful in endemic areas but may be useful in those with no prior exposure.

The initial intensive phase of therapy is typically done with ceftazidime or meropenem. Meropenem is recommended in severe cases (i.e., septic shock). Trimethoprim/sulfamethoxazole (TMP/SMX) can be added if there is involvement of the CNS, bone/joints, skin, or prostate. The intensive phase is given for at least 10 to 14 days (longer in more deep-seated infections). After that, an eradication phase is given for at least 3 months. The drug of choice for eradication is TMP/SMX. Source control should be achieved whenever possible (i.e., drainage of abscesses).

M. tuberculosis (**option A**) infection (tuberculosis) can present similarly to chronic melioidosis infection, but the acute presentation in this case, and gram-stain findings argue against tuberculosis. *B. mallei* (**option C**) is a gram-negative, aerobic, oxidase-positive rod that causes glanders. Glanders is a highly contagious disease that can be acquired from horses, mules, and donkeys. It is also a potential bioterror agent. Glanders can present very similar to melioidosis, but the lack of animal exposure in this case makes glanders unlikely. Treatment of glanders is the same as that for melioidosis. *T. marneffei* (**option D**), formerly *Penicillium marneffei*, is a mycosis that is endemic to Southeast Asia. Infection is typically seen in patients with advanced HIV. Talaromycosis can present similarly to disseminated histoplasmosis, and the skin lesions (umbilicated papules) classically resemble those of molluscum contagiosum or disseminated cryptococcosis. The host and the presentation in this case are not consistent with talaromycosis. Primary lung malignancy (**option E**) could be a consideration in a smoker, but it does not explain the gram stain and skin lesion.

KEY LEARNING POINT

Melioidosis should be suspected in a patient residing in or recently traveling to an endemic region (Southeast Asia or Northern Australia) and presenting with a severe pneumonia.

REFERENCES AND FURTHER READING

- Bennet JE, Dolin R, Blaser MJ, eds. *Mandell, Douglas, and Bennett's Principles and Practice of Infectious Diseases*. 9th ed. Elsevier; 2020.
- Cohen J, et al., eds. *Infectious Diseases*. 4th ed. Elsevier; 2017.
- Thompson GR 3rd, Le T, Chindamporn A, et al. Global guideline for the diagnosis and management of the endemic mycoses: an initiative of the European Confederation of Medical Mycology in cooperation with the International Society for Human and Animal Mycology. *Lancet Infect Dis*. 2021;21(12):e364–e374. https://doi.org/10.1016/S1473-3099(21)00191-2.

A 22-year-old male presents to the emergency room with a 4-day history of fevers, chills, sore throat, and right-sided neck pain. He is otherwise healthy and takes no medications. He has no allergies. Vital signs show temperature 103° F, heart rate 125 beats per minute, blood pressure 95/60 mmHg, respiratory rate 22, and oxygen saturation 92% on room air. On examination, he appears ill. There is no conjunctival injection or sinus tenderness. External ear canals and tympanic membranes appear normal bilaterally. There is pharyngeal erythema with tonsillar enlargement and exudate. Palpation over the anterolateral right neck elicits discomfort. Heart exam shows a regular tachycardia with no murmur. Lung exam shows increased work of breathing but no focal abnormalities. The remainder of the examination is unremarkable. White blood cell count is 16,000 cells/uL (80% neutrophils, 12% band forms). Contrast CT of the neck reveals a filling defect in the right internal jugular vein.

Which of the following best describes the most likely causative organism?

A. An anaerobic gram-positive rod.

B. An anaerobic gram-negative rod.

C. An anaerobic gram-positive coccus.

D. An aerobic, oxidase-positive, gram-negative rod.

E. A branching filamentous gram-positive rod.

The best answer is an anaerobic gram-negative rod (**option B**). This patient's presentation is highly concerning for Lemierre's syndrome. Lemierre's syndrome is a suppurative septic thrombophlebitis of the internal jugular vein that occurs in the setting of *Fusobacterium* spp. (most commonly *Fusobacterium necrophorum*) infection. Fusobacteria are anaerobic gram-negative rods. Rarely, other bacteria may cause this syndrome as well including streptococci, anaerobes, and *Staphylococcus aureus*.

The infection classically develops in healthy young adults in the setting of acute pharyngitis, but it can also develop following otitis, mastoiditis, and dental infections. It classically occurs 1 to 3 weeks after the primary infection. The bacteria invade the pharyngeal mucosa and extend to the neighboring tissues/vasculature to produce septic thrombophlebitis of the internal jugular vein. This thrombophlebitis is often accompanied by bacteremia and septic emboli. Septic embolic most commonly go to the lungs to produce pneumonia, cavitary lesions and/or empyema, but emboli can travel many other places as well (i.e., brain and epidural abscesses, endocarditis, joints, etc.).

The diagnosis requires a high index of suspicion. High fevers and neck pain/tenderness in the setting of recent acute pharyngitis should prompt consideration of Lemierre's syndrome. Contrast CT of the neck and chest is best diagnostic test to detect the jugular venous thrombosis and complications of the infection. CT may show a filling defect in the internal jugular vein (Fig. 72.1), soft-tissue swelling, or enhancement along the vein.

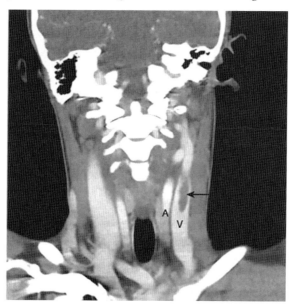

Figure 72.1 – Lemierre's syndrome computed tomography scan *(arrow)* venous thrombosis.
A, Artery; *V*, vein.
Reproduced with permission of the Ochsner Clinic Foundation, 2017. From Harper LK et al: Lemierre syndrome: the forgotten disease. *Ochsner J.* 2016;16(1):7–9.

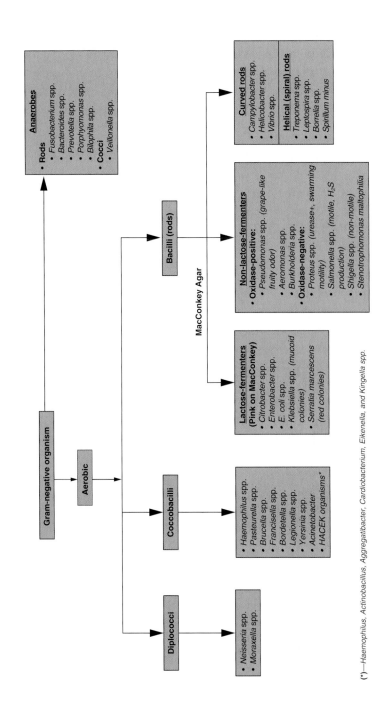

Figure 72.2 – Overview of selected gram-negative bacteria

(*)—*Haemophilus, Actinobacillus, Aggregatibacter, Cardiobacterium, Eikenella, and Kingella spp.*

Ultrasound and MRI are considered alternatives. Imaging of other potential sites may be warranted as well (i.e., MRI brain). Blood cultures (before antibiotics) should be obtained, although the organism may take some time to identify, in light of its anaerobic nature. Culture of the throat and other involved areas (i.e., pleural fluid in empyema) should be obtained as well.

A multidisciplinary approach to management is recommended. Treatment should involve antimicrobials and source control (i.e., drainage of an empyema). Antimicrobial therapy should cover fusobacteria and other oral bacteria (i.e., streptococci, anaerobes, etc.). *F. necrophorum* is intrinsically resistant to macrolides, tetracyclines, and fluoroquinolones. In addition, it may produce beta-lactamases as well. Consequently, initial therapeutic options include ceftriaxone plus metronidazole, piperacillin/tazobactam, or meropenem. If central nervous system (CNS) infection is suspected, then piperacillin/tazobactam should be avoided because it does not have reliable CNS penetration. If using ceftriaxone for CNS infection, then a higher dose may be necessary (i.e., 2 grams IV every 12 hours). Clinical response is characteristically slow, but once the patient has improved and infection has been controlled appropriately, then therapy may be de-escalated to an oral regimen. Treatment duration is typically 3 to 6 weeks. Anticoagulation is controversial but is not unreasonable to use if the clot propagates despite appropriate antibiotic therapy.

An anaerobic gram-positive rod (**option A**) could represent *Actinomyces* spp., *Clostridium* spp., or *Cutibacterium acnes*. An anaerobic gram-positive coccus (**option C**) could represent *Peptostreptococcus* spp. An aerobic, oxidase-positive, gram-negative rod (**option D**) could represent *Pseudomonas* spp., *Aeromonas* spp., or some *Burkholderia* spp. A branching filamentous gram-positive rod (**option E**) could represent either *Actinomyces* spp. or *Nocardia* spp. Fig. 72.2 reviews the microbiologic identification of some common gram-negative bacteria.

KEY LEARNING POINT

The most common cause of Lemierre's syndrome is an anaerobic, gram-negative bacillus (rod) called **Fusobacterium necrophorum.**

REFERENCES AND FURTHER READING

- Cohen J, ed. *Infectious Disease.* 4th ed. Elsevier; 2017.
- Fort GG. Lemierre syndrome. In: *Ferri's Clinical Advisor 2022.* Elsevier; 2022:919.
- Klembczyk K, McAleese S. Microbiology and infectious disease. In: *Harriet Land Handbook.* 22nd ed. Elsevier; 2021:408–446.
- Kuppalli K, Livorsi D, Talati NJ, Osborn M. Lemierre's syndrome due to *Fusobacterium necrophorum. Lancet Infect Dis.* 2012;12(10):808–815. https://doi.org/10.1016/S1473-3099(12)70089-0.
- Lee WS, Jean SS, Chen FL, Hsieh SM, Hsueh PR. Lemierre's syndrome: a forgotten and re-emerging infection. *J Microbiol Immunol Infect.* 2020;53(4):513–517. https://doi.org/10.1016/j.jmii.2020.03.027.

A 40-year-old male is referred to the infectious disease clinic for a positive tuberculosis-interferon gamma release assay (TB-IGRA). He denies fevers, night sweats, weight loss, anorexia, shortness of breath, cough, and hemoptysis. He has no other symptoms. He has no medication allergies. He has a history of chronic HIV infection, for which he takes efavirenz, tenofovir disoproxil fumarate, and emtricitabine (Atripla). He denies any history of liver disease or peripheral neuropathy. He does not drink alcohol. He was born in Sudan and immigrated to the United States 10 years ago. Vital signs are within normal limits. Lungs are clear. The remainder of the examination is within normal limits. HIV viral load (quantitative PCR) was undetectable 6 months prior. CD4 count at that time was 700 cells/μL. Chest x-ray done 1 month prior showed no evidence of active TB.

What is the best initial therapy for this patient?

A. Isoniazid (INH), rifampin, pyrazinamide, and ethambutol.

B. INH for 6 months.

C. INH for 9 months.

D. INH and rifapentine (both weekly) for 3 months.

E. Rifampin for 4 months.

The best initial treatment is once weekly isoniazid (INH) and rifapentine (**option D**). This patient has latent tuberculosis infection (LTBI). LTBI is defined as a positive immune response to TB testing (i.e., positive tuberculin skin test [TST] or IGRA such as the T.SPOT test or the QuantiFERON-Gold) but no evidence of active TB (symptoms, signs, or imaging evidence). Screening for LTBI (with TST or IGRA) is indicated in populations that are either at high risk for LTBI or are at high risk for progression to active TB in the setting of LTBI. These populations include:

- Close contacts of a known pulmonary TB case
- Immigrants (especially in the past 5 years) from areas with a high burden of TB
- Immune-suppressed individuals (i.e., HIV-positive patients, transplant candidates or recipients, patients on tumor necrosis factor alpha [TNF-α] inhibitor treatment, dialysis patients, patients with a history of silicosis, or individuals who are homeless, incarcerated, injection drug users, or healthcare workers).

Patients with a positive screening test (i.e., TST or IGRA) should be evaluated by providers experienced in managing TB. Evaluation should include a detailed review of systems (because TB can affect virtually any organ), medication reconciliation (especially if using rifamycin-based therapy), review of comorbid conditions (i.e., liver disease, alcohol use, etc.), and detailed review of TB risk factors (see earlier). In addition, patients should be asked about prior Bacillus–Calmette–Guerin (BCG) vaccination and prior TB testing. Physical examination should also be very thorough, including the easily overlooked areas such as a detailed lymph node examination and spinal percussion. All patients should be screened for HIV. Women of childbearing age should be screened for pregnancy. Baseline liver function testing (LFT) is often done but is probably most useful for those with baseline liver disease or other risk factors for hepatotoxicity (i.e., alcohol use). Chest x-ray (ideally a posteroanterior/lateral approach) should also be done to look for radiographic evidence of active TB. The approach to the management of a positive TB screening test is shown in Fig. 73.1.

The induration (48–72 hours after placement of TST) cut-off values for a positive TST are summarized in Table 73.1.

Table 73.2 compares the TST and IGRA tests.

The treatment options are shown in Fig. 73.1. Untreated latent TB carries a 5% to 10% lifetime risk of reactivation, and the majority of these events occur in the first few years after

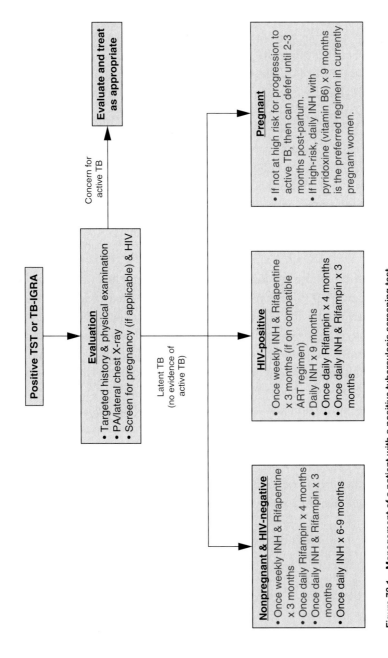

Figure 73.1 – Management of a patient with a positive tuberculosis screening test.
Regimens in red are the preferred regimens. *ART*, antiretroviral therapy; *INH*, Isoniazid; *PA*, posteroanterior; *TB-IGRA*, tuberculosis interferon-gamma release assay (i.e., QuantiFERON-Gold or T.SPOT); *TST*, Tuberculin skin test.

Within the figure:

Positive TST or TB-IGRA

Evaluation
- Targeted history & physical examination
- PA/lateral chest X-ray
- Screen for pregnancy (if applicable) & HIV

Concern for active TB → **Evaluate and treat as appropriate**

Latent TB (no evidence of active TB)

Nonpregnant & HIV-negative
- Once weekly INH & Rifapentine x 3 months
- Once daily Rifampin x 4 months
- Once daily INH & Rifampin x 3 months
- Once daily INH x 6-9 months

HIV-positive
- Once weekly INH & Rifapentine x 3 months (if on compatible ART regimen)
- Daily INH x 9 months
- Once daily Rifampin x 4 months
- Once daily INH & Rifampin x 3 months

Pregnant
- If not at high risk for progression to active TB, then can defer until 2-3 months post-partum.
- If high-risk, daily INH with pyridoxine (vitamin B6) x 9 months is the preferred regimen in currently pregnant women.

Table 73.1 – Induration Cut-Off Values for a Positive Tuberculin Skin Test

≥5 mm	≥10 mm	≥15 mm
• Recent contact with an individual with untreated TB • Fibrotic lesions on chest imaging • Immune-suppressed individuals (i.e., HIV, organ transplant, some malignancies and/or chemotherapy, TNF-α inhibitors, steroids at dose ≥15 mg/day for ≥1 month)	• Recent immigrant (last 5 years) from TB-endemic area • High-risk employee or resident—correctional facility, homeless shelter, nursing home, healthcare facility, mycobacterial lab personnel • Children <5 years of age	• Everyone else

TB, Tuberculosis; *TNF-α*, tumor necrosis factor alpha.

Table 73.2 – Tuberculin Skin Test and Interferon Gamma Release Assay Compared

Factor	Tuberculin Skin Test	Interferon Gamma Release Assay
Description	• Subcutaneous injection (typically in the anterior forearm) of a purified protein derivative (PPD) from heat-killed cultures of *Mycobacterium tuberculosis* • The size of induration (not erythema) in millimeters is read after 48–72 hours (see Table 73.1)	• Common types—T.SPOT and QuantiFERON Gold • Blood tests that measure interferon-gamma released from memory T-cells stimulated by previously encountered *M. tuberculosis* antigens • Results may be positive, negative, or indeterminate/uninterpretable
Preferred use	• Children <5 years of age (because these children have high rates of uninterpretable interferon gamma release assay [IGRA] results)	• Prior Bacillus–Calmette–Guerin (BCG) vaccination • Patients with high risk of being lost to follow-up (i.e., would not return to have tuberculin skin test [TST] read)
False positives	• **Prior BCG vaccination** (if >10 years since BCG vaccine, then a positive TST should not be attributed to BCG) • **Nontuberculous mycobacterial (NTM) infections** • **Allergic reaction** (immediate hypersensitivity) to PPD • **Boosting phenomenon** (seen with prior remote *M. tuberculosis* infection) • **Technical issues**—incorrect interpretation, etc.	• **Some NTM infections**—*M. marinum, M. szulgai, M. kansasii,* and *M. flavescens* • **IGRA boosting phenomenon (related to prior TST)**—avoid by obtaining IGRA within 3 days of TST or 3 months after TST • **IGRA conversion seen with serial testing**—defined as conversion from negative to positive within 2 years of last test • **Technical issues**
False negatives	• **Recent tuberculosis (TB) infection**—may need to repeat test in 8–10 weeks • **Overwhelming TB infection** • **Immune suppression** • **Recent live virus vaccination** • **Natural waning of immunity**	• **Same as for TST**

M, Mycobacterium.

the infection. This number is substantially higher in immune-compromised individuals. Treatment for latent TB is highly effective at preventing the emergence of active TB. The choice of therapy will depend on patient preference and comorbid conditions (including HIV and pregnancy status). The dosing and adverse effects of the chosen regimen should always be discussed with patients (and always let the patient know about the red-orange bodily fluid discoloration seen with rifamycin therapy). In addition, the signs and symptoms of active TB and liver injury (a common adverse effect with all the drugs used to treat LTBI) should be discussed. The local department of public health may be helpful for ongoing monitoring and may provide the medications at reduced (or no) cost. Patients who are started on LTBI treatment should be seen routinely to assess medication adherence and adverse effects. Lab testing is not routinely necessary unless otherwise clinically indicated. LFTs should only be checked in those with abnormal baseline LFTs or those at risk for hepatotoxicity. If patients develop symptoms or signs of active TB, then an appropriate evaluation for active TB (i.e., chest x-ray, sputum analysis, etc.) should be done.

INH, rifampin, pyrazinamide, and ethambutol (**option A**) is the initial regimen for active TB. This patient does not have active TB, so it would not be an appropriate treatment. INH for 6 months (**option B**) is not recommended in HIV patients. In HIV patients, INH should be given for 9 months. INH for 9 months (**option C**) can be used, but it can be difficult to take and tolerate for the required duration. Weekly INH plus rifapentine has been shown to be noninferior to INH in HIV patients who are not on antiretroviral therapy (ART). This regimen is easier to take and may have a higher treatment completion rate. In light of this, it can be given safely in patients on ART with a raltegravir- or efavirenz-based regimen. Rifampin for 4 months (**option E**) is not recommended in individuals with HIV due to lack of data. In addition, rifampin has many drug-drug interactions that make it difficult to take with ART. It should only be used if there is no available alternative.

An all-too-common situation in the management of LTBI is the issue of the non-HIV immune-compromised patient (i.e., transplant candidates, patients on biologic therapy, etc.). The transplant candidate with LTBI should ideally be treated before transplant (similar regimens can be used as for non-HIV, nonpregnant individuals), because rifamycin-based therapy is very difficult to give post-transplant (due to drug-drug interactions). Post-transplant, INH may be the best choice. If a patient requiring biologic therapy (usually a TNF-α antagonist) is found to have LTBI, then treatment should be provided prior to starting the biologic. The American College of Rheumatology recommends that patients be on at least 1 month of LTBI treatment prior to starting or resuming the biologic. If there is a choice in TNF-α therapy, then etanercept may have the lowest risk of TB reactivation.

KEY LEARNING POINT

In HIV-positive patients on certain antiretroviral therapy regimens (i.e., raltegravir- or efavirenz-based regimen), the combination of isoniazid and rifapentine (each given once weekly) is as effective as isoniazid monotherapy but is much easier to complete.

REFERENCES AND FURTHER READING

- Godfrey MS, Friedman LN. Tuberculosis and biologic therapies: anti-tumor necrosis factor-α and beyond. *Clin Chest Med.* 2019;40(4):
721–739. https://doi.org/10.1016/j.ccm.2019.07.003.
- Huaman MA, Sterling TR. Treatment of latent tuberculosis infection—an update. *Clin Chest Med.* 2019;
40(4):839–848. https://doi.org/10.1016/j.ccm.2019.07.008.
- Snow KJ, Bekkar A, Huang GK, Graham SM. Tuberculosis in pregnant women and neonates: a meta-review of current evidence. *Paediatr Respir Rev.* 2020;36:27–32. https://doi.org/10.1016/j.prrv.2020.02.001.
- Orazulike N, Sharma JB, Sharma S, Umeora OUJ. Tuberculosis (TB) in pregnancy—a review. *Eur J Obstet Gynecol Reprod Biol.* 2021;259:167–177. https://doi.org/10.1016/j.ejogrb.2021.02.016.
- Yoon C. Positive screening test for tuberculosis. In. *Murray & Nadel's Textbook of Respiratory Medicine.* 7th ed. Elsevier; 2022:559–568.

A 35-year-old male is referred to the infectious disease clinic for evaluation of recurrent fevers. The fevers started 3 weeks ago, and they can get as high as 104° F. He notes that the week prior to the fever onset he was staying at a cabin in the woods of Cascades National Park in Washington for a hiking trip. The initial fever lasted a few days and was associated with rigors, myalgias, headaches, and nausea. He denies ever having a rash or joint swelling. Since the initial fever, he has had these same symptoms occurring once a week and lasting for a couple days at a time. In between fever episodes, he says he feels fine. He has seen multiple doctors over this time and has not received a definitive diagnosis. He does not consume unpasteurized dairy and denies any large animal (i.e., farm animal) exposures. He feels well today. Vital signs reveal temperature 98° F, heart rate 80 beats per minute, blood pressure 120/80 mmHg, and respiratory rate 16. He appears well overall. There is no icterus. Heart and lung exam are normal. A spleen tip is felt below the left costal margin. There is no spinal tenderness, joint swelling, lymphadenopathy, or rash. Review of recent laboratory studies has shown platelet count as low as 30,000 cells/µL, hemoglobin as low as 9 g/dL, normal white blood cell count, and mildly elevated transaminases (less than three times the upper limit of normal). Lactate dehydrogenase and haptoglobin levels have been normal.

What is the most likely diagnosis?

A. Adult-onset Still disease.

B. Tick-borne relapsing fever (TBRF).

C. Louse-borne relapsing fever (LBRF).

D. Brucellosis.

E. Babesiosis.

The most likely diagnosis is TBRF (**option B**). Endemic TBRF is caused by various *Borrelia* spp. that are transmitted by *Ornithodoros* soft ticks. This infection is found almost world-wide (excluding Australia and Antarctica). In the United States, infection is most often acquired in the highlands (i.e., mountains) of the Western United States (Rocky Mountains distribution) in association with old wood cabins that are often rodent-infested.

The incubation period is 3 to 18 days. Patients initially present with a febrile influenza-like illness (i.e., high fevers, rigors, myalgias, etc.). The febrile episodes often last a few days (and are associated with rigors and sweats) and then remit for approximately 1 week. This pattern repeats several times, but each subsequent episode is less severe. The fever pattern is explained by the fact that the organism changes its surface antigen approximately every 7 days (antigenic variation). Associated manifestations may include gastrointestinal symptoms, hepatosplenomegaly, bleeding, an erythematous or petechial skin rash, acute respiratory distress syndrome, neurologic dysfunction (i.e., lymphocytic meningitis resembling Lyme disease, cranial neuropathies, paresthesia, etc.), and ocular inflammation (i.e., iritis, optic neuritis, etc.). Rarely, patients can develop myocarditis. Laboratory studies may reveal anemia, thrombocytopenia, and/or elevated transaminases.

The diagnosis is made by examination of Wright–Giemsa–stained peripheral blood smears, particularly during a febrile episode. An example of a positive smear is shown in Fig. 74.1.

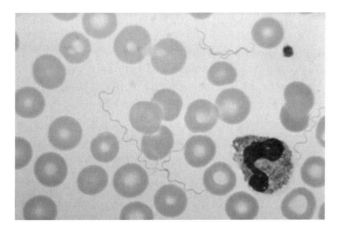

Figure 74.1 – *Borrelia recurrentis* on blood smear
Warrell DA. Chapter 131 Relapsing fever. In: Cohen J, Powderly WG, Opal SM, eds. *Infectious Diseases*. 4th ed. Elsevier; 2017. Copyright David A. Warrell.

A negative blood smear does not rule out the diagnosis, as the test is only approximately 70% sensitive. Alternatively, the diagnosis can be made by serology (acute and convalescent samples needed) or PCR. Differential diagnosis can be broad, but considerations in the United States include (but are not limited to) other tick-borne illnesses (i.e., Colorado tick fever), leptospirosis, tularemia, and rat-bite fever.

Treatment for TBRF depends on whether the central nervous system (CNS) is involved or not. If there is no CNS involvement, then either doxycycline (or tetracycline) or erythromycin can be given for 10 days. If the CNS is involved, then treatment should be intravenous penicillin-G or intravenous ceftriaxone for 10 to 14 days. Treatment is associated with a severe, potentially life-threatening Jarisch–Herxheimer reaction; thus, post-treatment observation is necessary. The treatment for this reaction is supportive, and pre-treatment with steroids is not helpful.

Epidemic LBRF (**option C**) is caused by *Borrelia recurrentis*, which is spread by the human body louse (*Pediculus humanus*). This infection is typically seen in poor socioeconomic areas or in times of war or famine. It is endemic to parts of Africa (South Sudan, Somalia, Ethiopia), Yemen, Peru, and Bolivia. LBRF is often more severe than TBRF and also carries a higher rate of mortality. It presents similarly to TBRF, but these patients more commonly get bleeding, bruising, jaundice, shock, hepatosplenomegaly, and CNS involvement. Patients with LBRF tend to have fewer relapses than those with TBRF. Treatment involves a single dose of tetracycline or erythromycin. Treatment is associated with a severe, potentially life-threatening Jarisch–Herxheimer reaction (more common than with TBRF); thus, post-treatment observation is necessary.

Adult-onset Still disease (**option A**) is a relatively rare inflammatory disorder characterized by high-grade fevers, pharyngitis, lymphadenopathy, arthritis, hepatosplenomegaly, and a classic evanescent, salmon-colored truncal rash. Patients often have a marked leukocytosis and a strikingly elevation serum ferritin. Still disease is unlikely, because many of the clinical features of Still disease are not seen in this case. Brucellosis (**option D**) can cause a protracted febrile illness, but the lack of animal exposure or consumption of unpasteurized dairy makes this diagnosis less likely. Babesiosis (**option E**) is unlikely in this case because babesiosis typically occurs in the northeast and upper midwest United States. In addition, the lack of hemolysis argues against babesiosis.

Table 74.1 summarizes some common vector-borne infectious diseases.

Table 74.1 – Vector-Borne Diseases

Vector or Exposure	Association
Hard ticks	• *Borrelia burgdorferi* (Lyme disease), various *Rickettsia* spp. (i.e., Rocky Mountain spotted fever, African tick-bite fever, etc.), *Babesia* spp., *Anaplasma phagocytophilum, Ehrlichia* spp., *Borrelia miyamotoi* (hard-tick relapsing fever), *Francisella tularensis* (tularemia), Colorado tick fever, Heartland virus, Powassan virus
Soft ticks	• *Borrelia* spp. (endemic tick-borne relapsing fever), arboviruses
Chiggers	• *Orientia tsutsugamushi* (scrub typhus)
Mites	• *Rickettsia akari* (rickettsial pox), scabies
Lice	• *Bartonella quintana* (trench fever), *Rickettsia prowazekii* (epidemic typhus), *Borrelia recurrentis* (epidemic louse-borne relapsing fever)
Fleas	• *Yersinia pestis* (plague), *Rickettsia typhi* (murine [endemic] typhus), *Rickettsia felis* (flea-borne spotted fever), *Bartonella henselae* (cat-scratch disease), *Tunga penetrans* (tungiasis)
Reduviid (triatomine) bug	• *Trypanosoma cruzi* (Chagas disease)
Mosquitos	• *Anopheles*—*Plasmodium* spp. (malaria), *Wuchereria bancrofti* and *Brugia* spp. (lymphatic filariasis), arboviruses • *Aedes*—chikungunya, Zika, dengue, yellow fever • *Culex*—West Nile virus
Tsetse flies	• *Trypanosoma brucei* spp. (African trypanosomiasis, sleeping sickness)
Sand flies	• *Leishmania* spp. (leishmaniasis), *Bartonella bacilliformis* (Oroya fever)
Horse flies or deer flies	• *Francisella tularensis* (tularemia), *Loa Loa* (filariasis)
Black flies	• *Onchocerca volvulus* (onchocerciasis, river blindness), *Mansonella ozzardi* (mansonelliasis)

KEY LEARNING POINT

Tick-borne relapsing fever should be suspected in patients presenting with a prolonged/recurrent febrile illness after exposure to rodent-infested areas (classically wood cabins) in the Western United States.

REFERENCES AND FURTHER READING

• Berenger JM, Parola P. Arthropod vectors of medical importance. In: Cohen J, et al., eds. *Infectious Diseases*. 4th ed. Elsevier; 2017:104–112.
• Horton J. Relapsing fever caused by *Borrelia species*. In: Bennet JE, Dolin R, Blaser MJ, eds. *Mandell, Douglas, and Bennett's Principles and Practice of Infectious Diseases*. 9th ed. Elsevier; 2020:2906–2910.
• Warrell D. Relapsing fevers. In: Cohen J, et al., eds. *Infectious Diseases*. 4th ed. Elsevier; 2017:1105–1109.

A 60-year-old male is referred to the infectious disease clinic for evaluation of fever. He has intermittently been experiencing fevers and fatigue for the past 2 months. Associated symptoms have included myalgias and occasional headaches. He has seen his primary care provider several times without a diagnosis. Work-up to date has shown:

- Hemoglobin—10 g/dL
- Platelet count—460,000 cells/uL
- White blood cell count—10,000 cells/uL (60% neutrophils, 30% lymphocytes)
- Normal renal, hepatic function, and urinalysis with microscopy
- C-reactive protein—10 mg/dL (normal <0.8 mg/dL)
- Erythrocyte sedimentation rate—65 mm/h (normal 0–15 mm/h)
- HIV p24 antigen/antibody test—negative
- Three sets of blood cultures—no growth after 5 days
- Chest x-ray—normal

- Respiratory film array (including SARS CoV-2)—negative
- Tuberculosis QuantiFERON—negative
- Epstein–Barr virus–specific-serology—consistent with past infection
- Ferritin—500 ng/mL (normal <336 ng/mL)
- Thyroid-stimulating hormone—normal
- Rheumatoid factor—normal
- Antinuclear antibody—normal
- Creatine kinase—normal
- Lactate dehydrogenase—normal

He has not received any antibiotics or steroids. He has taken acetaminophen and ibuprofen, which have provided only minimal relief of his symptoms. He is otherwise healthy and does not take any medications. He denies family history of infections, malignancy, or autoimmune disease. He lives in Illinois with his wife. He works as a lawyer. He denies any recent travel or known sick contacts. He does not have any pets and denies animal exposure. He does not spend much time outdoors. He does not consume unpasteurized dairy. He is sexually active with his wife. He denies any prior tuberculosis exposures. He drinks a glass of wine with dinner most days of the week. He does not smoke, vape, or use illicit drugs. Vital signs are within normal limits except for a temperature of 101° F. He looks well overall. There is no scalp tenderness, icterus, or conjunctival injection. Conjunctiva is slightly pale. Ear, nose, and mouth exam is normal. There is no palpable lymphadenopathy. There is tenderness to palpation over the shoulders bilaterally. Heart and lung exams are normal. There is no hepatosplenomegaly, joint swelling, or skin rash. The remainder of the examination is unremarkable. The patient says he "wants you to be straight with him and tell him what he can expect with this illness."

Which of the following responses is most appropriate?

A. You most likely have a rare illness that we have yet to diagnose.

B. The longer you have fevers without a diagnosis, the more likely you are to have a serious illness with poor prognosis.

C. The longer you have fevers without a diagnosis, the less likely you are to have an infection.

D. It is very uncommon for patients to go undiagnosed when they have fevers this long.

E. I don't know what is going on, but maybe we could try an antibiotic to see how you respond.

Table 75.1 – Etiologies of Fever of Unknown Origin

Etiology	More Common	Less Common
Infection	• Viral infections—Epstein–Barr virus, cytomegalovirus, HIV, respiratory viruses (esp. COVID) • Endovascular infections (i.e., endocarditis) • Intra-abdominal abscesses • Osteomyelitis (especially vertebral and mandibular) • Tuberculosis	• Typhoid fever • Malaria • Cat-scratch disease (*Bartonella henselae*) • Toxoplasmosis • Brucellosis • Q fever • Tick-borne illness • Endemic mycoses (esp. histoplasmosis)
Malignancy	• Leukemia • Lymphoma • Renal cell carcinoma	• Multiple myeloma • Hepatocellular carcinoma • Liver metastases • Atrial myxoma
Inflammatory	• Adult-onset Still's disease • Giant cell (temporal) arteritis ± polymyalgia rheumatica	• Systemic lupus erythematosus • Polyarteritis nodosa • Sarcoidosis • Crohn disease
Miscellaneous	• Idiopathic • Drug fever • Alcoholic hepatitis	• Factitious fever • Hyperthermia syndromes • Endocrinopathy—adrenal insufficiency, pheochromocytoma, thyrotoxicosis • Periodic fever syndromes

The most appropriate response is **option C**. This patient is presenting with a fever of unknown origin (FUO). The contemporary definition of FUO includes:

- Temperature greater than 101° F (38.3° C) that lasts at least 3 weeks, and
- No diagnosis despite 3 days of inpatient stay/work-up or at least two outpatient visits

FUO has many causes, and the relative frequency of each cause varies between sources. Approximately 20% of cases are idiopathic (which is why **option D** is incorrect). Some of the more common etiologies of FUO (in all comers) are shown in Table 75.1. Please note that this list is not an exhaustive list by any means.

A detailed discussion of each of these etiologies is beyond the scope of this book. There are additional rarer etiologies that are not discussed here. More detailed explanations can be found in the references later.

The overall approach to the evaluation of FUO is summarized in Fig. 75.1.

A few generalizations about the approach to FUO are worth noting:

- Before committing to an evaluation of FUO, it is important to confirm that the patient meets criteria for FUO and that they actually have fevers measured objectively. This can often be clarified based on the history and review of prior visits.

- The medical history and physical examination (H&P) are arguably the most important parts of the evaluation for FUO. The H&P and clinical circumstances (see "Additional Evaluation" box in Fig. 75.1) should guide the subsequent evaluation and management. AVOID just using a shotgun approach!

- Important aspects of the medical history include fever characteristics (onset, pattern, duration, etc.), associated symptoms, a detailed general review of systems, review of medications (including supplements, herbals, etc.), family history, and a comprehensive social history. A useful mnemonic for the social history in infectious disease is **HE IS TOAST**:

    - **H**—HIV (exposure or prior testing)
    - **E**—Environmental exposure (i.e., hiking, etc.)
    - **I**—Ingestions (i.e., unpasteurized dairy)
    - **S**—Substance abuse (vaping, alcohol, illicit drugs)
    - **T**—Travel history
    - **O**—Occupation
    - **A**—Animal exposures (humans, large animals, pets, and critters like ticks and mosquitos)
    - **S**—Sexual history
    - **T**—Tuberculosis (TB) risk factors—prior TB exposure, prior TB testing, homelessness, incarceration, healthcare work, etc.

- Easily overlooked aspects of the physical examination include the lymph node exam, dermatologic exam (including the hair and nails), joint exam (including spinal percussion), and genital exam.

- Patients with a prolonged, undiagnosed FUO are more likely to have a benign and/or noninfectious etiology. This is why **option C** is correct and **option B** is incorrect.

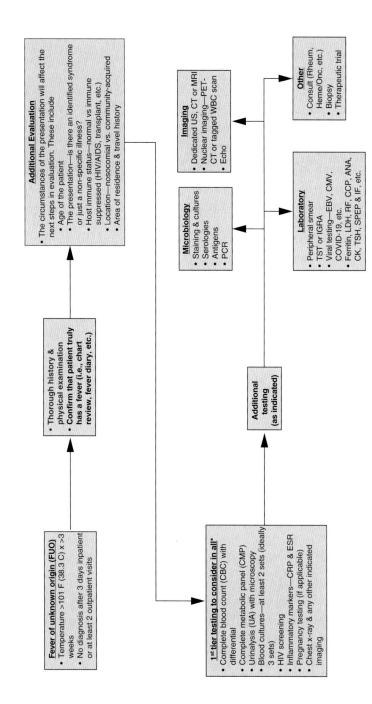

Figure 75.1 – Approach to fever of unknown origin. *Most of these should already have been done, but need to verify. ANA, Antinuclear antibody; CCP, cyclic citrullinated peptide; CK, creatine kinase; CMV, cytomegalovirus; COVID-19, novel coronavirus disease 2019; CRP, C-reactive protein; EBV, Epstein-Barr virus; ESR, erythrocyte sedimentation rate; IF, immunofixation; IGRA, interferon gamma release assay; LDH, lactate dehydrogenase; PCR, polymerase chain reaction; RF, rheumatoid factor; SPEP, serum protein electrophoresis; TSH, thyroid-stimulating hormone; TST, tuberculin skin test.*

- An atypical or uncommon presentation of a common illness is much more likely than any presentation of a rare illness. This is why **option A** is incorrect.

- Do not routinely administer antibiotics to "see what happens" or to make yourself feel better (**option E**). This approach may cloud the diagnostic work-up and put the patient at risk for adverse effects without really gaining much. Antibiotics should only be considered if the patient is severely ill (i.e., hemodynamically unstable) or there is strong clinical evidence of an infection.

- Do not routinely administer steroids unless there is a clear indication for steroids (i.e., refractory shock, clear-cut steroid-responsive inflammatory disorder). Although steroids may be helpful to manage some symptoms, they may cloud the diagnostic process as well (i.e., suppress fever, decrease yield of biopsy in cases of lymphoma, etc.).

- A trial of naproxen may differentiate infection (fever does not respond to naproxen) from malignancy (rapid decline in fever with naproxen), although this is not perfect by any means (studies are weak and mixed).

- Age-appropriate malignancy screening should always be considered.

KEY LEARNING POINT

The longer a patient with fever of unknown origin goes undiagnosed, the less likely they are to have an infectious cause (i.e., prognosis is generally favorable).

REFERENCES AND FURTHER READING

- Cunha BA. Fever of unknown origin: clinical overview of classic and current concepts. *Infect Dis Clin North Am.* 2007;21(4):867-915, vii. https://doi.org/10.1016/j.idc.2007.09.002. Erratum in: *Infect Dis Clin North Am.* 2008 Jun;22(2):xv.
- Cunha BA. Fever of unknown origin: focused diagnostic approach based on clinical clues from the history, physical examination, and laboratory tests. *Infect Dis Clin North Am.* 2007;21(4):1137–1187, xi. https://doi.org/10.1016/j.idc.2007.09.004.
- Hayakawa K, Ramasamy B, Chandrasekar PH. Fever of unknown origin: an evidence-based review. *Am J Med Sci.* 2012;344(4):307–316. https://doi.org/10.1097/MAJ.0b013e31824ae504.
- Wright WF. Fever of unknown origin. In: Bennet JE, Dolin R, Blaser MJ, eds. *Mandell, Douglas, and Bennett's Principles and Practice of Infectious Diseases.* 9th ed. Elsevier; 2020.

A 40-year-old male presents to the HIV clinic for follow-up. For the past 2 months, he has felt unwell. He complains of fevers, malaise, anorexia, weight loss, and unresolving skin lesions. He has a history of poorly-controlled HIV related to poor adherence to antiretroviral therapy (ART). At the last visit 9 months ago, his CD4 count was 70 cells/uL (6% CD4 cells). He does not take any medications and has no medication allergies. Vital signs reveal temperature 100.8° F. The remaining vital signs are within normal limits. On examination, he appears malnourished. Skin examination is shown in Fig. 76.1.

A biopsy of the lesion reveals vascular proliferation with predominant neutrophilic infiltration. Warthin–Starry silver stain shows dark-appearing organisms. Fungal and acid-fast stains are negative. What is the next best step in the management of this patient?

A. Doxycycline.

B. Chemotherapy.

C. Restart antiretroviral therapy.

D. Itraconazole.

E. Isoniazid, rifampin, pyrazinamide, and ethambutol.

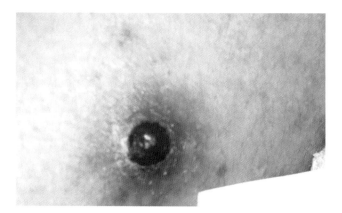

Figure 76.1 – Skin examination
Rolain J, Raoult D. Chapter 299 Bartonella infections. In: Goldman L, Schafer AI, eds. *Goldman-Cecil Medicine*. 26th ed. Elsevier; 2020.

The best next step in management is doxycycline (**option A**). This patient most likely has bacillary angiomatosis (BA), which is typically caused by *Bartonella henselae* (and less commonly *Bartonella quintana*).

Bartonella spp. are fastidious, pleomorphic, gram-negative coccobacilli that are best visualized with the Warthin–Starry Silver stain (Fig. 76.2). There are many different *Bartonella* species, and the manifestations of *Bartonella* infections depend on the host immune status and the infecting species. The more common species are summarized in Table 76.1.

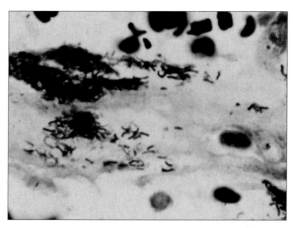

Figure 76.2 – Warthin–Starry stain
Koehler J. *Bartonella* infections in HIV-infected individuals. In: *Sande's HIV/AIDS Medicine*. 2nd ed. Elsevier; 2012:421–432. Reprinted with permission from Elsevier. Steed D, Collins J, et al., Haemophagocytic lymphohistiocytosis associated with bartonella peliosis hepatis following kidney transplantation in a patient with HIV. *Lancet Infect Dis*. 2022; 10:e303–e309.

Table 76.1 – *Bartonella* Infections

Species	Epidemiology	Disease Association(s)
B. henselae	• Acquired by cat bite or scratch • Vector—cat flea	• Cat-scratch disease • Bacillary angiomatosis (BA) • Peliosis hepatis • Culture-negative endocarditis
B. quintana	• Vector—human body louse	• Trench fever • Less common cause of BA • Culture-negative endocarditis
B. bacilliformis	• Vector—sand fly • Acquired in higher elevations of Peru, Ecuador, and Colombia	• Oroya fever—acute Carrion disease • Peruvian warts ("verruga peruana")—chronic Carrion disease

Infections may be acute or chronic in nature. Table 76.2 summarizes the various manifestations of *Bartonella* infections, including their diagnosis and management.

Chemotherapy (**option B**) would be an appropriate consideration in the management of Kaposi sarcoma (KS). KS can present very similar to BA, but the biopsy in KS more commonly shows a lymphoplasmacytic infiltrate. Restarting antiretroviral therapy (**option C**) should be done, but starting doxycycline is more important. In most cases, ART can be started right away, but if there is concern for detrimental effects from immune-reconstitution inflammatory syndrome, as could occur with neurologic *Bartonella* infections, ART start should be delayed for a few weeks. Itraconazole (**option D**) would be a good choice for a patient with disseminated fungal infection (i.e., *Cryptococcus* and endemic mycoses most commonly). These infections can cause skin lesions in disseminated infection, but the appearance and biopsy in this case are not consistent. Umbilicated papules can be seen with molluscum contagiosum, disseminated cryptococcosis, and talaromycosis. Verrucous lesions are classically seen with blastomycosis. Isoniazid, rifampin, pyrazinamide, and ethambutol (**option E**) would be the regimen of choice for cutaneous tuberculosis (TB). Cutaneous TB has various morphologies, but the biopsy findings in this case are not supportive of this diagnosis.

ADVANCED HIV (AIDS) EVALUATION

Generally speaking, advanced HIV patients present to the hospital (often due to development of an opportunistic infection [OI]) in one of two ways:

- New diagnosis of HIV that the patient was not aware of
- Worsening of known HIV infection, most commonly due to poor adherence to ART

Infectious disease specialists are often consulted in these cases. Therefore, it is worth knowing how to approach these patients. The following are some important considerations.

Important elements of the history

- A detailed review of systems should be performed, because these patients are at risk for diseases involving virtually any body system (see Table 76.3). In addition, they can have more than one process going on at any given time (i.e., Occam's razor does not apply)

Table 76.2 – Manifestations of *Bartonella* Infections

Manifestation	Presentation	Diagnosis[a]	Management[c]
Oroya fever	• Incubation 1–3 months • Flu-like illness + hemolytic anemia • May get meningoencephalitis and superinfection (esp. *Salmonella* spp.)	• Microscopy (Giemsa-stained peripheral blood smear) to detect intraerythrocytic organisms	• High mortality if untreated • Ciprofloxacin + ceftriaxone for 14 days • If more severe → chloramphenicol + ceftriaxone for 14 days
Trench fever	• Incubation 2–3 weeks • Typically homeless patients • Fevers (often fever of unknown origin), headache, bone pain • Can be severe and protracted	• Culture, PCR, or microscopy	• Doxycycline for 28 days + gentamicin for 14 days • Alternative to gentamicin is rifampin for 14 days
Cat-scratch disease (CSD)	• History of cat bite or scratch (especially kittens) • Papulopustular skin lesions develop ~1 week postexposure, and then 1–3 weeks later patients get regional lymphadenitis • May get bacteremia or endocarditis, erythema nodosum, neuroretinitis, encephalitis or various musculoskeletal manifestations (i.e., osteomyelitis), granulomatous hepatosplenic lesions, etc.	• Serology[b]—IgG by immunofluorescence (IF) ≥1:256 strongly suggestive	• Azithromycin (Z-pak) for 5 days • Lymphadenopathy may take several months to resolve despite treatment • If disseminated (i.e., hepatosplenic, neurologic, etc.) → doxycycline (or azithromycin) + rifampin for 4–6 weeks
Bacteremia and endocarditis (typically subacute)	• Often have preexisting valvular disease • Fever and vegetations seen in 90% • Often have glomerulonephritis (anti-PR3 or C-ANCA vasculitis), which limits use of gentamicin in treatment	• Immunohistochemistry (IHC; Warthin–Starry stain) of valve tissue • Serology[b]—IgG by IF ≥1:256 (often ≥1:800) • Transesophageal echo	• Valve surgery often necessary • Doxycycline + gentamicin for 2 weeks, then doxycycline alone for: • 4 weeks (if bacteremia but no endocarditis) • 6 weeks (if endocarditis + valve replacement) • 3 months (if no valve replacement) • Alternative to gentamicin is rifampin • Serial serology may help to determine treatment end-point
Neurologic and ophthalmic	• Oculoglandular (Parinaud) syndrome—conjunctivitis and preauricular lymphadenopathy • Meningoencephalitis • Neuroretinitis	• Culture or PCR	• (Doxycycline or azithromycin) + rifampin • 4–6 weeks' duration in most cases

(Continued)

Table 76.2 – Manifestations of *Bartonella* Infections *(Cont'd)*

Manifestation	Presentation	Diagnosis[a]	Management[c]
Peliosis hepatis (PH)	• Typically seen in immune-compromised patients (i.e., advanced HIV/AIDS, etc.) • Multiple blood-filled (vascular proliferation) cystic lesions in the liver, spleen, bone marrow, and abdominal nodes	• IHC • Imaging (Fig. 76.3— hypodense liver lesions on CT)	**Treatment of *Bartonella* infections in immune-compromised patients:** • Doxycycline or azithromycin • If disseminated or severe infection, then add rifampin and may need longer treatment • Rifampin may be difficult to tolerate with antiretroviral therapy or immune-suppressant medications • Duration = at least 3 months • BA responds quickly, whereas PH responds very slowly • If relapse occurs after initial treatment course, then retreat (often for longer duration) and consider long-term prophylaxis (HIV—continue until CD4 >200 cells/uL for ≥6 months)
Bacillary angiomatosis (BA)	• Typically seen in immune-compromised patients (i.e., advanced HIV/AIDS, etc.) • Skin lesions (red-purple papule or nodule) resembling Kaposi sarcoma (KS). May involve viscera as well	• Biopsy with IHC—will show inflammation (macrophages, neutrophils) and vascular proliferation, with staining showing organisms • Rule out KS	
Verruga peruana	• Angioproliferative cutaneous tumors (may bleed easily)	• PCR or IHC	• Azithromycin for 7–14 days • Alternatives—ciprofloxacin for 14 days or rifampin for 3–4 weeks
SENLAT	• Stands for "scalp eschar with neck lymphadenopathy" • Associated with tick bite	• PCR or IHC	• Treat like CSD

[a]Culture can be used for most manifestations, but the organism can be difficult and time-consuming to isolate. In addition, PCR can be very useful for all of these manifestations.

[b]Serology may be limited by crossreactivity with other *Bartonella* spp. In addition, it can take several weeks to develop antibodies, so convalescent sample may be necessary.

[c]In immune-compromised individuals (i.e., HIV/AIDS, transplant), treatment duration should always be at least 3 months.

- If the patient was on ART before, then the details of the regimen should be clarified. These may include the specific drugs/regimens that the patient has taken, the rationale for changing regimens or for poor adherence, and prior resistance testing (and timing in relation to the ART)

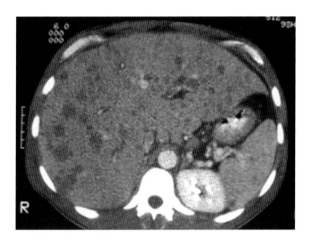

Figure 76.3 – Peliosis hepatis on computed tomography scan
Reproduced with permission from Koehler JE, Tappero JW. Bacillary angiomatosis and bacillary peliosis in patients infected with human immunodeficiency virus. *Clin Infect Dis.* 1993;17:612–624.

- Prior use of pre-exposure prophylaxis (PrEP)

- Prior history of OIs and associated prophylaxis and treatments. Prior history of sexually transmitted infections and associated treatment specifics

- Detailed social history as discussed in case 75 ("HE IS TOAST" mnemonic). Patients with HIV have a high incidence of substance abuse, mental health disorders, and other socioeconomic issues that affect their care

Important elements of the physical examination

- A thorough head-to-toe physical examination should be performed

- Most patients with advanced HIV will appear cachectic (i.e., loss of muscle mass, temporal wasting, etc.)

- Look closely for findings suggestive of the diseases discussed in Table 76.3

- Do not forget the lymph node and genital examinations

Ancillary data considerations

- AIDS is defined by a CD4 count <200 cells/uL (or <14%) or the presence of an OI

- For patients with a known diagnosis of HIV:

  - **Review the prior CD4 T-lymphocyte counts**. They will often be reported as an absolute number (i.e., 200 cells/uL) and a percentage (i.e., 14%). In general, the % and the absolute value should correlate. Certain factors may cause discordant results, and these more often affect the absolute value (i.e., the % is minimally changed). These factors include infections, medications, alcohol use, and pregnancy. If this situation occurs, it can be helpful to review ART adherence and the prior CD4 values to see if the decline makes clinical sense or not. For example, if a patient had a CD4 count of 600 cells/uL (40%) 6 months ago but is now admitted with a pneumonia, and the repeat CD4 count (which probably should not have been done) is 200 cells/uL (35%), then the drop is likely the result of the acute infection. As a general rule, the CD4 count declines by approximately 50 cells/uL per year (on average) in patients with untreated HIV.

- **HIV viral load (quantitative serum RNA by PCR).** If a patient is taking ART reliably, then the viral load should be undetectable (i.e., <20 copies/mL in most modern assays). The viral load is the usual marker we follow to assess HIV control in patients taking ART

- **Viral resistance testing (genotype assay)** may be considered, depending on what the previous regimen was. Some regimens have higher barriers to resistance development, and resistance is unlikely to develop with these regimens. The genotype test is only run if there is viremia (requires at least 500–1,000 copies/mL). To detect a resistance mutation, the test should be done while the patient is on the "failing ART regimen" or within 4 weeks of stopping it. The rationale is that the mutant strain is only seen in the setting of selective drug pressure. If the genotype is done outside of these parameters, then the virus will have reverted to the wild-type strain, and any new mutations may not be detected

- **Tropism assay** should be done if planning to use the CCR5 antagonist Maraviroc

- **See next section ("newly diagnosed patients") because many of those tests will apply to these patients**

- For newly diagnosed patients, the following should be considered:
  - **Documentation of the positive HIV test** with HIV p24 antigen/antibody screen and confirmatory assay
  - **HIV viral load (serum RNA/PCR)**
  - **CD4 T-lymphocyte count (absolute and percentage are both nice to see)**
  - **Viral resistance testing (genotype assay)** should be done but is only run if there is viremia (requires at least 500–1,000 copies/mL)
  - **Metabolic evaluation**—This includes complete blood count with differential, complete metabolic profile, urinalysis with microscopy, serum lipid profile, and diabetes screening (fasting blood glucose or hemoglobin A1c)

- **Hepatitis screening**
  - Hepatitis A virus (HAV) total antibody (IgM and IgG)
  - Hepatitis B virus (HBV) serology (HBV surface antigen, surface antibody, and total core antibody)—These are very useful to know when managing HIV/HBV coinfected patients, who typically need to be on two active anti-HBV drugs
  - Hepatitis C serology
- **Sexually transmitted illness testing**
  - Multisite testing for gonorrhea and chlamydia. This is typically done by swabbing any exposed site (for pharyngeal or rectal exposures) or obtaining a urinary sample (for genital exposures). These specimens are typically tested using nucleic-acid amplification testing
  - Syphilis screening—The choice of test is often institution-specific. Most institutions start with a treponemal specific test (syphilis IgG, FTA-ABS, etc.) with reflex nontreponemal testing (i.e., RPR) only if the treponemal-specific test is positive
- **Tuberculosis screening**—This may include tuberculin skin test (≥5 mm is considered positive) or interferon-gamma release assay (T-SPOT or QuantiFERON Gold)
- *Toxoplasma* **IgG** helps guide prophylaxis and potentially treatment in the setting of suspected toxoplasmosis
- **Pregnancy testing (if applicable)**
- **Testing done only in select situations**
  - HLA-B*5701 should be checked if planning to start an abacavir (ABC)-based regimen. HLA-B*5701–positive patients are at increased risk of developing a severe hypersensitivity reaction with ABC, so if positive, ABC should be avoided
  - Glucose-6-phosphate dehydrogenase (G6PD) level may be useful if planning to use drugs associated with hemolysis in G6PD deficiency (i.e., primaquine, dapsone, etc.).

Additional work-up should be guided by presentation, clinical suspicion, and CD4 count. More than one infection may be present at one time (i.e., oral thrush plus *Pneumocystis* pneumonia). Table 76.3 summarizes the manifestations of advanced HIV in a systematic fashion. It is important to remember that these patients also get run-of-the-mill infections and disorders (not included in the table), so do not forget about these. Prophylaxis is available for some infections, but it is important to remember that prophylaxis does not completely eliminate the possibility of a given infection. Similar to solid-organ transplant patients

Table 76.3 – Manifestations of Advanced HIV (Untreated)

Presentation	Comments
Fevers	• Infection is very common and must be ruled out. The work-up is guided by CD4 count, signs/symptoms, and exposures • Noninfectious—malignancy, drug reactions, etc.
Ophthalmologic	• Toxoplasmosis, cytomegalovirus (CMV) retinitis, progressive outer retinal necrosis caused by varicella-zoster virus (VZV) or less commonly herpes simplex virus (HSV), ocular tuberculosis (TB), ocular syphilis
Oral lesions	• Infectious—candidiasis (oral/thrush), oral hairy leukoplakia (Epstein–Barr virus [EBV]), HSV, histoplasmosis oral ulcerations, Kaposi sarcoma • Noninfectious—aphthous ulceration
Dermatologic	• Infectious—warts (human papilloma virus [HPV]), HSV, VZV, scabies, disseminated molluscum contagiosum, disseminated fungal infection (*Cryptococcus*, talaromycosis [penicilliosis], histoplasmosis, blastomycosis), bacillary angiomatosis (*Bartonella henselae* or *Bartonella quintana*), Kaposi sarcoma (HHV-8) • Noninfectious—seborrheic dermatitis, eosinophilic folliculitis, psoriasis (often severe), prurigo nodularis
Endo/metabolic	• Adrenal insufficiency (mostly infectious)—CMV, *Mycobacterium avium complex* (MAC), TB, HIV, histoplasmosis • Wasting disease (protein calorie malnutrition), osteopenia, avascular necrosis of bone
Cardiovascular	• Uncontrolled inflammation in poorly controlled HIV → accelerated atherosclerosis → higher risk for stroke, coronary artery disease/myocardial infarction, and venous thromboembolism
Pulmonary	• Infectious—*Pneumocystis jirovecii* pneumonia, disseminated fungal infection, mycobacterial infections (tuberculosis and nontuberculous mycobacteria), *Nocardia* spp., *Rhodococcus* spp., CMV (rarely), Kaposi sarcoma • Noninfectious—malignancy (primary effusion lymphoma, Castleman disease, etc.)
Gastrointestinal	• Esophagitis—*Candida* spp., CMV, HSV, aphthous ulcers • Enterocolitis—MAC, CMV, parasitic infections (i.e., *Giardia, Cryptosporidium*, Microsporidium, *Cystoisospora, Cyclospora*), histoplasmosis, AIDS enteropathy, Kaposi sarcoma and other malignancies (lymphoma) • Cholangiopathy—AIDS cholangiopathy, *Cryptosporidium*, Microsporidia
Renal	• HIV-associated nephropathy—typically nephrotic syndrome related to the collapsing variant of focal segmental glomerulosclerosis
Hematologic and oncologic	• Anemia—chronic disease, bone marrow infiltration (infection, malignancy), drug toxicity • Leukopenia—typically see mild leukopenia (with lymphopenia) in advanced HIV • Thrombocytopenia—infections (HIV, hepatitis viruses), idiopathic thrombocytopenic purpura, thrombotic thrombocytopenic purpura • Pancytopenia—CMV, MAC, histoplasmosis, leishmaniasis, malignancy • Lymphoma—non-Hodgkin's lymphoma, including EBV-associated central nervous system (CNS) lymphoma • Kaposi sarcoma (HHV-8)—can be cutaneous or visceral • Cervical or anal cancers (HPV)

Table 76.3 – Manifestations of Advanced HIV (Untreated) *(Cont'd)*

Presentation	Comments

Neurologic	• **Meningoencephalitis**
	  • Bacterial—tuberculosis, syphilis, *Listeria*
	  • Viral—HIV-related, HSV, VZV, CMV (ventriculoencephalitis or polyradiculopathy)
	  • Fungal—*Cryptococcus*, endemic mycoses
	  • Parasitic—Toxoplasmosis
	• **Space-occupying lesions**
	  • Cerebral toxoplasmosis—often multiple enhancing basal ganglia lesions, positive *Toxoplasma* IgG
	  • Primary CNS lymphoma—often single enhancing lesion, cerebrospinal fluid (CSF) PCR may be positive for EBV
	  • Progressive multifocal leukoencephalopathy—often multiple nonenhancing white matter lesions, may have positive JC virus PCR in CSF
	  • Other—cryptococcoma, tuberculoma, nocardiasis
	• **Cognitive**—HIV-associated neurocognitive disorder
	• **Myelopathy**—vacuolar myelopathy (HIV), CMV, HSV, VZV, human T-lymphotropic virus, cord compression (infectious, malignancy)

(discussed in case 64), these patients may require more invasive work-ups than immune-competent patients.

KEY LEARNING POINT

Bacillary angiomatosis (BA) classically presents in advanced HIV patients with skin lesions that appear similar to Kaposi sarcoma (KS). BA is characterized by neutrophilic inflammation (also macrophages), and KS is characterized by lymphoplasmacytic inflammation. BA is treated with at least 3 months of doxycycline.

REFERENCES AND FURTHER READING

- Algahtani SA, Sulkowski MS. Gastrointestinal, hepatobiliary, and pancreatic manifestations of human immunodeficiency virus infection. In: Bennet JE, Dolin R, Blaser MJ, eds. *Mandell, Douglas, and Bennett's Principles and Practice of Infectious Diseases.* 9th ed. Elsevier; 2020:1684–1689.
- Garland JM, et al. Human immunodeficiency virus infection. In: *Cecil Essentials of Medicine.* 10th ed. Elsevier; 2022:944–962.
- Koehler J. *Bartonella* infections in HIV-infected individuals. In: *Sande's HIV/AIDS Medicine.* 2nd ed. Elsevier; 2012:421–432.

- Patel P, et al. Human immunodeficiency virus infection. In: *Hunter's Tropical Medicine and Emerging Infectious Diseases*. 10th ed. Elsevier; 2020.
- Rolain J-M, et al. *Bartonella* infections. In: *Goldman-Cecil Medicine*. 26th ed. Elsevier; 2020:1967–1971.
- Rose ST, Koehler JE. *Bartonella*, including cat-scratch disease. In: Bennet JE, Dolin R, Blaser MJ, eds. *Mandell, Douglas, and Bennett's Principles and Practice of Infectious Disease*. 9th ed. Elsevier; 2020:2824–2843.
- Siddiqi OK, et al. Neurologic diseases caused by human immunodeficiency virus type 1 and opportunistic infections. In: Bennet JE, Dolin R, Blaser MJ, eds. *Mandell, Douglas, and Bennett's Principles and Practice of Infectious Diseases*. 9th ed. Elsevier; 2020:1690–1706.
- Sterling TR, Chaisson RE. General clinical manifestations of human immunodeficiency virus infection (including acute retroviral syndrome and oral, cutaneous, renal, ocular, metabolic, and cardiac diseases). In: Bennet JE, Dolin R, Blaser MJ, eds. *Mandell, Douglas, and Bennett's Principles and Practice of Infectious Diseases*. 9th ed. Elsevier; 2020:1658–1674.

A 35-year-old female is admitted to the hospital with a new diagnosis of acute myelogenous leukemia. She received induction chemotherapy, which resulted in complete remission. She then underwent consolidation with an allogeneic hematopoietic stem cell transplant 14 days ago. Current medications include acyclovir, cefepime, and fluconazole. Today, she developed fevers and chills. Vital signs reveal temperature 101° F, heart rate 105 beats per minute, blood pressure 100/70 mmHg, respiratory rate 18, and oxygen saturation 96% on room air. Examination is fairly unremarkable. She has a peripherally inserted central catheter in her right brachial region, and there is no insertion site erythema, discharge, or tenderness. Laboratory studies show white blood cell count 0 cells/uL, hemoglobin 7.3 g/dL, platelets 12,000 cells/uL, creatinine 1.0 mg/dL (creatinine clearance >60 mL/min), and normal liver function tests. Blood cultures are obtained.

Which of the following processes is this patient most at risk for?

A. Candidemia.
B. Nocardiosis.
C. Graft-versus-host disease (GVHD).
D. *Pneumocystis* pneumonia.
E. Hemorrhagic cystitis due to BK virus.

She is most at risk for candidemia (**option A**) because she is in the pre-engraftment phase post–stem cell transplant. The other options (**options B, C, D**, and **E**) are all more likely to occur postengraftment.

This patient's presentation is concerning for an infection in the post–hematopoietic stem cell transplantation (HSCT) patient. The risk for infections post-HSCT largely depends on the conditioning regimen (myeloablative regimens are higher risk than reduced intensity regimens), the type of stem cell transplant (allogeneic HSCTs are at higher risk than autologous HSCTs), and timing in relation to the transplant (discussed later). Other factors that modify the risk are the use of prophylactic antimicrobials, the type of stem cells that were used, epidemiologic exposures, and the need for more intensive immune suppression (i.e., prophylaxis or treatment of GVHD). Three post-HSCT periods are typically defined, and each is associated with particular syndromes and infections:

- **Pre-engraftment period**
  - Time from transplant to neutrophil recovery (day 20–30 approximately).
  - Major risks are prolonged neutropenia (from underlying disease and/or the conditioning regimen) and disruption of skin and mucosal barriers (i.e., catheters, mucositis, etc.).
  - Most of the issues that arise in this period are related to hospitalization (i.e., hospital-acquired infections, volume overload, catheter-related complications, etc.), viral infections (i.e., herpes simplex virus, respiratory viruses, etc.), neutropenia pathogens (i.e., invasive *Candida* and mold infections), or complications of the underlying disease and its treatment.

- **Early postengraftment period**
  - Time from day of engraftment to day 100.
  - Both cellular and humoral immunity are impaired. Natural killer cells are first to recover followed by CD8+ (cytotoxic) T-lymphocytes.
  - Major risks include complications of acute GVHD and its therapy, along with many of the same risks as for pre-engraftment.
  - In this phase, opportunistic pathogens are more common, including herpes viruses like cytomegalovirus (CMV; especially problematic if stem cell donor is CMV-seronegative and stem cell recipient is CMV-seropositive), *Pneumocystis*, molds, polyoma viruses (BK virus and JC virus), respiratory viruses, and, in rare cases, disseminated strongyloidiasis and disseminated toxoplasmosis.

- **Late postengraftment period**
  - Time after day 100.
  - This period is mostly seen with allogeneic transplants.
  - Both cellular and humoral immunity are impaired. B-lymphocytes and CD4+ (helper) T-lymphocytes slowly recover out to 2 years.
  - Major risks are ongoing issues with GVHD and its therapy, which results in delayed immune reconstitution (i.e., hyposplenism, reduced opsonization, etc.).
  - In the period, we see many of the same pathogens as for early postengraftment but also encapsulated bacteria and herpes viral infections (i.e., varicella-zoster virus infections).

The infections associated with each post-transplant phase in autologous and allogeneic transplants are shown in Figs. 77.1 and 77.2.

The post-HSCT periods and associated complications are not absolute, but they do serve as a useful guide when seeing these patients and building a differential. It is important to remember that full immunologic recovery may not be seen until 6 to 12 months for autologous HSCT and 12 to 24 months for allogeneic HSCT. These durations may be even more prolonged depending on the post-transplant course (i.e., GVHD treatment). In addition, as with all immune-compromised individuals, presentations may be more subtle, and more than one infection or disease process may occur at any one time. HSCT patients can also get the usual infections or diseases that non–immune-compromised patients get, so do not overlook these. Furthermore, many noninfectious conditions can mimic infection, including the underlying malignancy, GVHD, engraftment syndrome, and drug adverse effects/reactions. When trying to diagnose these patients, it can be difficult to obtain more invasive testing (i.e., biopsy) because of the risk for infection and bleeding that can be seen with severe neutropenia and thrombocytopenia, respectively. Lastly, when treating infections in these patients, reduction of the overall immune suppression should always be considered.

There are some conditions that are seen more commonly or exclusively in post-HSCT patients. These include:

Hepatic sinusoidal obstruction syndrome (SOS; previously known as veno-occlusive disease)
- Typically manifests in the pre-engraftment period and is very rare to see after day 30.
- Risk factors include pre-existing liver disease and certain treatments for the underlying malignancy or transplant.

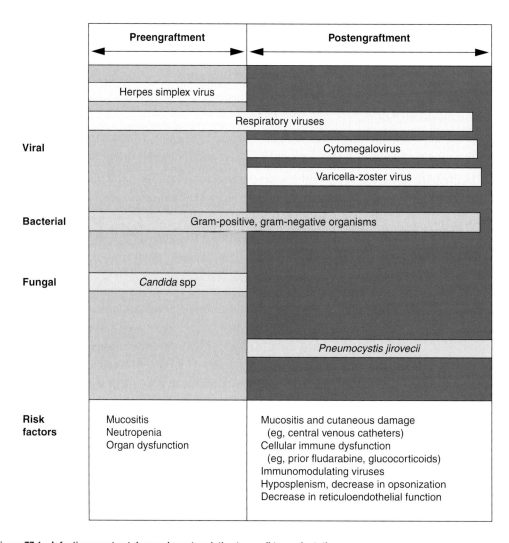

	Preengraftment	Postengraftment
	Herpes simplex virus	
	Respiratory viruses	
Viral		Cytomegalovirus
		Varicella-zoster virus
Bacterial	Gram-positive, gram-negative organisms	
Fungal	*Candida* spp	
		Pneumocystis jirovecii

Risk factors	Mucositis
	Neutropenia
	Organ dysfunction
		Mucositis and cutaneous damage
		  (eg, central venous catheters)
		Cellular immune dysfunction
		  (eg, prior fludarabine, glucocorticoids)
		Immunomodulating viruses
		Hyposplenism, decrease in opsonization
		Decrease in reticuloendothelial function

Figure 77.1 – Infections post autologous hematopoietic stem cell transplantation

- Presentation may consist of right upper quadrant pain, jaundice, hepatomegaly, and ascites.
- Hepatic SOS carries a high mortality. Management includes intensive supportive care and defibrotide. Transjugular intrahepatic portosystemic shunting or liver transplantation may be necessary in some cases.

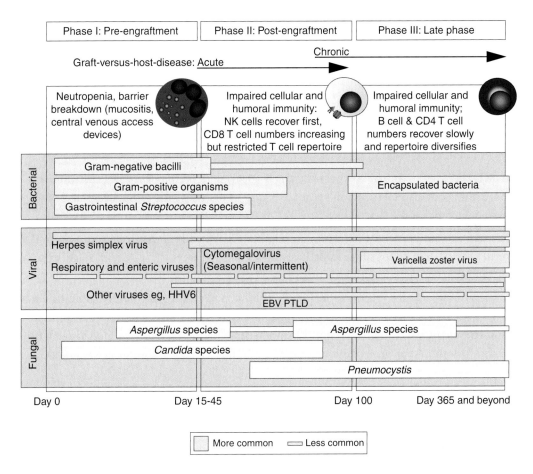

Figure 77.2 – Infections post allogeneic hematopoietic stem cell transplantation

Engraftment syndrome (ES)

- ES occurs in some HSCT patients at the time of engraftment (~day 20–30).
- ES may present with fevers, skin rash, diarrhea, hepatitis (elevated liver function testing [LFT]), acute kidney injury, encephalopathy, and capillary leakage (noncardiogenic pulmonary edema, weight gain, etc.).
- It is considered a diagnosis of exclusion. The biggest differential to exclude is infection.

- Treatment involves steroids. Most patients will be placed on antimicrobials similar to neutropenic fever management, but these can often be stopped if no evidence of infection is found after 2 to 3 days.

Neutropenic enterocolitis (typhlitis)

- A condition typically seen in patients with severe neutropenia that is thought to be related to invasion of intestinal bacteria into the gut wall (usually the cecum). The infection is typically polymicrobial in nature.

- It can present very similar to appendicitis (fevers, right lower abdominal pain, diarrhea, etc.), but it can also be subtle in some cases due to neutropenia. Thus, a high index of suspicion is needed.

- Evaluation should include abdominal imaging (CT typically shows inflammation of the cecal region), testing for other infectious causes of enterocolitis (i.e., *Clostridiodes difficile*, stool film-array, etc.), and blood cultures.

- Management includes volume repletion, bowel rest, and empiric antibiotics targeting enteric pathogens and febrile neutropenia (i.e., piperacillin-tazobactam, cefepime + metronidazole, or meropenem; vancomycin can be added in hemodynamically unstable individuals). Failure to improve should prompt consideration of antifungal therapy and surgical consultation.

GVHD

- GVHD is a phenomenon seen in allogeneic transplants only.

- Acute GVHD presents in the first 100 days post-transplant (most often in the early postengraftment phase) with skin lesions (maculopapular eruption), LFT abnormalities (typically cholestatic appearance), and gastrointestinal upset.

- Chronic GVHD can occur at any time post-transplant, and presentation may include:

  - Dermatologic—Skin lesions resembling lichen-planus, scleroderma, and systemic sclerosis; vaginal sclerosis; or dry eyes.

  - Gastrointestinal—May see oral lichen planus–like lesions, esophageal webs or strictures, and elevated LFT.

  - Musculoskeletal manifestations—May see muscle or joint fasciitis.

  - Pulmonary—May see bronchiolitis obliterans/obliterans syndrome and cryptogenic organizing pneumonia (used to be called bronchiolitis obliterans with organizing pneumonia).

- GVHD is confirmed with biopsy (either skin or gastrointestinal tract).

- Prevention and treatment involve immune suppression, which increases risk for infections and may delay immune reconstitution.
- GVHD patients have impaired cellular immunity and hypogammaglobulinemia, which puts them at risk for viral reactivation (especially herpes viruses) and infection by encapsulated organisms.

Hemorrhagic cystitis (HC)

- Early-onset HC (pre-engraftment) is typically associated with chemotherapy (i.e., cyclophosphamide). This may be prevented with hydration and mesna.
- Later-onset HC (post-engraftment) is typically caused by BK virus, adenovirus, or CMV.
- The predominant manifestation is hematuria.
- Management includes hydration, continuous bladder irrigation, and antivirals (i.e., cidofovir for BK virus and adenovirus or ganciclovir for CMV). Reduction of immune suppression may be necessary as well.

Diffuse alveolar hemorrhage (DAH)

- Risk factors include medications (i.e., chemotherapy), GVHD, and various infections including bacteria, viruses, and fungi.
- DAH presents with acute respiratory failure with diffuse pulmonary infiltrates.
- Diagnosis requires bronchoalveolar lavage (BAL), showing progressively bloodier BAL fluid.
- Treatment involves supportive care, steroids, and antimicrobials.

Posterior reversible encephalopathy syndrome (PRES)

- PRES is a syndrome associated with the use of calcineurin inhibitors (CNI; tacrolimus or cyclosporine) for GVHD management.
- PRES manifests with various neurologic signs and symptoms in conjunction with imaging showing edema involving the posterior cerebral white matter.
- Treatment is typically supportive. Discontinuing the CNI and treating underlying infections are important as well.

A summary of various medications used in hematologic malignancies and their infectious risk is presented in Table 77.1.

Table 77.1 – Infections Associated With Selected Oncologic Therapies

Medication	Infectious Considerations
High-dose steroids (≥20 mg/day)	• Increases risk for various infections, including bacteria, viruses, fungal organisms (particularly *Pneumocystis*), and even parasitic infections (i.e., strongyloidiasis)
Purine analogs (-arabine)	• Associated with prolonged neutropenia and prolonged suppression of cell-mediated immunity (i.e., CD4 recovery may take 40 months) • In combination with hypomethylating agents, increases risk of invasive fungal infections (IFIs) and herpes infections (varicella zoster virus [VZV] and herpes simplex virus [HSV])
Tyrosine kinase inhibitors (TKIs)	• TKIs affect multiple cells (neutrophils, T-cells, B-cells) • Dasatinib may have the highest risk of infection • Increased risk of hepatitis B virus (HBV) reactivation
JAK inhibitor (ruxolitinib)	• Affects function of natural killer (NK) cells and dendritic cells and reduces cytokine response (i.e., IL-1, IL-6, TNF-α) • Increased risk for VZV and HBV reactivation
BTK inhibitor (ibrutinib)	• Affects B-cell signaling and may increase risk for opportunistic infections (i.e., *Pneumocystis, Aspergillus*, or VZV)
BCL-2 inhibitor (venetoclax)	• ~3% of patients may get opportunistic infection—Pneumocystis, toxoplasmosis, nocardiosis, viral infections, and candidiasis
PI3-K inhibitor (idelalisib)	• Increased risk of *Pneumocystis* and cytomegalovirus (CMV) infections • Should be given with *Pneumocystis* prophylaxis and CMV monitoring
Anti-CD20 monoclonal antibodies (i.e., rituximab)	• Affect B-cells and plasma cells → hypogammaglobulinemia • Downstream effects on T-cells may result in impaired cellular immunity • Increased risk for viral infections (HBV reactivation)
Anti-CD30 monoclonal antibody (brentuximab)	• Affects B-cells, T-cells, and NK cells • Increased risk for CMV and JC virus reactivation.
Anti-CD38 monoclonal antibody (daratumumab)	• Predominantly affects plasma cells (drug is used in multiple myeloma)
Anti-CD52 monoclonal antibody (alemtuzumab)	• May cause profound immune suppression with reduction of monocytes, neutrophils, B-cells, and T-cells for 4–9 months after therapy • Increased risk of viral reactivation (esp. CMV and HSV) and IFI
Proteasome inhibitors (i.e., bortezomib)	• Increased risk of viral infections (esp. VZV and influenza)
Bispecific T-cell engager (blinatumomab)	• Associated with fevers, cytokine release syndrome, and fungal pneumonias
PD-1 inhibitor (pembrolizumab)	• Associated with tuberculosis reactivation, fevers, and autoimmune diseases (i.e., thyroiditis, adrenalitis, etc.)
Chimeric antigen receptor T-cells	• May have neutropenia ± lymphodepletion for weeks • Cytokine release syndrome is fairly common

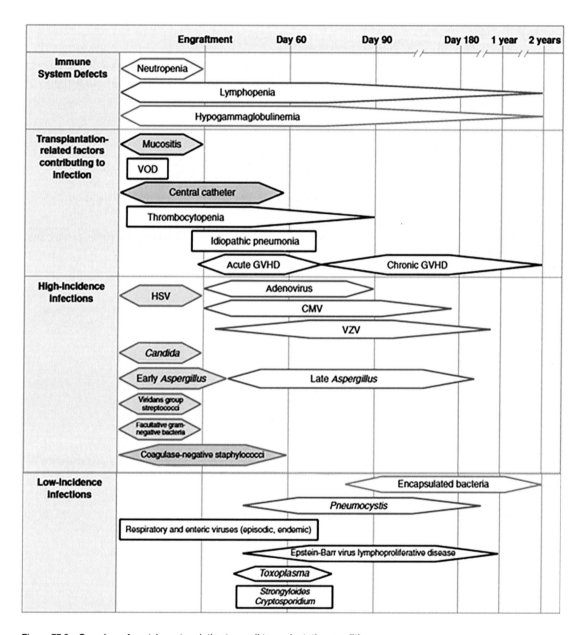

Figure 77.3 – Overview of post–hematopoietic stem cell transplantation conditions.
Immune defects predisposing to infection are bordered by color (pink, neutropenia; blue, lymphopenia; green, hypogammaglobulinemia). Barrier defects predisposing to infection are shaded in color (gold, mucosal breakdown; gray, skin breakdown). Contribution of defects to infections occurring with high incidence are designated by border color (for immune defects) or shading (for barrier defects) or both. *CMV*, Cytomegalovirus; *GVHD*, graft-versus-host disease; *HSV*, herpes simplex virus; *VOD*, veno-occlusive disease; *VZV*, varicella-zoster virus. From Niederhuber J, Armitage J, et al. *Abeloff's Clinical Oncology*. 6th ed. Elsevier Inc.; 2019.

KEY LEARNING POINT

Knowledge of the various post–hematopoietic stem cell transplantation (HSCT) periods can be very helpful when seeing patients post-HSCT. Each period/phase is associated with certain infections and disease processes. Another summary of the important points is shown in Fig. 77.3.

REFERENCES AND FURTHER READING

- Atkins S, He F. Chemotherapy and beyond: infections in the era of old and new treatments for hematologic malignancies. *Infect Dis Clin North Am.* 2019;33(2):289–309. https://doi.org/10.1016/j.idc.2019.01.001.
- Nathan S, Ustun C. Complications of stem cell transplantation that affect infections in stem cell transplant recipients, with analogies to patients with hematologic malignancies. *Infect Dis Clin North Am.* 2019;33(2): 331–359. https://doi.org/10.1016/j.idc.2019.01.002.
- Wingard JR, Bow E, Bond S, et al. Overview of infections following hematopoietic cell transplantation. In: Post TW, ed. *UpToDate.* Waltham: UpToDate; 2020.
- Young JH, Ustun C. Infections in recipients of hematopoietic stem cell transplants. In: Bennet JE, Dolin R, Blaser MJ, eds. *Mandell, Douglas, and Bennett's Principles and Practice of Infectious Diseases.* 9th ed. Elsevier; 2020: 3654–3671.

A 60-year-old-male is admitted to the hospital with a 2-day history of fevers and chills. He has a history of heart failure with reduced ejection fraction. Medications include aspirin, atorvastatin, lisinopril, metoprolol, and furosemide. He had a biventricular implantable cardioverter-defibrillator (ICD) placed for cardiac resynchronization a little over 1 month ago. He notes a penicillin allergy, which he describes as a rash when he was a child. Vital signs reveal temperature 101° F, heart rate 90 beats per minute, blood pressure 100/78 mmHg, respiratory rate 16, and oxygen saturation 98% on room air. He appears generally well. Heart exam reveals a regular rate and rhythm. There is a grade two holosystolic murmur heard over the apex. Lungs are clear. There is redness, warmth, and tenderness over the ICD pocket site. In addition, there is purulent material oozing out of the lower portion of the surgical incision. He has trace peripheral edema. The remainder of the physical examination is unremarkable. White blood cell count is 13,000 cells/uL. Creatinine is 1.0 mg/dL (clearance >60 mL/min). Blood cultures are obtained, and vancomycin is started. Blood cultures eventually grow methicillin-susceptible *Staphylococcus aureus*. Transesophageal echocardiogram reveals a small echodensity on the ICD lead but no valvular echodensity. The device is extracted, and follow-up blood cultures are clear. What is the most appropriate management for this patient?

A. Cefazolin for 4 weeks.

B. Cefazolin for 2 weeks.

C. Nafcillin for 4 weeks.

D. Nafcillin for 2 weeks.

E. No further therapy is necessary.

The most appropriate therapy is cefazolin for 4 weeks (**option A**). This patient has a cardiovascular implantable electronic device (CIED)–related infection, specifically an ICD pocket and lead infection.

CIED-related infections are fairly common. They are most commonly caused by staphylococci (coagulase-negative staphylococci [CoNS] and *S. aureus*). In congruence with their virulence, *S. aureus* infections are typically not subtle, but CoNS infections certainly can be subtle. From a pathophysiologic standpoint, the device pocket can become infected at the time of implantation, at replacement, or during any other surgical manipulation of the pocket. Rarely, pocket infection can be secondary to dissemination from a primary bacteremia. From the pocket, the infection can spread distally to become systemic (bacteremia, lead infection, or valvular infection/endocarditis).

There are various subtypes of CIED to be aware of, and these include:

- **Superficial incisional infection**—involves only the skin and subcutaneous tissue of the incision and not the deeper soft tissues
- **Isolated generator pocket infection**—localized erythema, swelling, pain/tenderness, warmth, or drainage with negative blood cultures
- **Isolated pocket erosion**—device and/or lead(s) visible through the skin (hardware exposure), exposed hardware is assumed to be infected
- **Bacteremia**—positive blood cultures with or without systemic illness
- **Lead infection**—lead vegetation and bacteremia
- **Valvular infection (endocarditis)**—valvular vegetation and bacteremia
- **Occult bacteremia with probable CIED infection**—absence of an alternative source of infection and resolution with CIED extraction
- **Combinations of the above**

The approach to diagnosis and management is shown in Fig. 78.1 and Table 78.1.

Cefazolin for 2 weeks (**option B**) could be considered in isolated pocket infection but is not appropriate for invasive infection due to *S. aureus*. Nafcillin for 4 weeks (**option C**) could be considered, but it would not be ideal for this patient in light of his penicillin allergy and history of heart failure. Nafcillin comes with a large sodium and fluid load, which could

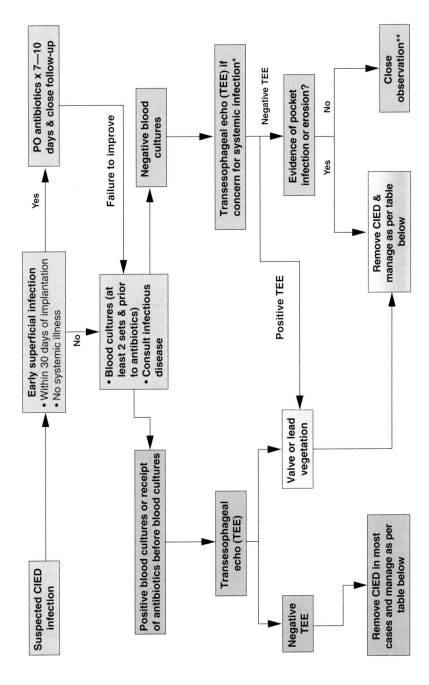

Figure 78.1 – Diagnosis of cardiovascular implantable electronic device-related infections.

*Bloodstream infections may be present even in patients without systemic signs or symptoms.

**If there is ongoing suspicion for CIED infection despite negative testing, then additional tests such as FDG-PET/CT or tagged white blood cell (WBC) scan may be helpful. PET/CT is most useful for defining pocket infection and extracardiac evidence of endovascular infection (i.e., discitis). Tagged WBC scan is more sensitive for detection of lead and/or valvular vegetation and may be helpful in excluding CIED-related infections. In addition, obtaining acid-fast bacillus and/or fungal blood cultures may be considered. *CIED*, Cardiovascular implantable electronic device; *CT*, computed tomography; *FDG*, (18) F-fluorodeoxyglucose; *PET*, positron emission tomography; *PO*, oral.

Table 78.1 – Management of Cardiovascular Implantable Electronic Device Infections

Situation	Recommended Management[a]	Duration of Treatment[b]	When to Reimplant Device[c]
Empiric therapy	• Vancomycin ± gram-negative coverage (i.e., cefepime)	• N/A	• N/A
Superficial incision site infection (erythema or stitch abscess)	• Can forgo removal of device only if not systemically ill and within 1 month of device implantation • Oral antibiotics covering skin organisms (staphylococci and streptococci) should be used—an example would be doxycycline + cephalexin	• 7–10 days with close follow-up • Failure to improve should prompt further evaluation (i.e., blood cultures, etc.)	• N/A
Pocket infection	• Remove (extract) entire device • Blood cultures and transesophageal echocardiogram should be negative • Antibiotic choice is guided by intraoperative pocket culture results	• 14 days	• Once blood cultures have been negative for at least 72 hours (3 days)
Bacteremia	• Remove (extract) entire device in most cases • Definitely remove if due *Staphylococcus aureus, Cutibacterium acnes,* coagulase-negative staphylococcus, or *Candida spp.* • Probably remove if due to *Enterococcus spp.* or *Streptococcus spp.* • Can forgo removal if due to gram-negative organism, but if fails to clear or recurs after treatment, then remove entire device	• At least 2 weeks • 4–6 weeks if *S. aureus* or complicated infection (i.e., metastatic foci of infection)	• Once blood cultures have been negative for at least 72 hours (3 days)
Lead infection	• Remove (extract) entire device	• At least 2 weeks • 4 weeks for *S. aureus*	• Once blood cultures have been negative for at least 72 hours (3 days)
Valvular infection (endocarditis)	• Remove (extract) entire device	• 4–6 weeks (per endocarditis guidance)	• Once blood cultures have been negative for at least 14 days

[a]Cardiovascular implantable electronic device (CIED) removal within 3 days of diagnosis is associated with reduced in-hospital mortality. Needle aspiration from the pocket for culture should not be done. When the CIED is removed, cultures from the pocket tissue and leads should be obtained. The sensitivity of tissue culture (69%) is higher than that of the swab culture (31%) of the pocket. Be aware that lead contamination can occur when leads are extracted through the generator pocket. The culture results are used to guide the choice of definitive antimicrobial therapy. If a device cannot be removed, then consider obtaining surveillance blood cultures after completion of antimicrobial therapy vs. long-term suppressive antibiotic therapy.

[b]Start day of therapy is the day of source control (either day of device extraction or blood culture clearance, whichever is most recent).

[c]Reimplantation should be done on contralateral side, assuming the device is still necessary and the infection has been sufficiently controlled (i.e., bacteremia cleared, metastatic abscesses drained, etc.).

potentially exacerbate heart failure. Of note, most "childhood penicillin allergies" are not true allergies, and patients often outgrow these reactions. In these situations, the risk of cross-reactivity with cephalosporins is extremely low. Nafcillin for 2 weeks (**option D**) is inappropriate for both reasons listed above. No further therapy (**option E**) would likely result in inadequate treatment and relapsed infection.

KEY LEARNING POINT

Treatment of cardiovascular implantable electronic device–related infections can be complicated and depends on various factors, including the specific type of infection, the degree of source control, and the offending organism. Nafcillin may cause exacerbations of heart failure due to the high sodium and volume load associated with nafcillin.

REFERENCES AND FURTHER READING

- Kusumoto FM, Schoenfeld MH, Wilkoff BL, et al. 2017 HRS expert consensus statement on cardiovascular implantable electronic device lead management and extraction. *Heart Rhythm.* 2021;18(10):1814. https://doi.org/10.1016/j.hrthm.2021.06.1174. Erratum in: *Heart Rhythm.* 2021. PMID: 28919379.

An 18-year-old male is brought into the emergency room by his girlfriend for evaluation of abrupt onset of fevers, chills, confusion and headache. He lives in a college dorm with one roommate. According to the roommate, he apparently went to bed early last night as he was feeling unwell. This morning, the girlfriend noted he was very confused, so she brought him in. He is otherwise healthy and does not take any medications. He has no medication allergies. Vital signs show temperature 103° F, heart rate 130 beats per minute, blood pressure 85/50 mmHg, and respiratory rate 20. On examination, he is somnolent and unable to follow basic commands. He appears toxic. There is nuchal rigidity. Heart exam shows regular tachycardia without murmur. Lungs are clear. Skin exam reveals petechiae and purpura. The remainder of the exam is unremarkable. Blood cultures are obtained, and the patient is started on vancomycin and ceftriaxone. He is intubated for airway protection. Noncontrast head CT is unremarkable. Cerebrospinal fluid (CSF) analysis reveals glucose 20 mg/dL, protein 500 mg/dL, and white blood cell (WBC) count 1,200 cells/uL (95% polymorphonuclear cells). Gram stain reveals gram-negative diplococci.

Which of the following individuals should be given chemoprophylaxis in this case?

A. The roommate.
B. The girlfriend.
C. The physician who intubated the patient.
D. The roommate, the girlfriend, and the physician who intubated the patient.
E. The roommate, and the physician who intubated the patient.

Chemoprophylaxis should be given to all three individuals (**option D**). This patient is presenting with classic meningococcal meningitis. Meningococcal meningitis is caused by a gram-negative diplococcus called *Neisseria meningitidis*. There are capsular and noncapsular subtypes, and capsular subtypes A, B, C, W, and Y are the most common. These five subtypes are the ones we have vaccinations for as well. *N. meningitidis* is transmitted by respiratory droplets. Acquisition results in asymptomatic carriage much more commonly than actual invasive infection. The carriage is most often transient/brief, but can be prolonged in some cases (i.e., up to ~1 year). Asymptomatic carriers are problematic because they can spread the infection readily. Risk factors for infection include asplenia, terminal complement deficiency (primary deficiency or due to eculizumab), travel to certain regions (i.e., African meningitis belt, Mecca pilgrimage) and close-quarter living (i.e., college dorms, military recruits, etc.).

The most common presentation of *N. meningitidis* infection is meningococcemia and meningitis. Patients often present abruptly (very soon after exposure) with symptoms and signs of acute meningoencephalitis and severe sepsis/shock, as portrayed in this case. A petechial or purpuric rash in the setting of meningitis should raise suspicion for meningococcal infection. An example of this finding is shown in Fig. 79.1.

Infection may result in multiorgan failure, amputations, and long-term neurologic injury. Adrenal gland infarction (Waterhouse–Friderichsen syndrome) and disseminated intravascular coagulopathy may compound the shock. Less common manifestations include primary

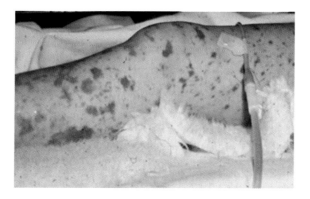

Figure 79.1 – Purpura in meningococcemia
Reprinted with permission from Elsevier. Stephens DS, Greenwood B, Brandtzaeg P. Epidemic meningitis, meningococcaemia, and Neisseria meningitidis. *Lancet.* 2007;369:2196–2210.

pneumonia, septic arthritis, purulent pericarditis, conjunctivitis, and urethritis. Certain *N. meningitidis* subtypes may cause a chronic meningococcemia characterized by low-grade fevers, arthralgia or arthritis, and a maculopapular rash.

The diagnosis is similar to most acute bacterial meningitis cases. Blood cultures and CSF analysis need to be obtained. Blood cultures are positive in about 50% of cases. The CSF findings often show a striking bacterial meningitis profile (i.e., very high WBC count, very low glucose, and high protein). CSF gram stain and/or culture are usually positive, especially if obtained prior to antibiotic administration. HIV screening should be done. Differential diagnoses to consider include Rocky Mountain spotted fever, vasculitis (i.e., Henoch–Schoenlein purpura), bacterial endocarditis, disseminated gonococcal infection, hemolytic uremic syndrome/thrombotic thrombocytopenic purpura, or acute hematologic malignancy.

The mortality of invasive meningococcal disease is very high. Antibiotic therapy should be started as soon as possible if the diagnosis is suspected. First-line treatment is ceftriaxone using the central nervous system dose (2 grams IV every 12 hours). Alternatives include meropenem or moxifloxacin. Steroids have not been shown to be beneficial in meningococcal meningitis. The duration of treatment will depend on the manifestation and clinical response. At least 7 days of therapy should be given in most cases. Respiratory isolation (i.e., droplet precautions) should be instituted and continued until the patient has received at least 24 hours of effective antibiotic therapy. Postexposure prophylaxis should always be considered. Chemoprophylaxis is more than 90% effective and should be initiated as soon as possible postexposure (ideally within 24 hours, but not after 14 days). It should be given to all respiratory contacts in the week before the diagnosis:

- Close contacts: household members, roommates, intimate contacts, child/daycare center workers, individuals seated next to an infected person on an airline for more than 8 hours, and so on.

- Persons directly exposed to respiratory or oral secretions (i.e., kissing, mouth-to-mouth resuscitation, endotracheal intubation, etc.)

Using these criteria for our case, prophylaxis should be given to the roommate, the girlfriend, and the intubating physician. The other options (A, B, C, and E) would leave at least one individual at risk. Prophylaxis options include ceftriaxone 250 mg IM once, ciprofloxacin 500 mg PO once, or rifampin 600 mg PO every 12 hours for 2 days.

As a corollary, another situation in which chemoprophylaxis should be considered is *Haemophilus influenzae* type B (HiB) meningitis. Prophylaxis is not necessary if the infection is due to other *H. influenzae* species. Chemoprophylaxis (typically rifampin for 4 days) should be given as soon as possible (up to 7 days postexposure) to:

- The index case patient if they were treated with ampicillin or chloramphenicol (note: those treated with ceftriaxone do not need prophylaxis).
- All household contacts in houses with a child less than 48 months (4 years) old who has not had the complete primary series of HiB vaccine.
- All immune-compromised household contacts under 18 years old.
- Daycare contacts 2 years and older, only if there have been two or more cases of HiB infection in the daycare within 60 days.

KEY LEARNING POINT

When managing meningococcal meningitis, it is important to provide chemoprophylaxis to all respiratory contacts (i.e., close contact or direct exposure to respiratory or oral secretions) of the index patient.

REFERENCES AND FURTHER READING

- Hasbun R, et al. Acute meningitis. In: Bennet JE, Dolin R, Blaser MJ, eds. *Mandell, Douglas, and Bennett's Principles and Practice of Infectious Diseases*. 9th ed. Elsevier; 2020:1183–1219.
- Overturf G. Bacterial meningitis. In: Kellerman R, et al., ed. *Conn's Current Therapy*. Elsevier; 2021:536–539.
- Stephens DS. *Neisseria meningitidis*. In: Bennet JE, Dolin R, Blaser MJ, eds. *Mandell, Douglas, and Bennett's Principles and Practice of Infectious Diseases*. 9th ed. Elsevier; 2020:2585–2607.
- Van de Beek D, Brouwer MC, Koedel U, Wall EC. Community-acquired bacterial meningitis. *Lancet.* 2021;398(10306):1171–1183. https://doi.org/10.1016/S0140-6736(21)00883-7.

A 55-year-old male is brought to the hospital by his family with a 4-month history of progressive cognitive decline with changes in behavior and personality. He has a history of type 2 diabetes mellitus. Medications include metformin, atorvastatin, and lisinopril. There is no family history of memory problems. He does not smoke. He drinks alcohol "socially." He does not use illicit drugs. Vital signs are within normal limits. Examination reveals a disheveled-appearing man. He does not respond to basic questioning. He occasionally exhibits jerking type motions in his right arm during the examination. He cannot walk on his own for the gait examination. Cranial nerves are intact. Babinski sign is positive. The remainder of the examination is unremarkable. Laboratory studies reveal normal serum vitamin B12 level and serum thyroid-stimulating hormone. HIV antigen/antibody screen is negative. Treponemal-specific syphilis screen is negative. Electroencephalogram (EEG) shows periodic sharp wave complexes. Contrast MRI of the brain shows basal ganglia hyperintensity on T2-weighted images and "cortical ribboning" on diffusion-weighted images.

Which of the following tests is most likely to establish the diagnosis?

A. Cerebrospinal fluid (CSF) 14-3-3 protein.

B. CSF real-time quaking-induced conversion (RT-QUIC) analysis.

C. Brain biopsy.

D. CSF total tau protein.

E. CSF neuron-specific enolase (NSE).

The test most likely to establish the diagnosis is brain biopsy (**option C**). This patient's presentation is highly concerning for a prion disease (PrD). PrDs are a group of rare fatal neurodegenerative diseases caused by the transformation of an endogenous normal protein (prion-related protein [PrP^C]) into an abnormal, misfolded protein called PrP^{SC} (Sc stands for scrapie). Prion is short for "proteinaceous infectious particle." The manifestations are a result of accumulation of PrP^{SC}, likely related to its ability to convert PrP^C to PrP^{SC}. PrDs can occur spontaneously (sporadic, 85%) or genetically (inherited, 14%) or can be transmitted (acquired, <1%). Several subtypes are defined, including:

- Creutzfeldt–Jakob disease (CJD), which can be sporadic CJD (sCJD), variant CJD, familial CJD, or iatrogenic CJD
- Fatal familial insomnia
- Gerstmann–Straussler–Scheinker syndrome
- Kuru

The characteristics of these subtypes are summarized in Table 80.1.

Table 80.1 – Comparison of Prion Diseases

Characteristic	sCJD	vCJD	fCJD	iCJD	FFI	GGS	Kuru
Avg. age of onset (years)	67	28	23–55	All ages	50	60	All ages
Avg. disease duration (months)	8	14	8–96	12	18	40	11
Most prominent early signs	Cognitive and/or behavioral	Psychiatric, sensory	Cognitive and/or behavioral	Cognitive, ataxia	Insomnia, autonomic instability	Ataxia, extrapyramidal	Ataxia, tremor
Cerebellar dysfunction (%)	>40	97	>40	>40	No	100 in P102I mutation	100
DWI/FLAIR MRI positive	Yes, >92%	Yes, pulvinar sign	Yes	Variable, some in deep nuclei or cerebellum	Unclear	Variable, most are negative	N/A
PSWCs on EEG	Yes, 65%	Rarely in end stage	Yes	Yes	No	No	N/A
Amyloid	Sparse plaques in 5%–10%	Severe	Sporadically seen	Sporadically seen	No	Severe	75% of cases

DWI, Diffusion-weighted imaging; EEG, electroencephalogram; fCJD, familial Creutzfeldt–Jakob disease; FFI, fatal familial insomnia; FLAIR, fluid-attenuated inversion recovery; GGS, Gerstmann–Straussler–Scheinker; iCJD, iatrogenic Creutzfeldt–Jakob disease; PSWC, periodic sharp wave complexes; sCJD, sporadic Creutzfeldt–Jakob disease; vCJD, variant Creutzfeldt–Jakob disease.

The quintessential PrD is CJD (usually the sporadic variant), so we will focus on this entity. More information on the other subtypes can be found in the reference below. In general, CJD should be suspected in patients presenting with a rapid onset of cognitive and/or behavioral change associated with sudden jerking movements called myoclonus (often a late finding), vision changes or loss, or extrapyramidal/cerebellar symptoms (ataxia, tremors, etc.). The end stage is often akinetic mutism, and death typically occurs from aspiration pneumonia.

The diagnosis is established by combining the clinical features and diagnostic tests (especially cerebrospinal fluid [CSF] analysis, imaging, and electroencephalogram [EEG]). Several diagnostic criteria exist, but most patients do not meet these criteria until late in the disease. The most definitive test is a brain biopsy. The biopsy will show the typical neuropathologic features: vacuolization (spongiform change), gliosis (astrocytic proliferation), and neuronal loss. EEG may show periodic sharp wave complexes (PSWCs) in approximately two-thirds of patients (more commonly in later disease stages). The EEG findings depend on the subtype, and the same EEG findings can be seen in other illnesses (i.e., Lewy body dementia, etc.). The CSF 14-3-3 protein (**option A**) is often discussed, but this test is actually not very sensitive or specific for CJD. Other CSF markers with widely variable sensitivity and specificity include CSF total tau protein (t-tau; **option D**), CSF neuron-specific enolase (NSE) (**option E**), and astrocytic protein S100β. Of these, t-tau testing may perform the best. CSF real-time quaking-induced conversion (RT-QUIC) analysis (**option B**) is a relatively new prion-specific test (unlike the aforementioned tests, which only show evidence of neuronal injury) that can be used on various tissues including brain, olfactory mucosa, skin biopsies, eye, and extraocular muscles. It cannot be run with blood or blood-contaminated CSF, though. The sensitivity is quoted to be up to 85%, and the specificity is greater than 98%. Consequently, a negative test cannot exclude CJD, but a positive test is highly suggestive. CSF analysis typically shows an isolated mild protein elevation. The presence of CSF pleocytosis, elevated CSF Immunoglobulin G (IgG) index, or oligoclonal bands actually suggests an alternative diagnosis.

MRI of the brain is highly sensitive and specific for the diagnosis of sCJD. Early findings include T2 hyperintensity in the basal ganglia. Later, one may see cortical gyral hyperintensities ("cortical ribboning") on fluid-attenuated inversion recovery (FLAIR) or diffusion-weighted imaging (DWI) sequences (DWI is more sensitive than FLAIR). These abnormalities are shown in Fig. 80.1.

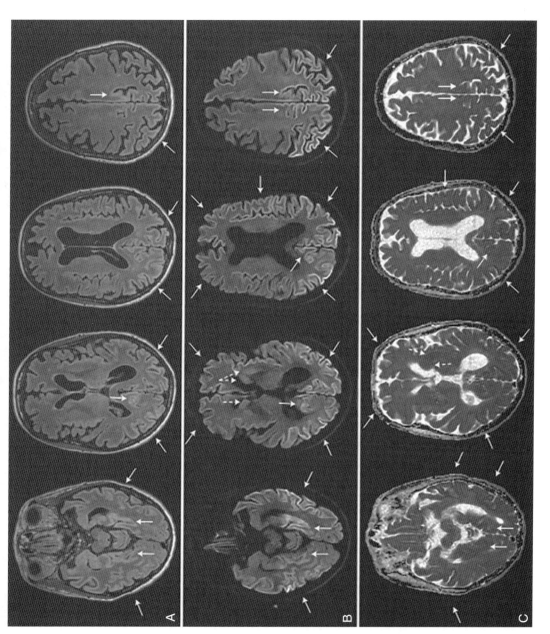

Figure 80.1 – Brain magnetic resonance images in sporadic Creutzfeldt–Jakob disease (sJCD) showing both cortical (solid arrows) and subcortical (dashed arrows) abnormalities on fluid-attenuated inversion recovery (FLAIR) (A), diffusion-weighted imaging (DWI) (B), and apparent diffusion coefficient (ADC) (C) sequences in sJCD. This MRI shows a common pattern in sJCD, including cortical gyral ("cortical ribboning"; solid arrows) and deep nuclei (dashed arrows) hyperintensities on FLAIR and DWI sequences and corresponding hypointensity on ADC sequences. The DWI hyperintensities with corresponding ADC hypointensity confirm that there is restricted diffusion of water molecules, which is found in more than 95% of sJCD cases. Note that, as seen in most brain MRIs in prion disease when restricted diffusion is present, the hyperintensities are much more evident on DWI than on FLAIR sequences. Tee B, et al. Prion diseases. In: *Bradley and Daroff's Neurology in Clinical Practice.* 8th ed. Elsevier; 2022:1430–1451.

Differential diagnosis includes other causes of dementia, severe depression, and other causes of delirium or encephalopathy. Reversible causes of cognitive dysfunction should be ruled out, including HIV, neurosyphilis, B12 deficiency (and maybe even copper deficiency that presents similarly), and hypothyroidism. Management is largely supportive because these diseases are uniformly fatal.

KEY LEARNING POINT

The most accurate test for the diagnosis of prion diseases is a brain biopsy.

REFERENCES AND FURTHER READING

• Tee B, et al. Prion diseases. In: *Bradley and Daroff's Neurology in Clinical Practice*. 8th ed. Elsevier; 2022:1430–1451.

A 60-year-old male is admitted to the hospital with fevers and chills. He has a history of atopic dermatitis, hypertension, and advanced chronic kidney disease (CKD) with baseline creatinine ranging from 2.5 to 3 mg/dL (creatinine clearance 25–30 mL/min). Medications include vitamin D, lisinopril, amlodipine, furosemide, and topical hydrocortisone. He denies alcohol use and IV drug use. Vital signs reveal temperature 102° F, heart rate 115 beats per minute, blood pressure 100/55 mmHg, and respiratory rate 16. Examination reveals an ill-appearing man. His skin is dry, and there are several excoriations present all over his body. The remainder of the examination is unremarkable. Laboratory analysis reveals white blood cell (WBC) count 16,000 cells/uL, hemoglobin 10 g/dL, platelet count 200,000 cells/uL, creatinine 4 mg/dL (creatinine clearance 15 mL/min), and creatine kinase 70 U/L (normal range: 55–170 U/L). Blood cultures are obtained. Vancomycin and piperacillin/tazobactam are started. The next day, the patient feels better. The blood cultures are growing methicillin-resistant *Staphylococcus aureus* (MRSA). The minimum inhibitory concentration (MIC) with respect to vancomycin is 2 ug/mL. The isolate is read as susceptible to daptomycin, ceftaroline, and linezolid. Blood cultures are repeated.

What is the next best step in management?

A. Continue vancomycin and piperacillin/tazobactam.

B. Continue vancomycin and stop piperacillin/tazobactam.

C. Change to daptomycin monotherapy.

D. Change to ceftaroline monotherapy.

E. Change to linezolid monotherapy.

The next best step is to change to daptomycin monotherapy (**option C**). This patient has *S. aureus* bacteremia (SAB). The major considerations in this case include his history of CKD and the high vancomycin MIC of 2 ug/mL. These two factors make vancomycin a much less attractive option.

SAB is very common and carries a significant rate of mortality (20%–40%, depending on where you look). Management of SAB by infectious disease (ID) physicians has been shown to improve outcomes. Therefore it is very important for ID physicians to know SAB in and out. An overall approach to the management of SAB is shown in Fig. 81.1.

Rule number 1—Don't dismiss it!

S. aureus in the blood should always be considered a real pathogen, even if it only grows in a single blood culture bottle. Because *S. aureus* is notoriously aggressive, and SAB carries a high mortality, failure to appropriately recognize SAB may result in detrimental consequences. The adage in ID is "respect *S. aureus*."

Rule number 2—Involve the infectious disease physician!

Formal ID consultation has been shown in multiple studies to improve outcomes and reduce mortality. In fact, some hospital systems mandate ID consultation in the setting of SAB and may even utilize the pharmacists involved in antimicrobial stewardship to facilitate ID consultation in the setting of SAB.

Rule number 3—Treat with the right drug!

If *S. aureus* is identified in a blood culture, but it is unknown if the isolate is MRSA or MSSA, then coverage for both (i.e., vancomycin) should be provided. Once the isolate is confirmed to be either MRSA or MSSA, then targeted therapy (Table 81.1) should be instituted, because these first-line drugs have been shown to be the most beneficial agents. There are several rapid methods for differentiating MRSA from MSSA. These include:

- Matrix-assisted laser desorption/ionization time-of-flight mass spectrometry—relatively new and now much more widely available.
- Penicillin-binding protein (PBP) 2A detection—MRSA carries the *mecA* gene, which encodes an altered PBP protein (PBP-2A) that is resistant to antistaphylococcal penicillins

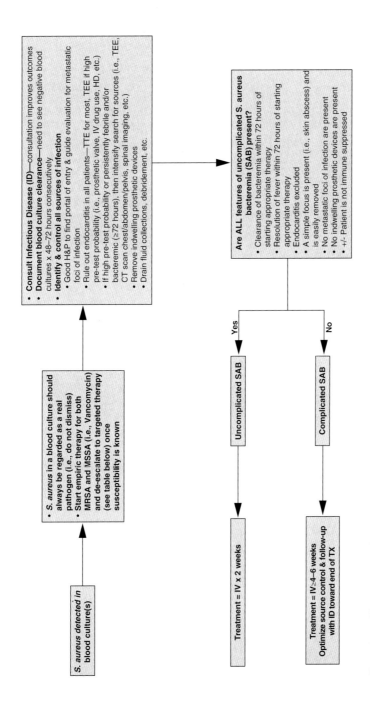

Figure 81.1 – Management of *Staphylococcus aureus* bacteremia

HD, Hemodialysis patient; *H&P*, history and physical; *IV*, intravenous; *MRSA*, methicillin-resistant *S. aureus*; *MSSA*, methicillin-susceptible *S. aureus*; *TEE*, transesophageal echo; *TTE*, transthoracic echo; *TX*, treatment.

Table 81.1 – *Staphylococcus aureus* Bacteremia Antibiotics

MSSAᵃ

First-line therapyᵇ	Cefazolin(Ancef)	• **Dose (if normal renal function)**—2 grams IV every 8 hours (or continuous infusion at 6 grams/day) • **Advantages**—very well-tolerated, easy to administer, including with dialysis • **Disadvantages**—requires renal dose adjustment, no CNS penetration (do not use for meningitis), less efficacious with larger burden of infection (inoculum effect)
	Nafcillin or oxacillin	• **Dose**—2 grams IV every 4 hours (or via continuous infusion at 12 grams/day) • **Advantages**—CNS penetration, potentially more effective with larger burden of infection, no renal dose adjustment • **Disadvantages**—less well-tolerated (see adverse effects), inconvenient dosing schedule → often need infusion pump for outpatient therapy • **Adverse effects (AEs)**—drug rashes, acute interstitial nephritis, hepatitis, high sodium content can cause sodium and/or volume overload in some patients
Alternative therapy	Vancomycin or daptomycin	• See respective sections below

MRSA

First-line therapy	IV vancomycin	• Dosing depends on patient age, weight, and renal function. Previously, we would target trough level 15–20 ug/mL for severe infections, but newest recommendation is to target AUC/MIC of 400–600 ug/mL (assumes MIC of 1 ug/mL by broth microdilution) • **Advantages**—long track record (best data with this drug), relatively easy to administer, relatively cheap, can be given with dialysis • **Main disadvantage is the AE profile**—nephrotoxicity, infusion reactions (red-man syndrome), drug rashes, cytopenia • **Avoid if vancomycin MIC is >2 ug/mL**—some experts stay away from vancomycin even when the MIC is 2, although data does not show detrimental outcomes with MIC of 2 • Vancomycin is slowly bactericidal and may take time to become therapeutic, so it is more common to see persistent MRSA bacteremia with vancomycin

	Daptomycin (Cubicin)	• Considered noninferior to vancomycin
		• Dosing is weight-based (use adjusted body weight if obese) and depends on renal function and the type of infection.
		• **Advantages**—very easy to administer (given once daily if CrCl ≥30 mL/min or every 48 hours if CrCl <30 mL/min), very well-tolerated
		• **Disadvantages**—cost, cannot be used for primary pneumonia (inactivated by surfactant)
		• **Adverse effects**
		  • Muscle injury—need to check baseline CK and monitor CK weekly while on the medication, consider holding statin medication while on daptomycin as well
		  • Rare reports of eosinophilic pneumonia

(Continued)

Table 81.1 – *Staphylococcus aureus* Bacteremia Antibiotics *(Cont'd)*

Alternative therapy	Ceftaroline (Teflaro)	• Fifth-generation cephalosporin with spectrum analogous to **ceftriaxone + MRSA coverage** • **Advantages**—well-tolerated, typically dosed twice daily • **Disadvantages**—cost, less available data, renal dose adjustment necessary
	Linezolid (Zyvox)	• **Advantages**—highly bioavailable (PO = IV), convenient twice daily dosing • **Disadvantages**—cost, adverse effects with use >2 weeks (i.e., myelosuppression and neuropathy), risk of serotonin syndrome especially with other serotonergic agents, bacteriostatic so not a great choice for SAB upfront but may be useful for oral step-down in the latter portion of the treatment course • **Tedizolid** is a closely related drug that may be less toxic
	Less commonly used agents	• These agents are not recommended for routine use. • IV trimethoprim/sulfamethoxazole, long-acting lipoglycopeptides (i.e., oritavancin, etc.), quinupristin/dalfopristin

ᵃGenerally speaking, ceftriaxone should be avoided in SAB because studies (not very high quality) have shown that it may be inferior to cefazolin in MSSA bacteremia.
ᵇFor all intents and purposes, cefazolin and the antistaphylococcal penicillins (i.e., nafcillin and oxacillin) are considered equivalent in terms of efficacy. Both of these agents outperform vancomycin in MSSA bacteremia.
AUC, Area under the curve; *CK*, creatine kinase; *CNS*, central nervous system; *CrCl*, creatinine clearance; *IV*, intravenous; *MIC*, minimum inhibitory concentration; *MRSA*, methicillin-resistant *Staphylococcus aureus*; *MSSA*, methicillin-sensitive *S. aureus*; *PO*, oral; *SAB*, *S. aureus* bacteremia.

(i.e., methicillin, oxacillin). There are rapid bench tests that can detect the presence of PBP-2A in minutes.

- Cefoxitin disc screen—Cefoxitin is a potent inducer of the *mecA* gene, and a positive cefoxitin screen is suggestive of MRSA.
- PCR detection of the *mecA* gene—This testing is often a part of multiplex blood culture identification panels (i.e., Biofire, Verigene, etc.).

The drugs of choice and alternative options for MSSA and MRSA are shown in Table 81.1.

Rule number 4—Document blood culture clearance!

Blood cultures should be repeated either daily (typically one set is all that is necessary if using this approach) or every other day (obtain two sets if using this approach). Persistent bacteremia (i.e., positive blood cultures for ≥72 hours) and/or fever (lasting ≥72 hours) despite appropriate therapy is highly suggestive of metastatic infection. Persistent bacteremia is also associated with higher mortality. It is not uncommon to see many days of bacteremia in patients with invasive *S. aureus* infections (i.e., endocarditis). In addition, the bacteremia may be intermittent in some cases, which is why we like to see several days of negative blood cultures before deeming the bacteremia cleared.

Rule number 5—Identify and control all sources of infection!

As shown in Fig. 81.1, this step is very complicated, and this is why the ID physician is such a vital part of the management. Once a patient has SAB, the bacteria have a free ride to every area of the body. Therefore the infection can seed any location in the body. The first step in evaluation is a thorough history and physical (H&P). Important historical features include a good review of systems (with particular focus on areas of pain or discomfort that are new to the patient) and asking about substance abuse (especially IV drug abuse). Important elements of the physical examination include assessing for stigmata of endocarditis, close skin examination (looking for portals of *S. aureus* entry), spinal percussion, and close assessment of all large joints including the acromioclavicular joint, the sternoclavicular joint, pubic symphysis, and sacroiliac joint. In addition, if any prosthetic devices are in place (i.e., IV lines, pacemakers, etc.), these should be closely examined for signs of infection. In most cases, the portal of entry (often a skin disruption such as the excoriations in this case patient) and additional foci of infection should be evident from the H&P. This assessment will guide the subsequent evaluation and management.

Any obvious foci of infection (i.e., skin abscess) should be drained, and any prosthetic devices that can be removed safely should be removed. An exception is peripheral IVs, unless they appear infected or there is evidence of thrombophlebitis. Failure to remove an infected prosthesis or drain/debride an area of infection (i.e., abscess) is associated with treatment failure and relapse.

Endocarditis is fairly common in the setting of SAB. Almost every patient with SAB should get a transthoracic echocardiogram (TTE). Echo may not be necessary in the rare case of nosocomial-onset SAB that clears quickly (within 48–72 hours) and has no other characteristics of complicated infection (i.e., nosocomial SAB due to peripheral IV thrombophlebitis). TTE alone misses a significant percentage (~15%–20%) of endocarditis cases in the setting of SAB, especially with small vegetations (<5 mm) or vegetations on the mitral or aortic valves. If there is a low pretest probability of endocarditis, then a good-quality TTE may be helpful to rule out endocarditis. In these cases, it can be helpful to consider using 4 weeks of therapy as the duration, because this will adequately treat most native valve endocarditis due to *S. aureus*. Most echocardiographers (cardiologists) who interpret TTE exams will actually note in their echo report that "a transesophageal echocardiogram should be pursued if there is significant concern for endocarditis." TEE is probably the best test for excluding valvular vegetation. TEE is more sensitive than TTE, but the specificities of both of these tests are fairly similar. There is a lot of interprovider variability with respect to the approach to echocardiography (especially TEE) in SAB. In general, a TEE should be obtained in patients with a high pretest probability of endocarditis. The following are considered to have a significant pretest probability of endocarditis in SAB:

- Patients with clinical stigmata of endocarditis (i.e., heart murmur, embolic phenomena, etc.)
- Prior history of infective endocarditis
- Patients with persistent fevers and/or bacteremia (≥72 hours) despite appropriate antibiotic therapy
- Intravenous drug abusers
- Patients with cardiac devices—implantable cardioverter-defibrillator, pacemaker, prosthetic valves, etc.
- Patients on hemodialysis
- Presence of another metastatic focus of infection (i.e., spinal infection, septic pulmonary or cerebral emboli, etc.) or no identified source of infection
- Community-onset SAB—this one is a bit controversial, but the thought is that one cannot tell exactly when the SAB started in community-onset cases; therefore, these patients were likely bacteremic for longer than meets the eye (thus the higher risk of endocarditis)

Echocardiography may be the most useful when done approximately 1 week following the onset of bacteremia/symptoms (if known). Consequently, if the initial TEE is negative in a patient with a high pretest probability of endocarditis, then repeat TEE in 1 week may be considered.

Risk factors for more complicated infection (i.e., metastatic foci) include community-onset SAB, persistent bacteremia and/or fever as noted above, presence of indwelling devices, immune suppression (i.e., HIV, malignancy, renal failure, etc.), presence of a metastatic focus of infection (i.e., psoas abscess), and lack of identifiable source. The time to culture positivity (faster onset = higher risk) is considered by some providers, but this one is a bit controversial. If a patient fails to clear the bacteremia and defervesce by 72 hours, or there is high clinical suspicion for a particular infection, then additional work-up should be pursued. This work-up may include TEE (if not already done), CT scan of the chest, abdomen, and pelvis with contrast, MRI of the entire spine with contrast, and in some cases nuclear imaging (PET/CT or tagged WBC scanning). If any foci of infection are discovered, they need to be addressed if possible (i.e., drain an abscess).

Rule number 6—Treat for the appropriate duration!

Management is relatively straightforward in most cases. As shown in Fig. 81.1, patients should be stratified into one of two groups: complicated SAB or uncomplicated SAB. It can be very difficult to meet all the criteria for uncomplicated SAB, but if the criteria are all met, then treatment duration can be 2 weeks. For complicated SAB, the duration is typically at least 4 to 6 weeks. The range exists because certain infections (i.e., vertebral osteomyelitis/discitis, endocarditis, etc.) may require a longer duration (typically at least 6 weeks). The duration starts from the day of blood culture clearance or definitive source control (whichever is most recent). Treatment should generally be IV for the entire duration of the therapy (see Table 81.1 for the drug choices). Long-term IVs (i.e., peripherally inserted central catheters) should not be placed until the bacteremia has cleared definitively. There are not much data for oral therapy in SAB, but in uncomplicated cases the use of linezolid for the tail end of therapy (the second week) can be considered. In general, most patients should be followed up with by an ID provider toward the end of therapy. Repeat imaging may be necessary to monitor progress in certain situations (i.e., an undrained visceral abscess).

Combination therapy has been shown to shorten the duration of bacteremia by an average of approximately 1 day, but this often comes at the risk of increased nephrotoxicity. In addition, studies have not shown significantly improved outcomes with combination therapy. Combination therapy often comes into play in patients with persistent/prolonged SAB despite appropriate therapy. If the patient has ongoing bacteremia for at least 1 week despite appropriate therapy, the following should be considered (roughly in the listed order):

- Ensure that source control is optimized as much as possible
- Review the isolate susceptibility (initial and subsequent isolates) to look for MIC creep that can be seen with some drugs (i.e., vancomycin in some MRSA cases)
- Consider salvage therapy, for example:
  - MSSA SAB—if on cefazolin, change to nafcillin
  - MRSA SAB—if on vancomycin, change to daptomycin plus or minus ceftaroline

Rifampin (if the *S. aureus* isolate is susceptible) for biofilm penetration is only beneficial in *S. aureus* infections associated with retained prosthetic material (i.e., prosthetic joint infection). Rifampin should not be used alone and should not be started until the infection is well-controlled (i.e., bacteremia cleared, source control optimized) in order to avoid rapid development of resistance seen with rifampin in *S. aureus* infections. Drug-drug interactions and liver function always need to be considered when using rifampin. Lastly, patients should be warned about the red-orange discoloration of bodily fluids that rifampin causes.

Continuing vancomycin and piperacillin/tazobactam (**option A**) would not be appropriate, as this combination has been associated with an increased incidence of acute kidney injury, which may be detrimental to this patient with underlying renal dysfunction. In addition, there are enough data to allow us to de-escalate therapy. Continuing vancomycin and stopping piperacillin/tazobactam (**option B**) could be considered, but vancomycin may not be the best choice for a patient with underlying renal dysfunction. furthermore, the vancomycin MIC is on the higher end of susceptibility, and some experts shy away from using vancomycin in these cases (although the available data do not support doing this). Changing to ceftaroline monotherapy (**option D**) could also be done, but this agent is considered second-line therapy for MRSA bacteremia. Changing to linezolid monotherapy (**option E**) would not be appropriate, as this agent is bacteriostatic and typically not used upfront for MRSA bacteremia.

KEY LEARNING POINT

Staphylococcus aureus bacteremia should typically be managed by an infectious disease physician. Important management considerations include:

- *Not ignoring* S. aureus *in the blood (i.e., do not dismiss as a contaminant)*
- *Documenting blood culture clearance*
- *Identifying all sources of infection and controlling them*
- *Treating with the correct drug for the correct duration*

REFERENCES AND FURTHER READING

- Holubar M, Meng L, Alegria W, Deresinski S. Bacteremia due to methicillin-resistant *Staphylococcus aureus*: an update on new therapeutic approaches. *Infect Dis Clin North Am.* 2020;34(4):849–861. https://doi.org/10.1016/j.idc.2020.04.003.
- Keynan Y, Rubinstein E. *Staphylococcus aureus* bacteremia, risk factors, complications, and management. *Crit Care Clin.* 2013;29(3):547–562. https://doi.org/10.1016/j.ccc.2013.03.008.
- Thwaites GE, Edgeworth JD, Gkrania-Klotsas E, et al. Clinical management of *Staphylococcus aureus* bacteraemia. *Lancet Infect Dis.* 2011;11(3):208–222. https://doi.org/10.1016/S1473-3099(10)70285-1.

A 55-year-old female is admitted to the hospital with a large subarachnoid hemorrhage complicated by intraventricular hemorrhage and hydrocephalus. Consequently, she was intubated on arrival, and an external ventricular drain (EVD) was placed. She was placed on cefazolin prophylaxis with plan to continue cefazolin while the drain was in place. On hospital day 7, she develops a fever to 102° F. The remainder of her vital signs are unchanged. Blood cultures are obtained and vancomycin and cefepime are started. On examination, the patient develops agitation when the sedation is weaned. There is no nuchal rigidity. The shunt entry site appears clean, and the drain appears to be functioning normally. Oxygenation and ventilation parameters have been stable, and there are minimal secretions noted when the endotracheal tube is suctioned. Heart is regular (rate and rhythm), and lungs are clear. There is no abdominal distension or tenderness. A right internal jugular central line shows no erythema or purulent discharge. Several peripheral intravenous catheters (IVs) are in place and show no insertion site abnormalities. A Foley catheter is in place and draining yellow urine. Per the bedside nurse, the patient has not had any diarrhea, rash, or decubitus wounds. Head CT shows intraventricular blood with an appropriately positioned ventricular catheter. On hospital day 10, the patient continues to have intermittent fevers, but is otherwise hemodynamically stable. The blood cultures have been without any growth. The serial cerebrospinal fluid (CSF) analyses are shown here:

CSF Parameter	Hospital Day 1	Hospital Day 4	Hospital Day 7	Hospital Day 10
Protein (mg/dL)	200	150	100	80
Glucose (mg/dL)	70	68	65	72
White blood cell count (neutrophil %) in cells/uL	100 (90%)	70 (80%)	45 (70%)	40 (70%)
Culture	No growth	No growth	Rare *Cutibacterium acnes*	No growth

What is the next best step in the management of this patient?

A. Deescalate to penicillin monotherapy and treat for 10 to 14 days.
B. Stop vancomycin and cefepime and restart cefazolin prophylaxis.
C. Stop all antibiotic therapy.
D. Obtain a respiratory culture.
E. Exchange the EVD catheter.

The next best step in management is to stop all antibiotic therapy (**option C**). The patient's cerebrospinal fluid (CSF) parameters have been serially improving, while the remaining clinical status has largely been unchanged despite appropriate antibiotic therapy. The *Cutibacterium acnes* growth was rare and likely represents contamination given the overall clinical picture. The agitation and ongoing fevers are likely secondary to the central nervous system (CNS) bleed.

The types of CNS devices commonly seen are ventriculoperitoneal (VP) shunts and external ventricular drains (EVDs). Less commonly, patients may have deep-brain stimulators, spinal cord stimulators, or VP and ventriculoatrial (VA) shunts. The main concern in this case is for a CNS device–associated infection (CDAI; hospital-acquired meningitis/ventriculitis). The organisms that typically cause CDAI are staphylococci (coagulase-negative staphylococci most commonly, but also *Staphylococcus aureus*), various gram-negative organisms (including *Pseudomonas* spp.), *C. acnes*, and rarely *Candida* spp. Interestingly, these patients may become infected with the usual community-acquired meningitis organisms as well. Infection occurs by one of the following mechanisms:

- Infection at the time of implantation (most common and occurs soon after surgery)
- Retrograde infection from the distal end of a VP shunt (i.e., intra-abdominal infection)
- Percutaneous contamination (i.e., during shunt tap)
- Hematogenous seeding of the shunt from a primary bacteremia (especially for VA shunts)

Biofilm formation is a problematic feature of these infections, which makes them difficult to treat with antibiotics alone. This problem is compounded by the fact that most of the antibiotics we use for CDAI have poor CNS penetration in the setting of CDAI.

The diagnosis of CDAI can be very difficult, especially when it occurs in the setting of an acute neurologic injury (such as in this patient). The reasoning behind this is that CDAI manifestations overlap with the manifestations of various neurologic injuries (especially CNS bleeds) and postsurgical abnormalities (i.e., chemical meningitis). In addition, positive cultures may represent contamination and not actual infection. Therefore, the entire clinical picture has to be taken into consideration. This includes the symptoms and signs, the laboratory findings (especially the CSF analysis), CNS imaging, and microbiologic data (blood and CSF cultures in particular). In addition, serial CSF values may be more useful than isolated values, as demonstrated in this case.

The presentation of CDAI is not specific and may include fevers, chills, altered mental status, nausea and/or vomiting, lethargy, shunt malfunction, or abnormalities surrounding the shunt tubing (i.e., erythema, tenderness, erosion, etc.). Nuchal rigidity and other meningeal signs are not very common. In patients with distal VP shunt infections, abdominal pain or signs of peritonitis may occur. In VA shunts, bacteremia or glomerulonephritis (shunt nephritis related to immune complex deposition) may be the presentation. Patients may have leukocytosis, although this finding is also nonspecific. Blood cultures should be obtained, although yield is fairly low. Imaging should be considered as well, including MRI of the brain with contrast and, in the case of VP shunts, abdominal imaging to look for intra-abdominal fluid collections (these are typically CSF collections near the catheter). CSF parameters including CSF white blood cell (WBC) count and differential, glucose, and protein are not very helpful either (i.e., normal findings do not exclude infection, and abnormal findings do not prove infection). CSF Gram stain and culture (obtained before antibiotics) are the most important test to establish the diagnosis. The culture is obtained directly from the shunt ("shunt tap") or drain. If the shunt is removed due to concern for infection, then the shunt components should be cultured as well. There is a recommendation to hold cultures longer (up to 10 days) to isolate *C. acnes*. Nowadays, most cultures will easily identify *C. acnes*, and this prolonged hold is no longer necessary. Lastly, the evaluation should include an assessment for other infections that can be seen in hospitalized patients.

Empiric antibiotics should provide coverage for methicillin-resistant *S. aureus* (MRSA) and *Pseudomonas* spp. A typical regimen would be vancomycin plus either cefepime or meropenem. For penicillin-allergic patients, aztreonam can be used for the gram-negative coverage. An important component of management is removal of the infected device and replacement (bridging) with an EVD. Targeted therapy and timing of reimplantation are shown in Table 82.1. One should remember to always use the CNS dosing for these agents. Drugs that should be avoided (due to poor CNS penetration) include piperacillin/tazobactam and cefazolin. Periodic CSF analysis and gram stain/culture should be obtained to assess the response to therapy (i.e., should see improving parameters, culture becoming negative, etc.).

Deescalating to penicillin monotherapy and treating for 10 to 14 days (**option A**) would be appropriate if this patient actually had meningitis/ventriculitis due to *C. acnes*. Stopping vancomycin and cefepime and restarting cefazolin prophylaxis (**option B**) is not recommended. Prolonged (i.e., past the periprocedural period) prophylactic antimicrobials are offered by some centers, but there is not great evidence to support this practice. Periprocedural (i.e., at the time of shunt or drain placement) antimicrobial prophylaxis is recommended. In

Table 82.1 – Definitive Therapy for Central Nervous System Device-Associated Infection

Organism	Primary Treatment	Alternative Treatment[c]	Treatment Duration[b]	When It Is Okay to Reimplant Shunt (If Still Necessary)
CoNS—methicillin-resistant[a]	• Vancomycin	• Linezolid or daptomycin or TMP/SMX	• No CSF abnormalities → 10 days • If CSF abnormalities → 14 days	• No CSF abnormalities → once CSF culture is negative for 72 hours • CSF abnormalities → once CSF culture is negative for 1 week
CoNS—methicillin-sensitive[a]	• Nafcillin	• Vancomycin		
Cutibacterium acnes	• Penicillin-G	• Ceftriaxone		
MSSA[a]	• Nafcillin	• Vancomycin	• 10–14 days	• Once CSF culture is negative for 10 days
MRSA[a]	• Vancomycin	• Linezolid or daptomycin or TMP/SMX		
Corynebacterium spp.	• Vancomycin	• Linezolid	• Similar to CoNS	• Similar to CoNS
Pseudomonas spp.	• Cefepime	• Meropenem or aztreonam or ciprofloxacin	• 21 days	• Once CSF culture is negative for 10–21 days
ESBL- or Amp-C–producing GNR	• Meropenem (prolonged infusion)	• Ciprofloxacin or TMP/SMX • Cefepime may be considered for Amp-C organisms		
Acinetobacter baumanii	• Meropenem (prolonged infusion)	• Colistin or polymyxin B		
Most other GNR	• Ceftriaxone	• Cefepime, meropenem, aztreonam, or ciprofloxacin		
Candida spp.	• Amp-B + 5-FC	• Fluconazole (if susceptible isolate) or • Voriconazole	• Continue Amp-B/5-FC for at least 2 weeks and until improved clinically and on CSF (improved parameters, clearance) • Can then consider changing to high-dose fluconazole (400–800 mg/day) if susceptible species or voriconazole • Treatment is continued until all symptoms/signs have resolved, CSF parameters have normalized, and there is no radiographic evidence of ongoing infection	
Aspergillus or Exserohilum spp.	• Voriconazole	• Posaconazole or Amp-B	• At least 3 months (potentially longer in immune-compromised)	• N/A

[a] If the hardware is retained, then consider using rifampin (if the isolate is susceptible) concurrently.
[b] Duration start date is the day of CSF culture clearance.
[c] If there is inadequate response to systemic therapy, then intraventricular therapy may be considered.

Amp-C, a beta-lactamase; CoNS, Coagulase negative staphylococci; CSF, cerebrospinal fluid; ESBL, extended-spectrum beta-lactamase; 5-FC, flucytosine; GNR, gram-negative rod; MSSA, methicillin-susceptible Staphylococcus aureus; MRSA, methicillin-resistant S. aureus; N/A, not available or not applicable; TX, treatment; TMP/SMX, trimethoprim/sulfamethoxazole.

addition, the use of antimicrobial impregnated shunts/drains is recommended. Obtaining a respiratory culture (**option D**) would be unnecessary because there is no clinical concern for tracheobronchitis or pneumonia in this patient. It would likely end up growing an organism that most likely was just a colonizer and not causing actual infection. Exchanging the EVD catheter (**option E**) is not routinely recommended.

KEY LEARNING POINT

Central nervous system device–associated infection can be very difficult to diagnose. The approach to diagnosis requires taking the entire clinical picture into consideration, and serial testing is often helpful.

REFERENCES AND FURTHER READING

- Bayston R, Pelegrin I. Infections in hydrocephalus shunts. In: Cohen J, ed. *Infectious Diseases*. 4th ed. Elsevier; 2017:221–224.
- Tunkel AR, Hasbun R, Bhimraj A, et al. 2017 Infectious Diseases Society of America's clinical practice guidelines for healthcare-associated ventriculitis and meningitis. *Clin Infect Dis*. 2017;64(6):e34–e65. https://doi.org/10.1093/cid/ciw861.

A 30-year-old male presents to the emergency room with a 1-week history of fevers, anorexia, weight loss, and right upper quadrant pain. He has no major medical problems and does not take any medications. He went to Mexico 3 months ago for a weeklong vacation. He stayed at a resort, but also went off-site for some meals and activities. He notes that, soon after returning home, he had a mild self-limited diarrheal illness. Vital signs reveal temperature 100.6° F, heart rate 80 beats per minute, blood pressure 115/80 mmHg, and respiratory rate 16. On examination, he looks uncomfortable. There is mild scleral icterus. Abdominal examination reveals tenderness in the right upper quadrant but no rebound tenderness. The remainder of the examination is unremarkable. Laboratory studies reveal white blood cell count 12,000 cells/uL, ALT 125 U/L, AST 100 U/L, alkaline phosphatase 300 U/L, and total bilirubin 4 mg/dL. CT scan of the abdomen is shown in Fig. 83.1.

What is the most appropriate therapy for this patient?

A. Metronidazole followed by paromomycin.

B. Metronidazole alone.

C. Albendazole.

D. Ceftriaxone and metronidazole.

E. Percutaneous drainage.

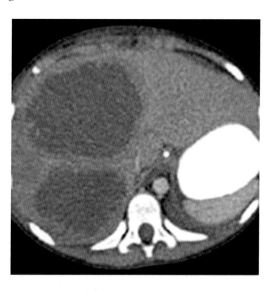

Figure 83.1 – Computed tomography scan of the abdomen.
Foong Ng K, Kee Tan K, et. al., Fatal case of amoebic liver abscess in a child. *Asian-Pac J Trop Med*. 2015; 8(10):878–880. https://doi.org/10.1016/j.apjtm.2015.09.018.

The most appropriate therapy is metronidazole followed by paromomycin (**option A**). Amebiasis is a parasitic infection caused by the protozoan *Entamoeba histolytica*. The infection (cyst form) is acquired by the fecal-oral route (i.e., ingestion of feces-contaminated food and/or water, or in the men who have sex with men population). The areas with the highest incidence are India, Mexico, Central and South America, and Africa. In the United States, the infection is typically seen in travelers or immigrants from endemic areas.

The initial infection can be asymptomatic/mild (~80%–90% of cases), or it can cause a full-blown colitis (a cause of bloody diarrhea). Colitis may cause toxic megacolon, perforation, peritonitis, appendicitis, and amebomas (granulation tissue resembling colon cancer). In some cases (<5%), the protozoa (the invasive trophozoite form) invade the bloodstream via the portal vein and cause extraintestinal infection. Hepatic abscesses are the most common extraintestinal infection. A major risk factor for hepatic abscess formation is alcohol use. The hepatic abscesses can develop years after the initial infection, which can make the diagnosis difficult. Amebic abscesses present similar to pyogenic liver abscesses, with fevers, right upper quadrant pain, hepatomegaly, and potentially even jaundice. Differential diagnosis of hepatic lesions should include echinococcosis, pyogenic liver abscess, and malignancy. Less common manifestations of amebiasis include brain abscesses, thoracic infections (lung abscesses/ empyema or pericardial infection), and cutaneous lesions.

Diagnosis can be difficult. Serology is only useful in areas where the infection is not endemic, because prior exposure is fairly common, and the antibodies remain positive for many years after exposure. In addition, serology may be negative early in the infection, so serology is probably most useful in chronic infections (including extraintestinal infection). Stool microscopy has very low sensitivity (<40%), but microscopy of drained abscess material may be helpful. Antigen testing can be done on stool or serum. Stool antigen is most useful in intestinal disease (~90% sensitivity), and serum antigen testing is most useful in extraintestinal infection (>95% sensitivity). PCR is part of most stool film-array panels now and is probably the most useful test. It can be done on stool or abscess material and is highly sensitive regardless of the location of the infection. Ultrasound (US) of the liver is the best initial imaging test. Lesions are typically solitary. US may show a rounded, homogeneous, hypoechoic lesion located near the liver capsule. The right hepatic lobe is the most common location. CT is most useful in the early phase of abscess formation and may show a rounded, hypoechoic lesion as well (see Fig. 83.1). Colon biopsy may show flask-shaped ulceration, as shown in Fig. 83.2.

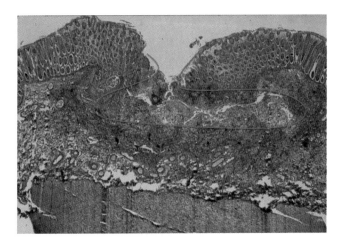

Figure 83.2 – Flask-shaped colonic ulceration in intestinal amebiasis.
Petri WA, et al. *Entamoeba species*, including amebic colitis and liver abscess. In: Bennet JE, Dolin R, Blaser MJ, eds. *Mandell, Douglas, and Bennett's Principles and Practice of Infectious Diseases*. 9th ed. Elsevier; 2020:3273–3286. Courtesy of Herman Zaiman and the H.W. Manter Laboratory of Parasitology.

Treatment of isolated asymptomatic intestinal disease (colonization) is done with a luminal agent such as paromomycin for 5 to 10 days or diloxanide for 10 days. Due to concern over adverse effects, iodoquinol is not really used much anymore. Treatment of symptomatic intestinal disease (colitis) or extraintestinal disease consists of a systemic agent (metronidazole for 10 days or tinidazole for 5 days) and an intraluminal agent (as previous) to eradicate the intestinal infection. Medical therapy is often successful in eradicating the hepatic abscess, but in 15% of cases medical therapy alone is not enough. Percutaneous drainage is superior to aspiration. The drained material is often described as "anchovy paste." Drainage can also be considered if:

- There is no improvement after approximately 1 week of medical therapy—can also consider adding pyogenic liver abscess coverage in this case
- The abscess is large—greater than 10 cm in any location or greater than 5 cm in the left hepatic lobe (risk of rupture into pericardium)
- The abscess is subcapsular or close to rupture
- There is concern for superinfection

Complications of inadequately treated amebic infections include rupture into neighboring organs and bacterial superinfection. Other family members and/or household contacts should also be screened for infection and treated as indicated.

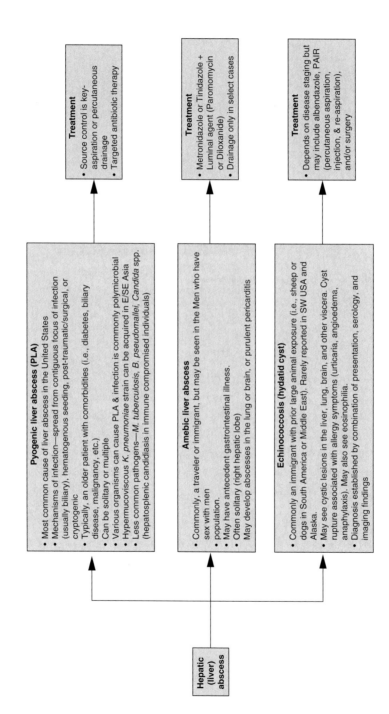

Hepatic (liver) abscess

Pyogenic liver abscess (PLA)
- Most common cause of liver abscess in the United States
- Mechanisms of infection—spread from contiguous focus of infection (usually biliary), hematogenous seeding, post-traumatic/surgical, or cryptogenic
- Typically, an older patient with comorbidities (i.e., diabetes, biliary disease, malignancy, etc.)
- Can be solitary or multiple
- Various organisms can cause PLA & infection is commonly polymicrobial
- Hypermucoviscous *K. pneumoniae* strain can be acquired in E/SE Asia
- Less common pathogens—*M. tuberculosis, B. pseudomallei, Candida* spp. (hepatosplenic candidiasis in immune compromised individuals)

Treatment
- Source control is key-aspiration or percutaneous drainage
- Targeted antibiotic therapy

Amebic liver abscess
- Commonly, a traveler or immigrant, but may be seen in the Men who have sex with men population.
- May have antecedent gastrointestinal illness.
- Often solitary (right hepatic lobe)
- May develop abscesses in the lung or brain, or purulent pericarditis

Treatment
- Metronidazole or Tinidazole + Luminal agent (Paromomycin or Diloxanide)
- Drainage only in select cases

Echinococcosis (hydatid cyst)
- Commonly an immigrant with prior large animal exposure (i.e., sheep or dogs in South America or Middle East). Rarely reported in SW USA and Alaska.
- May see cystic lesions in the liver, lung, brain, and other viscera. Cyst rupture associated with allergy symptoms (urticaria, angioedema, anaphylaxis). May also see eosinophilia.
- Diagnosis established by combination of presentation, serology, and imaging findings

Treatment
- Depends on disease staging but may include albendazole, PAIR (percutaneous aspiration, injection, & re-aspiration), and/or surgery

Figure 83.3 – Hepatic abscesses

Metronidazole alone (**option B**) would not eradicate the intestinal infection. Albendazole (**option C**) is the drug of choice for echinococcosis. Echinococcosis is a parasitic infection caused by various species of tapeworm called *Echinococcus*. This infection may present similar to extraintestinal amebiasis. Unlike amebiasis, echinococcosis is associated with exposure to certain animals (classic vignette involves dogs and sheep in South America) and is very uncommon in Mexico. Ceftriaxone and metronidazole (**option D**) would provide coverage for a community-acquired pyogenic liver abscess. This could be considered if the patient fails to respond to the treatment for amebiasis. The history in this case is not consistent with pyogenic liver abscess. Percutaneous drainage (**option E**) for amebiasis may be considered based on the indications listed above. If this were a pyogenic liver abscess, then every effort should be made to drain the abscess as soon as possible.

KEY LEARNING POINT

The treatment of amebic liver abscess involves systemic therapy (metronidazole or tinidazole) and intraluminal therapy (paromomycin or diloxanide).
An overview of the approach to hepatic (liver) abscesses is shown in Fig. 83.3.

REFERENCES AND FURTHER READING

- Bouton TC, Chan PA. Echinococcosis. In: *Ferri's Clinical Advisor 2022*. Elsevier; 2020.
- Ferri FF. Liver abscess. In: *Ferri's Clinical Advisor 2022*. Elsevier; 2020:921–922.
- Petri WA, et al. *Entamoeba* species, including amebic colitis and liver abscess. In: Bennet JE, Dolin R, Blaser MJ, eds. *Mandell, Douglas, and Bennett's Principles and Practice of Infectious Diseases*. 9th ed. Elsevier; 2020:3273–3286.
- Roediger R, Lisker-Melman M. Pyogenic and amebic infections of the liver. *Gastroenterol Clin North Am.* 2020;49(2):361–377. https://doi.org/10.1016/j.gtc.2020.01.013.

A 30-year-old male is admitted to the hospital with a 2-day history of fevers, nausea, vomiting, and abdominal pain. He is otherwise healthy and takes no medications. He has no medication allergies. Vital signs reveal temperature 102° F, heart rate 125 beats per minute, blood pressure 92/55 mmHg, and respiratory rate 20 on room air. On examination, he appears ill. Oral mucosa is dry. Heart exam shows a regular tachycardia but no murmur. Lungs are clear. Abdomen is mildly distended and firm. Rebound tenderness is present over the right lower quadrant. Bowel sounds are hypoactive. The remainder of the examination is unremarkable. Laboratory studies reveal white blood cell count of 18,000 cells/uL (90% neutrophils) and creatinine 1.4 mg/dL. CT of the abdomen reveals inflammation around the appendix with a small amount of free air in the abdomen. Blood cultures are obtained, and fluid resuscitation is initiated. Emergent surgery is planned.

What is the most appropriate initial antibiotic therapy?

A. Cefoxitin.

B. Ampicillin/sulbactam.

C. Piperacillin/tazobactam.

D. Moxifloxacin.

E. Ceftriaxone plus metronidazole.

The most appropriate initial therapy in this case would be piperacillin/tazobactam (**option C**). This patient is presenting with perforated appendicitis. In the grand scheme of things, this is just an example of secondary peritonitis. An overview of intra-abdominal infections (IAIs) is shown in Fig. 84.1.

Primary (spontaneous) peritonitis and peritoneal dialysis (PD)-associated peritonitis are less commonly managed by infectious disease (ID) specialists. Most primary physicians (i.e., internal medicine specialists) are capable of managing primary (spontaneous) peritonitis. In most medical systems, nephrologists manage PD-associated peritonitis. More complicated cases may be referred to ID. The International Society for Peritoneal Dialysis (ISPD) has created guidelines for the management of PD-associated peritonitis, and these can be accessed at: https://www.ISPD.org/guidelines/. This case discussion will focus on secondary peritonitis, as it is much more commonly managed with the help of ID specialists.

In general, the number of microorganisms increases as you descend the gastrointestinal (GI) tract. In the upper GI tract (stomach and duodenum), there are small amounts of bacteria (typically transient organisms from the oral cavity such as viridans-group streptococci and lactobacilli) and *Candida* spp. In the distal small intestine and colon, additional organisms become more prevalent including the enteric gram-negative rods (Enterobacteriaceae), enterococci, and various anaerobes. With antimicrobial exposure, use of antacid medications (i.e., proton pump inhibitors), and healthcare exposure, the flora changes significantly—the amounts of *Enterobacter* spp., *Enterococcus* spp., *Pseudomonas* spp., and *Candida* spp. increase significantly. With GI organ stasis or obstruction, the number of organisms may increase and become problematic (i.e., small intestinal bacterial overgrowth in gastroparesis). The most common microbes causing IAI overall are *Escherichia coli* and *Klebsiella* spp. The most common and significant anaerobes are the *Bacteroides* spp. (especially *B. fragilis*).

With such a wide array of organisms in the GI tract, it should not be surprising that most secondary peritonitis infections are polymicrobial. The presentation may consist of fevers, chills, anorexia, nausea, vomiting, and severe abdominal pain that is made worse with any movement. Patients will often appear toxic and septic (i.e., febrile, tachycardia, hypotension, etc.). Examination may show abdominal distension, hypoactive or absent bowel sounds, abdominal wall rigidity, tenderness with palpation and rebound tenderness. Some patients have more subtle presentations, including those with lax abdominal wall muscles (i.e., postoperative patients, cirrhotic patients, etc.), those with deep abscesses that are not contacting the peritoneum, or those who are on steroids.

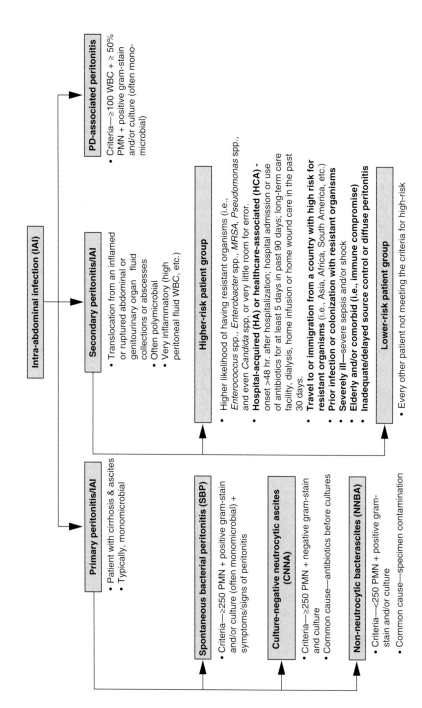

Figure 84.1 – Intra-abdominal infections

MRSA, Methicillin-resistant *Staphylococcus aureus*; *PD*, peritoneal dialysis; *PMN*, polymorphonuclear cells; *WBC*, white blood cell.

Intra-abdominal infection (IAI)

Primary peritonitis/IAI
- Patient with cirrhosis & ascites
- Typically, monomicrobial

Secondary peritonitis/IAI
- Translocation from an inflamed or ruptured abdominal or genitourinary organ fluid collections or abscesses
- Often polymicrobial
- Very inflammatory (high peritoneal fluid WBC, etc.)

PD-associated peritonitis
- Criteria—≥100 WBC + ≥ 50% PMN + positive gram-stain and/or culture (often mono-microbial)

Spontaneous bacterial peritonitis (SBP)
- Criteria—≥250 PMN + positive gram-stain and/or culture (often monomicrobial) + symptoms/signs of peritonitis

Culture-negative neutrocytic ascites (CNNA)
- Criteria—≥250 PMN + negative gram-stain and culture
- Common cause—antibiotics before cultures

Non-neutrocytic bacterascites (NNBA)
- Criteria—<250 PMN + positive gram-stain and/or culture
- Common cause—specimen contamination

Higher-risk patient group
- Higher likelihood of having resistant organisms (i.e., *Enterococcus* spp., *Enterobacter* spp., *MRSA*, *Pseudomonas* spp., and even *Candida* spp. or very little room for error.
- **Hospital-acquired (HA) or healthcare-associated (HCA)** - onset >48 hr. after hospitalization; hospital admission or use of antibiotics for at least 5 days in past 90 days; long-term care facility, dialysis, home infusion or home wound care in the past 30 days.
- **Travel to or immigration from a country with high risk for resistant organisms** (i.e., Asia, Africa, South America, etc.)
- **Prior infection or colonization with resistant organisms**
- **Severely ill**—severe sepsis and/or shock
- **Elderly and/or comorbid (i.e., immune compromise)**
- **Inadequate/delayed source control or diffuse peritonitis**

Lower-risk patient group
- Every other patient not meeting the criteria for high-risk

Laboratory evaluation should include complete blood count with differential, a complete metabolic panel (i.e., electrolytes, renal function, hepatic function), urinalysis with microscopy, serum lactic acid, serum lipase, coagulation parameters, and pregnancy testing. Blood cultures should be obtained. The best initial imaging test is often plain radiography of the abdomen and/or chest to look for free air (i.e., subdiaphragmatic air). The best test to localize the source is a CT abdomen/pelvis with oral and intravenous contrast. Ultrasound may be preferred in lesions of the right upper quadrant, retroperitoneum, or pelvis. Probably the most important test to obtain is a sample of the infected area (ideally before administering antibiotics). This may include paracentesis to sample infected ascites fluid, or aspiration or drainage of a fluid collection or abscess. Peritoneal fluid analysis at the minimum should include cell count with differential and microbiologic studies (stain and culture including aerobic, anaerobic, and fungal components). Abscess samples are typically only sent for the microbiologic studies (i.e., cell counts are not typically done). Of note, cultures should only be obtained from a fresh aspirate or during drain placement and not from an existing drain. The rationale for this is that cultures from existing drains may reveal organisms that are colonizing the drain tubing and may not actually be causing the peritoneal infection. Conversely, a peritoneal fluid analysis (i.e., cell count with differential) can be obtained from an existing drain and can potentially be used as a marker of treatment response.

The management of these infections can be very complicated. The most important aspect of management is source control. Source control involves addressing the focus (or foci) of infection (i.e., surgery to remove an inflamed organ or repair a perforation; draining abscesses, etc.). Failure to achieve source control is associated with increased mortality and treatment failure. Antimicrobial therapy alone (i.e., without source control) is often unsuccessful in managing most IAIs. Therefore, antimicrobial therapy is given as an adjunctive measure to source control.

Empiric antimicrobial therapy will depend on local antibiotic resistance patterns and risk stratification (i.e., high-risk vs. low-risk), as shown in Fig. 84.1. No single regimen has been shown to be more effective than any other regimen.

- **Low-risk patients:**
  - The coverage typically includes Enterobacteriaceae, anaerobes, and aerobic streptococci
  - Commonly used regimens include ceftriaxone + metronidazole (**option E**), a fluoroquinolone (FQ; typically ciprofloxacin or levofloxacin) + metronidazole, ertapenem monotherapy, or less commonly, moxifloxacin monotherapy (**option D**)
  - FQs should only be used if the local *E. coli* resistance is less than 10%

- **High-risk patients:**
  - Coverage is typically broader and depending on the clinical context, may include further coverage for:
    - Gram-positive organisms—methicillin-resistant *Staphylococcus aureus* (MRSA) and *Enterococcus* spp., including vancomycin-resistant *Enterococcus* spp. (VRE)
    - Gram-negative organisms—Amp-C beta-lactamase producers (i.e., *Enterobacter* spp., *Citrobacter* spp., etc.), *Pseudomonas* spp., and more resistant pathogens like extended-spectrum beta-lactamase (ESBL) producers (i.e., often *E. coli* or *Klebsiella* spp.) and carbapenem-resistant Enterobacteriaceae (CRE)
    - Candida spp.—coverage for *Candida* spp. may be considered in upper GI infectious sources or in patients with risk factors for invasive candidiasis (i.e., immune-suppressed, postsurgical (especially abdominal surgery), pancreatitis-associated IAI, prolonged hospital stays, extensive prior antibiotic exposure, etc.)

- Options for routine coverage for high-risk patients:
  - **Piperacillin/tazobactam (pip/tazo; Zosyn)**—broad coverage including most streptococci, methicillin-sensitive *S. aureus* (MSSA), *Enterococcus faecalis*, anaerobes (including *B. fragilis*), and many gram-negatives including *Pseudomonas* spp.
  - **Cefepime plus metronidazole**—coverage is fairly similar to pip/tazo, but cefepime covers Amp-C beta-lactamase producers more reliably; this regimen does not cover *Enterococcus* spp. (if suspicion for *Enterococcus* spp., then can add vancomycin or daptomycin)
  - **Meropenem**—very broad coverage including streptococci, MSSA, anaerobes (including *B. fragilis*), and many gram-negatives including *Pseudomonas* spp., Amp-C beta-lactamase producers, and ESBL-producing organisms; the major gaps in coverage are MRSA and many *Enterococcus* spp. (if suspicious for these organisms, then can add vancomycin or Daptomycin) and CRE
  - **Vancomycin + aztreonam + metronidazole**—mainly used in patients with severe penicillin allergy

- If empiric antifungal coverage (i.e., *Candida* spp.) is indicated:
  - An echinocandin (i.e., caspofungin, micafungin, or anidulafungin) is usually the best initial choice, because this class of antifungal will cover most *Candida* spp. reliably

- If the patient is hemodynamically stable and is not at risk for resistant *Candida* spp. (i.e., no prior azole antifungal exposure, no prior isolation of *C. krusei, C. glabrata,* or *C. auris*), then fluconazole can be considered as initial therapy

- Empiric coverage for other resistant pathogens (i.e., ESBL, VRE, CRE) should only be provided in the appropriate clinical context (i.e., prior isolation of these organisms, extensive antibiotic exposure, exposure to endemic region for CRE, hepatobiliary infection in liver transplantation for VRE, etc.). The options for these infections are discussed in the definitive management section below

Certain pathogen and antibiotic associations deserve mention here. Due to rising resistance in isolates of *B. fragilis*, clindamycin and the cephamycins (cefoxitin [**option A**] and Cefotetan) are no longer recommended for IAIs. Similarly, ampicillin/sulbactam (**option B**, Unasyn) is not very useful anymore because of the rise in resistance seen in *E. coli* and Enterobacteriaceae. Lastly, FQ resistance in *E. coli* has been on the rise; consequently, FQ should only be used if the local *E. coli* isolates are greater than 90% susceptible (i.e., local resistance <10%) to FQ.

Definitive therapy will depend on the organism(s) isolated and their susceptibility profile, the degree of source control, and the clinical response. What follows is a discussion of some useful principles for managing IAIs.

1. In general, one should use the narrowest regimen possible that will provide adequate coverage based on the available data (i.e., Gram stain and culture results).

2. Certain pathogens may not grow either due to antibiotics being given before obtaining the culture or due to their fastidious nature (i.e., anaerobes). Sometimes a pathogen may be evident on just the Gram stain in these situations. This principle always needs to be considered when designing a definitive regimen, because failing to cover a potential organism may be detrimental.

3. Regardless of whether or not they grow, anaerobes should always be covered, because failure to cover anaerobes has been associated with treatment failure. Routinely used antibiotics with reliable anaerobic coverage (i.e., will cover *B. fragilis* reliably) include:
   - Ampicillin/sulbactam (Unasyn)—IV
   - Amoxicillin/clavulanate (Augmentin)—essentially a PO formulation of ampicillin/sulbactam
   - Pip/tazo (Zosyn)—IV

- Metronidazole (Flagyl)—PO bioavailability is equivalent to the IV formulation, so use PO form whenever possible (unless concerned for ability to absorb/tolerate oral medication)
- Carbapenems—IV

4. In general, not every organism that is isolated needs to be covered. This is especially true in cases with excellent source control. When *Enterococcus* spp. and/or *Candida* spp. are isolated as part of a polymicrobial infection, coverage may or may not be necessary:

- *Enterococcus* spp.
    - In general, coverage should be considered in high-risk patients, patients with prosthetic heart valves, patients who have previously (recently) received FQ or cephalosporin therapy (these antibiotics select for *Enterococcus* spp.), situations where *Enterococcus* is the sole pathogen or a recurring pathogen, or patients who fail to improve despite appropriate treatment otherwise

- *Enterococcus* spp. (if penicillin- or ampicillin-susceptible)—options include:
    - Penicillin (typically IV formulation) or ampicillin
    - If desiring additional anaerobic coverage, then can use ampicillin/sulbactam (Unasyn) or pip/tazo (Zosyn)
    - If desiring oral options, then can use amoxicillin (or amoxicillin/clavulanic acid to get anaerobic coverage as well)

- *Enterococcus* spp. (if penicillin- or ampicillin-resistant, but vancomycin-susceptible)
    - First-line—vancomycin
    - Alternatives are similar to VRE options below

- VRE (*E. faecium*) that do not fit into one of the aforementioned *Enterococcus* spp. groups
    - First-line—daptomycin or linezolid
    - Alternatives—eravacycline

- *Candida* spp.
    - Coverage should be considered if the patient is high-risk, if *Candida* is the sole pathogen or a recurring pathogen, or if the patient fails to improve despite appropriate treatment otherwise

- If the subspecies is unknown, the patient is hemodynamically unstable, or the patient is at high risk for resistant *Candida* spp., then an echinocandin is the appropriate choice
- *C. krusei* is intrinsically resistant to fluconazole. The recommended treatment options are an echinocandin or an advanced generation azole (i.e., voriconazole)
- *C. glabrata* may be resistant to fluconazole, but more commonly, it is susceptible dose–dependent (SDD) to fluconazole. If the susceptibility is unknown, or the isolate is resistant, then an echinocandin is appropriate. If the isolate is SDD, then a higher dose (12 mg/kg/day) of fluconazole may be used
- *C. auris* is often very resistant to azoles, and the most appropriate therapy is often an echinocandin
- *C. guilliermondii* may have reduced susceptibility to fluconazole
- Most other *Candida* spp. (assuming no prior azole exposure) are predictably susceptible to fluconazole, but susceptibility testing should still be performed

5. Do not overlook Amp-C beta-lactamase–producing organisms

- Certain organisms carry either a chromosomal (inducible) or plasmid-mediated Amp-C beta-lactamase. These organisms can be remembered by the mnemonic "**MYSPACE**"
    - *M—Morganella morganii*
    - *Y—Yersinia* spp. *(some subspecies)*
    - *S—Serratia marcescens*
    - *P—Providencia stuartii, Proteus vulgaris, Pseudomonas* spp.
    - *A—Acinetobacter* spp., *Aeromonas* spp.
    - *C—Citrobacter* spp.
    - *E—Enterobacter* spp.
- In the presence of certain beta-lactams (classically third-generation cephalosporins like ceftriaxone), the Amp-C beta-lactamase may be induced (or more accurately stated, may become "derepressed"). When this happens, the organism becomes resistant to all penicillins (including the beta-lactamase inhibitors), most cephalosporins

(excluding cefepime), and aztreonam. Clinically, this may manifest as initial clinical improvement followed by clinical decompensation

- Of course, not all of the MYSPACE bugs are created equally. The most problematic (highest-risk) pathogens would be Enterobacter cloacae, Enterobacter (Klebsiella) aerogenes, and Citrobacter freundii.

- At times, these organisms may appear completely sensitive on the microbiology susceptibility report, but in the presence of the wrong antibiotic (i.e., ceftriaxone), they will show their true colors

- The keys to managing infections caused by these organisms are ensuring good source control (reduces the size of the inoculum) and choosing a drug that provides adequate coverage and achieves good concentration at the site of infection

- The best therapeutic choice in most cases is a carbapenem

- If there is good source control, then consideration can be given to using cefepime (if cefepime MIC ≤2; use higher dose, prolonged infusion cefepime – 2 g IV every 8 hours with each infusion given over 3 hours) or a non–beta-lactam (if susceptible), such as a FQ or, rarely, trimethoprim/sulfamethoxazole (TMP/SMX)

6. ESBL-producing organisms are considered resistant to most penicillins, most cephalosporins (including cefepime), and aztreonam. Resistance to ceftriaxone is sometimes used as a surrogate to identify ESBL producers. ESBL producers are often *E. coli, Klebsiella* spp., or *Proteus mirabilis.* The drug of choice in most cases is a carbapenem. An alternative in well-controlled infections may be a non–beta-lactam antibiotic (typically a FQ) if susceptible.

7. MRSA is very uncommon in IAIs but may be seen in the postoperative setting or in patients with certain conditions (i.e., chronic granulomatous disease). If identified, coverage options include:
   a. IV options—vancomycin, daptomycin, ceftaroline, or linezolid.
   b. PO options—linezolid, and potentially doxycycline (if susceptible), or TMP/SMX (if susceptible).

8. Lastly, CRE may rarely be recovered, and IAIs are where one is likely to see CRE. By definition, CRE are resistant to at least one carbapenem or produce a carbapenemase enzyme. CRE can be resistant to some carbapenems but not others. Knowledge of whether a CRE

isolate is carbapenemase-producing and, if it is, the specific carbapenemase produced (i.e., KPC, OXA-48, MBL) is important in guiding treatment decisions. The approach to the management of CRE in IAIs is shown in Fig. 84.2.

9. Oral therapy consideration

Appropriate patient response typically includes resolution of fevers, improvement of symptoms, and decline in markers of inflammation (i.e., improved leukocytosis and/or thrombocytosis, declining inflammatory markers, etc.). Transition to oral therapy can be considered if the patient has improved clinically, is tolerating oral intake, and has good source control and there is a highly bioavailable oral agent (see PO agents listed earlier) that can be used to treat the infection.

10. Treatment duration and follow-up

In patients with definitive source control, the duration of therapy is typically 4 to 7 days, based on several trials showing that shorter courses were no worse than longer courses. Unfortunately, many of the more complicated cases do not fit so nicely into this scheme. In cases with inadequate source control, the duration of therapy is not well-studied. The current practice is keeping patients on antimicrobial therapy while working to achieve the best possible source control. Often, these patients will have one or more intra-abdominal drains in place that will slowly decrease the amount of peritoneal contamination. Regardless of whether or not drains are placed, at some point imaging may need to be repeated to re-evaluate the clinical response. This is often done a few weeks after the most recent imaging, or when the drain(s) output drops off significantly (i.e., <5 cc/day for at least 2 days in a row). Patients are typically seen in follow-up at around the time of repeat imaging. Some providers may also repeat a paracentesis (i.e., if treating infected ascites) at some point during the therapy to assess response.

Treatment failure may show up as ongoing or recurrent sepsis or worsening/recurrent symptoms (i.e., abdominal pain, vomiting, etc.). The things to consider in these situations are:

- Is source control still appropriate?
  - Drains may become clogged or dislodged, which may manifest decreased drain output

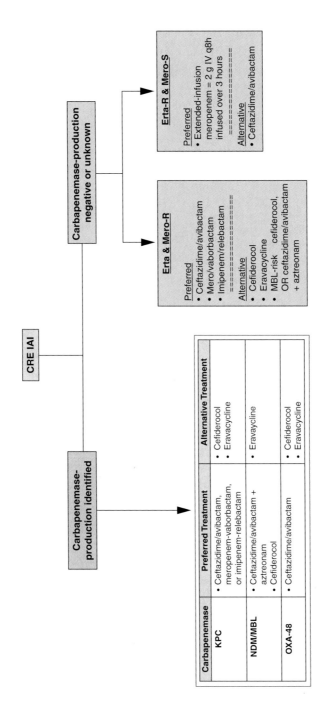

Figure 84.2 – Management of carbapenem-resistant Enterobacteriaceae (CRE) in intra-abdominal infections (IAIs)
Erta, Ertapenem; *Mero*, meropenem; *MBL*, metallo-beta-lactamase.

- • Sometimes, new foci of infection (i.e., abscesses) may develop that require drainage
  - • Repeat imaging may be helpful to answer this question
- • Are the appropriate organisms being covered?
  - • Review prior culture results
  - • Prolonged therapy with poor source control is a set-up for the development of resistant organisms. Ideally, culture should be repeated if possible before broadening antimicrobial therapy to cover resistant pathogens
- • Is there another infection present (i.e., *Clostridiodes difficile*, catheter-associated infection, etc.)?
- • Is there a noninfectious explanation (i.e., inflammation, necrosis, thrombus, etc.)?

KEY LEARNING POINT

The antimicrobial management of intra-abdominal infections can be very nuanced. The most important part of management is attaining good source control. The antimicrobials are usually just adjunctive (mop-up) measures, and if source control is adequate the antimicrobial therapy does not have to be perfect (i.e., covering everything).

REFERENCES AND FURTHER READING

- Bitar G, et al. Peritonitis, secondary. In: *Ferri's Clinical Advisor 2022*. Elsevier; 2022.
- Bush LM, et al. Peritonitis and intraperitoneal abscesses. In: Bennet JE, Dolin R, Blaser MJ, eds. *Mandell, Douglas, and Bennett's Principles and Practice of Infectious Diseases*. 9th ed. Elsevier; 2020:1009–1036.
- Kisat M, et al. Management of intra-abdominal infections. In: *Current Surgical Therapy*. 13th ed. Elsevier; 2020:1344–1346.
- Mazuski JE, Solomkin JS. Intra-abdominal infections. *Surg Clin North Am*. 2009;89(2):421–437, ix. https://doi.org/10.1016/j.suc.2008.12.001.
- O'Connell PR, et al. Intra-abdominal sepsis, peritonitis, pancreatitis, hepatobiliary, and focal splenic infection. In: *Infectious Diseases*. 4th ed. Elsevier; 2017:355–362.
- Tamma PD, Aitken SL, Bonomo RA, Mathers AJ, van Duin D, Clancy CJ. Infectious Diseases Society of America guidance on the treatment of extended-spectrum β-lactamase producing Enterobacterales (ESBL-E), carbapenem-resistant Enterobacterales (CRE), and *Pseudomonas aeruginosa* with difficult-to-treat resistance (DTR-*P. aeruginosa*). *Clin Infect Dis*. 2021;72(7):e169–e183. https://doi.org/10.1093/cid/ciaa1478.

A 70-year-old male is admitted to the hospital after suffering a right middle cerebral artery stroke. He did not qualify for thrombolytic therapy but did undergo mechanical thrombectomy. Despite these efforts, he continues to have dysphagia, aphasia, and left-sided hemiparesis, for which he requires ongoing hospitalization for rehabilitation. Medical history is significant for type 2 diabetes mellitus, hypertension, and dyslipidemia. Medications include metformin, insulin, atorvastatin, low-dose aspirin, and lisinopril. He has no medication allergies. He has not been hospitalized or received antibiotics in the past year. On hospital day 7, he develops fevers, cough, and shortness of breath. Vital signs at that time reveal temperature 101.5° F, heart rate 110 beats per minute, blood pressure 100/60 mmHg, respiratory rate 26, and oxygen saturation 92% on 4 L/min oxygen by nasal cannula. On examination, he appears to be working hard to breathe. He is aphasic. He has a nasal feeding tube in place. Heart exam shows an irregular tachycardia with no murmur. Lung exam reveals decreased breath sounds and crackles over the right lower lobe posteriorly. He has dense left-sided weakness. The remainder of the examination is unremarkable. Laboratory studies reveal white blood cell count 14,000 cells/uL (85% neutrophils) and creatinine 1.1 mg/dL (creatinine clearance 60 mL/min). Blood cultures and sputum cultures are ordered and pending. *Legionella* urine antigen is negative. Methicillin-resistant *Staphylococcus aureus* (MRSA) nasal swab (PCR testing) is negative. Chest x-ray shows a new opacity in the right lower lobe.

What is the next best step in the management of this patient?

A. Vancomycin and cefepime.
B. Vancomycin and ceftriaxone.
C. Cefepime monotherapy.
D. Ceftriaxone monotherapy.
E. Cefepime plus metronidazole.

The next best step in management is to start cefepime (**option C**). This patient has a hospital-acquired pneumonia (HAP). The approach to HAP and ventilator-associated pneumonia (VAP) is shown in Fig. 85.1.

HAP is defined as pneumonia (a combination of the symptoms, signs, labs, and imaging shown in Fig. 85.1) that starts after being hospitalized for at least 48 hours (i.e., after hospital day 2). VAP is defined as pneumonia that starts after being intubated for at least 48 hours. The pathogenesis typically involves aspiration of oropharyngeal or gastrointestinal secretions in the setting of impaired respiratory defenses (i.e., mucociliary clearance, etc.). The major organisms to be concerned about include *Staphylococcus aureus* (including MRSA), various gram-negative organisms including the enteric gram-negative rods and resistant gram-negatives like *Stenotrophomonas, Acinetobacter* spp., and *Pseudomonas* spp., and, at times, viruses and *Legionella* spp. The symptoms, signs, and ancillary data (labs, imaging, etc.) should all be utilized when deciding if a patient has HAP/VAP. The diagnosis can be difficult to make in some cases, so clinical judgment is often necessary (i.e., there is no specific number of these criteria that the patient has to meet to be diagnosed with HAP/VAP).

The initial evaluation should include blood cultures, a lower respiratory tract sample, MRSA nasal swab for PCR testing, and, depending on the clinical situation, a *Legionella* urine antigen and a respiratory viral panel (film-array). Blood cultures are fairly low-yield but may assist in narrowing therapy down the line. Noninvasive respiratory sampling (i.e., sputum culture, endotracheal aspirate) with semiquantitative culture is typically preferred over invasive testing due to ease of acquisition and lower risk associated with acquisition. A good sample should have minimal epithelial cells and plenty of polymorphonuclear cells. A more invasive sample (i.e., bronchoscopy with bronchoalveolar lavage) may be used if failing to respond to therapy or if there is concern for an odd pathogen (i.e., opportunistic organism). Isolation of *Candida* spp. almost always represents colonization, as primary *Candida* pneumonia is incredibly uncommon. MRSA nasal swab/PCR is not specific, but it has a high negative predictive value. Therefore, a negative test makes MRSA coverage unnecessary, especially in a patient with low pretest probability for MRSA pneumonia. The typical initial imaging test is a chest x-ray, but it is not very sensitive. The most sensitive imaging test is the chest CT. Chest CT is not done in every patient, but it may be helpful in equivocal cases. Additional etiologies of respiratory failure and/or pulmonary opacities should always be considered. Pulmonary opacities can be caused by the presence of blood, fluid, or pus in the lungs or lack of air in the lungs. With this in mind, differential considerations may include pulmonary edema, alveolar hemorrhage, acute respiratory distress syndrome, effusion, atelectasis/mucus plugging, or aspiration pneumonitis.

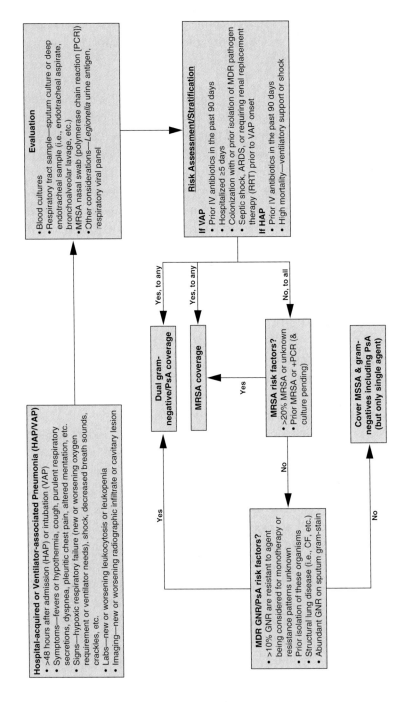

Figure 85.1 – Approach to hospital-acquired pneumonia/ventilator-associated pneumonia. *ARDS,* Acute respiratory distress syndrome; *CF,* cystic fibrosis, *GNR,* gram-negative rods; *MDR,* Multi-drug resistant; *MRSA,* methicillin-resistant *Staphylococcus aureus; MSSA,* methicillin-susceptible *S. aureus; PsA, Pseudomonas.*

Treatment depends on the local antibiogram and risk stratification, as shown in Fig. 85.1. All patients with suspected HAP/VAP should have coverage for methicillin-sensitive *S. aureus*, enteric gram-negatives, and *Pseudomonas* spp. Antimicrobial options include cefepime, piperacillin/tazobactam, or meropenem. The Infectious Diseases Society of America guidelines recommend levofloxacin as an option, but we try to reserve this agent, because it is the only oral option we have to treat *Pseudomonas* spp. Patients with certain risk factors (see Fig. 85.1) should also be provided coverage for MRSA and/or double coverage for resistant gram-negatives, including *Pseudomonas* spp. The drugs of choice for MRSA pneumonia are vancomycin or linezolid. Daptomycin should not be used, as it is inactivated by pulmonary surfactant. Typical options for gram-negative (including *Pseudomonas* spp.) coverage include piperacillin/tazobactam, cefepime, or meropenem. In penicillin-allergic patients, aztreonam is an option. Dual gram-negative coverage is fairly controversial, and if it is done, then it should be limited to a few days. The rationale for this is that data have shown that dual coverage is not any better than monotherapy for the definitive management of susceptible organisms. The typical second agent is a non–beta-lactam such as a levofloxacin or an aminoglycoside. If the patient has a prior history of a resistant pathogen (i.e., extended spectrum beta-lactamase organism), then appropriate coverage should be provided.

Clinical re-evaluation should be performed after 48 to 72 hours. If the patient has improved clinically and an organism is isolated, therapy should be narrowed to target the organism (choice depends on the organism and susceptibility profile). If no organism is isolated (assuming the culture was obtained prior to antibiotic administration) and/or the patient fails to improve, then additional differentials should be considered and/or additional work-up (i.e., CT scan if not already done) should be done to assess for complicated disease (i.e., abscess, empyema, etc.). Treatment duration for most cases of HAP/VAP is 7 days, but duration may be longer in some cases depending on clinical response or complications.

Vancomycin and cefepime (**option A**) would provide excessive coverage in light of the negative MRSA PCR. Similarly, vancomycin and ceftriaxone (**option B**) would provide excessive gram-positive coverage while providing suboptimal gram-negative coverage. Ceftriaxone monotherapy (**option D**) would provide suboptimal gram-negative coverage. Cefepime plus metronidazole (**option E**) would add unnecessary anaerobic coverage, which is really only necessary in cases of lung abscess or empyema.

KEY LEARNING POINT

Empiric therapy for hospital-acquired pneumonia/ventilator-associated pneumonia involves coverage for methicillin-susceptible Staphylococcus aureus *and gram-negatives including* Pseudomonas. *Adding coverage for methicillin-resistant* Staphylococcus aureus *and/or double coverage for gram-negatives/*Pseudomonas *is indicated only in certain situations.*

REFERENCES AND FURTHER READING

- Ansari E, Klompas M. *What is ventilator-associated pneumonia? How do I diagnose it? How do I treat it?* In: *Evidence-Based Practice of Critical Care*. 3rd ed. Elsevier; 2020:325–331.
- Kalil AC, Metersky ML, Klompas M, et al. Management of adults with hospital-acquired and ventilator-associated pneumonia: 2016 clinical practice guidelines by the Infectious Diseases Society of America and the American Thoracic Society. *Clin Infect Dis*. 2016;63(5):e61–e111.
- Meterskey ML, Kalil AC. Hospital-acquired pneumonia. In: *Murray & Nadel's Textbook of Respiratory Medicine*. 7th ed. Elsevier; 2022.

A 25-year-old male presents to the HIV clinic for follow-up. He thinks he may have a sexually transmitted illness. Two weeks ago, he noticed a small painless ulcer on the glans of his penis. The ulcer eventually went away, but recently he has developed painful "swellings" in his groin. He has a history of well-controlled chronic HIV infection. Medications include bictegravir, tenofovir alafenamide, and emtricitabine (Biktarvy). He has no medication allergies. He is sexually active with both male and female partners. He does not use condoms regularly. Vital signs are within normal limits. Examination of the genital region is shown in Fig. 86.1.

Appropriate diagnostic testing is sent off. What is the most appropriate next step in management?

A. Azithromycin once.

B. Doxycycline for 7 days.

C. Doxycycline for 21 days.

D. Benzathine penicillin-G once.

E. Ceftriaxone intramuscular once.

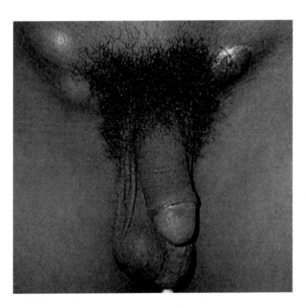

Figure 86.1 – Genital region examination
From Kleine C et al: Lymphogranuloma venereum. In: Ryan ET et al, eds: *Hunter's Tropical Medicine and Emerging Infectious Diseases*. 10th ed. Elsevier; 2020: 521–523, Figure 53.11.

This patient's presentation is most consistent with lymphogranuloma venereum. Therefore, the most appropriate next step is doxycycline for 21 days (**option C**). An overview of genital ulcer disease (GUD) is shown in Fig. 86.2.

In the United States, the most common infectious cause of GUD overall is herpes simplex virus. Syphilis is probably the next most common. Genital lesions can also be caused by noninfectious diseases such as Behçet syndrome, malignancy (especially squamous cell carcinoma), reactive arthritis (circinate balanitis), lichen planus, trauma, aphthous ulceration, and fixed drug eruptions. With the infectious etiologies, the lesion location often depends on the site of inoculation (i.e., genitals, rectum, oropharynx). Fig. 86.2 shows the manifestations of these illnesses. It is worth remembering that the history and physical examination are notoriously inaccurate. Consequently, diagnostic testing should always be considered.

As with other sexually transmitted illnesses (STIs), work-up should include screening for HIV and, in most cases, pregnancy testing (if applicable). In addition, testing for other STI should be performed (i.e., gonorrhea, chlamydia, syphilis, etc.). The diagnosis and management of the various causes of GUD are reviewed in Table 86.1. It is always important to counsel patients regarding the diagnosis and risk-reduction strategies. In addition, sexual partner management needs to be considered as well.

Azithromycin once (**option A**) is the treatment for chancroid and can be used for many uncomplicated *Chlamydia trachomatis* infections. Doxycycline for 7 days (**option B**) is now the first-line treatment for most *C. trachomatis* infections. Benzathine penicillin-G once (**option D**) is the treatment for early syphilis. Ceftriaxone intramuscular once (**option E**) can be used to treat chancroid or most gonococcal infections.

KEY LEARNING POINT

Common infectious causes of genital ulcer disease (and their first-line treatments):

- *Typically painful:*
    - *Herpes simplex virus—acyclovir, valacyclovir, or famciclovir*
    - *Chancroid (Haemophilus ducreyi)—azithromycin 1 g PO once or ceftriaxone 250 mg IM once*

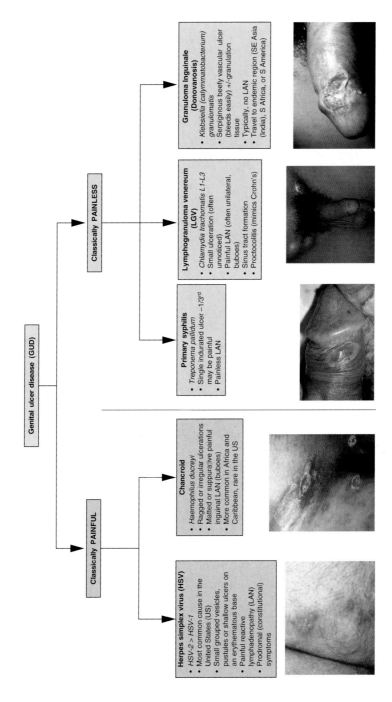

Genital ulcer disease (GUD)

Classically PAINLESS

Primary syphilis
- *Treponema pallidum*
- Single indurated ulcer –1/3rd may be painful
- Painless LAN

Lymphogranuloma venereum (LGV)
- *Chlamydia trachomatis L1-L3*
- Small ulceration (often unnoticed)
- Painful LAN (often unilateral, buboes)
- Sinus tract formation
- Proctocolitis (mimics Crohn's)

Granuloma Inguinale (Donovanosis)
- *Klebsiella (calymmatobacterium) granulomatis*
- Serpiginous beefy vascular ulcer (bleeds easily) +/-granulation tissue
- Typically, no LAN
- Travel to endemic region (SE Asia (India), S Africa, or S America)

Classically PAINFUL

Herpes simplex virus (HSV)
- *HSV-2 > HSV-1*
- Most common cause in the United States (US)
- Small grouped vesicles, pustules or shallow ulcers on an erythematous base
- Painful reactive lymphadenopathy (LAN)
- Prodromal (constitutional) symptoms

Chancroid
- *Haemophilus ducreyi*
- Ragged or irregular ulcerations
- Matted or suppurative painful inguinal LAN (buboes)
- More common in Africa and Caribbean, rare in the US

Figure 86.2 – Genital ulcer disease

411

Table 86.1 – Diagnosis and Management of Genital Ulcer Disease

Disease	Diagnosis	Management
Chancroid	• Specialized culture to identify *Haemophilus ducreyi* (<80% sensitive)—not widely available • Nucleic acid amplification testing (NAAT) can be used if available and locally verified • Must rule out herpes simplex virus (HSV) and syphilis	• First line—azithromycin 1-g PO once or ceftriaxone 250 mg IM once • Alternative—ciprofloxacin 500 mg PO BID for 3 days • Re-evaluate within 1 week. Slower response is seen in HIV patients and uncircumcised men. Lymphadenopathy may need aspiration or incision and drainage. Scarring may result despite appropriate treatment • Partners in the 10 days preceding onset of symptoms should be evaluated and treated
HSV[a]	• If genital lesions are present, then obtain swab from an unroofed lesion for NAAT (most sensitive) or, less commonly, viral culture. Both of these tests can differentiate HSV-1 from HSV-2 • If no genital lesions, then type-specific serology (IgG) may be used. IgM testing should not be used. False negatives can happen in early infections, so repeat testing in 12 weeks can be done. Due to the low specificity of serology, a second confirmatory test should be performed • Viral culture can be used to assess for resistant HSV • Tzanck prep/smear and direct immunofluorescence are not recommended	• Goals of treatment—treat or prevent symptomatic genital herpes recurrences, improve quality of life, and suppress virus to prevent transmission • Treatment regimens for first episode[b] • Acyclovir 400 mg PO TID • Valacyclovir 1 g PO BID • Famciclovir 250 mg PO TID • Duration—7–10 days (can extend past 10 days if healing is incomplete after 10 days) • HSV prophylaxis can be continuous (decreases recurrences by 70%–80% in patients with frequent recurrences) or episodic (to shorten duration of illness). Prophylaxis is probably most beneficial for HSV-2 (vs. HSV-1) due to higher risk of asymptomatic shedding and recurrences. It can be considered in HSV-1 if there are frequent recurrences. Episodic prophylaxis is most effective when given prior to lesion onset (i.e., during prodrome) or within 1 day of lesion onset. Prophylaxis should not be used for patients with positive serology but no symptomatic recurrences • Regimens for continuous suppression[b] • Acyclovir 400 mg PO BID • Valacyclovir 500–1000 mg PO daily • Regimens for episodic suppression[b] • Acyclovir 800 mg PO BID for 5 days, or 800 mg PO TID for 2 days • Valacyclovir 1-g PO daily for 5 days, or 500 mg PO BID for 3 days • Counseling—condom use reduces risk (but does not eliminate it), recurrent nature of infection, asymptomatic shedding and transmission risk, (antivirals reduce shedding and transmission in HIV-uninfected individuals) avoid sex when symptomatic, notify sex partners of HSV status, benefits of prophylaxis, asymptomatic sex partners can be tested with HSV-2 serology to assess risk • Resistant HSV treatment—options are IV cidofovir, IV foscarnet, topical cidofovir, or topical imiquimod

Table 86.1 – Diagnosis and Management of Genital Ulcer Disease *(Cont'd)*

Disease	Diagnosis	Management
Granuloma inguinale	• Biopsy or tissue crush preparation to identify Donovan bodies	• First-line—azithromycin 1 g PO weekly or 500 mg PO daily for at least 3 weeks (and until all lesions have completely healed) • Alternatives—doxycycline, trimethoprim-sulfamethoxazole, or erythromycin • Relapses are not uncommon, even months after successful treatment • Sex partners in the 60 days preceding symptom onset should be evaluated
Lymphogranuloma venereum (LGV)	• NAAT for *Chlamydia trachomatis*—this test will not tell you the exact subtype (LGV vs. non-LGV serotype), because the test just nonspecifically detects all *C. trachomatis* serotypes	• First-line—doxycycline 100 mg PO BID for 3 weeks (potentially longer in more complicated disease) • Alternative—azithromycin 1 g PO once weekly for 3 weeks (consider test-of-cure 4 weeks after completing this regimen, because it has not been validated) • Sex partners in the 60 days preceding symptom onset should be evaluated • Retesting for chlamydia 3 months after treatment
Syphilis	• Darkfield microscopy is the best test, but is not commonly done/available • Serology can be done—if negative, then consider repeating 2–4 weeks later	• Benzathine penicillin-G 2.4 million units IM once • Alternative—doxycycline for 14 days • Sex partners in the 90 days preceding the diagnosis of EARLY syphilis should be treated (regardless of serology result), while sex partners >90 days out should have serologic testing first • Close follow-up is necessary for serial syphilis testing (successful treatment → four-fold decline in nontreponemal [i.e. rapid plasma reagin] titer)

[a]Pregnancy considerations: Risk of transmission to the baby is highest (30%–50%) if infection is acquired around the time of labor/delivery. If asymptomatic at time of delivery, then can deliver vaginally. If symptomatic, then C-section is preferred. Acyclovir (and based on limited data, valacyclovir) is considered safe in all trimesters of pregnancy. Suppressive therapy is typically started at 36 weeks' gestation.

[b]Patients with HIV often have more severe, protracted, or atypical HSV infection. They often require longer durations of therapy for initial treatment and prophylaxis. Interestingly, HSV prophylaxis (in patients with HIV and HSV coinfection) does not reduce the risk of HSV or HIV transmission to susceptible partners. Antivirals mainly decrease the clinical manifestations.

- *Typically painless:*
  - *Primary syphilis (Treponema pallidum)—benzathine penicillin-G 2.4 million units IM once*
  - *Lymphogranuloma venereum (Chlamydia trachomatis L1–L3)—doxycycline for at least 21 days*
  - *Granuloma inguinale (Klebsiella granulomatis)—azithromycin for at least 21 days*

REFERENCES AND FURTHER READING

- Augenbraun MH. Genital skin and mucous membrane lesions. In: Bennet JE, Dolin R, Blaser MJ, eds. *Mandell, Douglas, and Bennett's Principles and Practice of Infectious Disease*. 9th ed. Elsevier; 2020.
- Clinical overview lymphogranuloma venereum. In: *Elsevier Point of Care*. Elsevier; 2021.
- McKiernan Borawski K. Sexually transmitted diseases. In: *Campbell-Walsh-Wein Urology*. 12th ed. Elsevier; 2021: 1251–1272.
- Workowski K, Bachmann L, Chan P, et al. Sexually transmitted infections guideline, 2021. *MMWR Recomm Rep.* 2021;70(4):27–39. https://doi.org/10.15585/mmwr.rr7004a1.

A 30-year-old female is referred to the infectious disease clinic for a positive syphilis screening test. She has no symptomatic complaints. She is currently pregnant, at 24 weeks' gestation. She has had inconsistent prenatal care. Her medications include a multivitamin and folic acid. She is allergic to amoxicillin and notes she developed hives when she was given amoxicillin 10 years ago. She does not recall ever having any symptoms of syphilis in the past. She has never been treated for syphilis in the past. She is sexually active with male partners. She does not use condoms consistently. Vital signs are within normal limits. On physical examination, she appears well. Neurologic examination is normal. Heart and lungs are normal. There are no rashes or genital lesions. Laboratory testing is significant for positive rapid plasma reagin with titer 1:32, positive fluorescent treponemal antibody absorption (FTA-ABS), negative nucleic acid amplification testing for gonorrhea and chlamydia, and negative HIV antigen/antibody test. No prior testing for these pathogens is available.

What is the most appropriate management of this patient?

A. Desensitize and administer benzathine penicillin-G once.

B. Desensitize and administer benzathine penicillin-G once weekly for three doses.

C. Desensitize and administer aqueous (intravenous) penicillin-G for 14 days.

D. Ceftriaxone for 14 days.

E. Doxycycline for 28 days.

The most appropriate management strategy for this pregnant patient with late latent syphilis is to desensitize and administer benzathine penicillin-G once weekly for three doses (**option B**).

Syphilis is a complicated infection caused by the spirochete bacterium *Treponema pallidum* subsp. *pallidum*. Infection is most often acquired/transmitted sexually, but vertical transmission can also occur. Incubation period is variable (median 3 weeks, range 10–90 days). The initial stage of infection (primary syphilis) is often characterized by a painless, often solitary, indurated ulceration at the site of exposure. In rare cases, the ulcer can be painful. The ulcer actually starts as a macule or papule in most cases. With genital infections, there may be bilateral painless inguinal lymphadenopathy. It is not uncommon for this stage to go unnoticed. The ulcer typically goes away after a few weeks. Secondary (disseminated) syphilis may present as an influenza-like illness, a diffuse maculopapular rash (often described as having a copper or bronze color) involving the palms and soles, lymphadenopathy (epitrochlear lymphadenopathy is highly suggestive), condyloma lata, gray oral mucous patches, alopecia, and hepatitis (especially disproportionately elevated alkaline phosphatase) (Fig. 87.1). Rarely, these patients may develop nephrotic syndrome.

Tertiary syphilis occurs 5 to 30 years after initial infection and is typically subdivided into neurosyphilis, cardiovascular syphilis, and gummatous syphilis. It may be characterized by chronic meningoencephalitis, tabes dorsalis, general paresis (neuropsychiatric disturbances), Argyll–Robertson pupil, gummas (necrotizing granulomatous lesions in skin, bones, brain, liver, gastrointestinal tract, or spleen), or aortitis/aortic aneurysm. Neurosyphilis can occur at any stage of syphilis. When it occurs earlier on in the disease process, neurosyphilis may

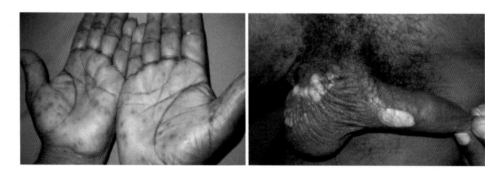

Figure 87.1 – Syphilis rash (left) and condyloma lata (right)
Radolf JD, et al. Syphilis (*Treponema pallidum*). In: Bennet JE, Dolin R, Blaser MJ, eds. *Mandell, Douglas, and Bennett's Principles and Practice of Infectious Diseases*. 9th ed . Elsevier; 2020:2865–2892. Courtesy Dr. Adriana Cruz, Centro Internacional de Entrenamiento e Investigaciones Médicas, Cali, Colombia.

manifest as meningoencephalitis, cranial neuropathy, vasculitis, or stroke. Later neurologic syphilis is more consistent with tertiary syphilis central nervous system manifestations. Ocular syphilis and otosyphilis can be thought of as a subset of neurosyphilis, because the management is very similar. Ocular syphilis can virtually affect any part of the eyeball and may result in permanent vision loss. Otosyphilis typically affects cranial nerve VIII and may cause permanent hearing loss. Latent syphilis is characterized by positive serologic testing but no signs or symptoms of primary, secondary, tertiary, or neurologic syphilis. The term "early latent syphilis" refers to latent syphilis that was acquired in the preceding year (i.e., unequivocal symptoms of primary, secondary, or neurologic syphilis, documented seroconversion, or a sex partner with confirmed syphilis). If these criteria are not satisfied, then patients are said to have late latent syphilis or latent syphilis of unknown duration. The natural history of untreated syphilis is shown in Fig. 87.2. As shown, syphilis is most infectious in the early syphilis phases (primary, secondary, and early latent syphilis).

When evaluating patients with concern for syphilis (especially in latent syphilis), there are several historical details that can be helpful. A good review of systems which should include questioning about constitutional symptoms, meningoencephalitis symptoms, ocular symptoms (i.e., vision loss, photophobia, etc.), otic symptoms (i.e., hearing loss, tinnitus, vertigo, etc.), genital or oral ulceration, alopecia, skin rashes, and lymphadenopathy. Patients should be asked about a prior history of syphilis and, if previously infected, when and how were they treated (documentation of the treatment should be acquired if possible). Important elements of the examination include examination of skin and mucus membranes (including oral and genital) and a good neurologic examination. Patients should be screened for HIV and pregnancy (women of childbearing age). Screening for other sexually transmitted illnesses (i.e., gonorrhea and chlamydia) should be done as well. Syphilis testing can be complicated, so a detailed discussion is warranted.

Diagnosis of syphilis should include synthesis of the history, physical examination, and the testing described next. Darkfield microscopy of lesion tissue or exudate is the best test for diagnosing primary syphilis infection. Unfortunately, this test is not commonly done, requires a certain level of expertise, and is not widely available. The most common way that syphilis is diagnosed these days is by serum serologic testing. Serologic testing can be treponemal-specific or treponemal-nonspecific. A combination of these tests is required for the diagnosis, and the order of the testing depends on whether the specific laboratory uses a traditional or reverse algorithm (Figs. 87.3 and 87.4). The serologic modalities are summarized in Table 87.1.

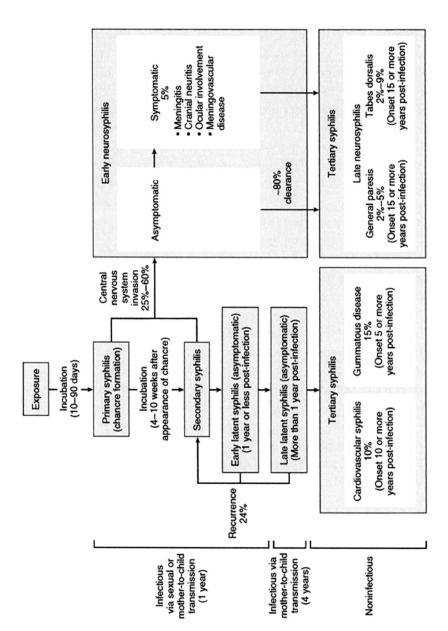

Figure 87.2 – Natural history of syphilis

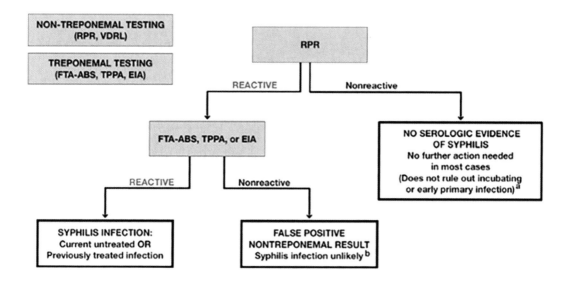

Figure 87.3 – Traditional algorithm. If suspected, then empiric treatment should be provided; if still suspicious, consider repeating RPR in several weeks

[a]if exposure in preceding 90 days or clear-cut manifestation of primary syphilis (i.e., chancre), then empiric treatmen should be considered.

[b]this could also represent early infection especially if history consistent so consider empiric treatment vs repeat serologic testing in 2-4 weeks

EIA, Enzyme immunoassay; *FTA-ABS*, fluorescent treponemal antibody absorption; *RPR*, rapid plasma reagin; *TPPA, Treponema pallidum* particle agglutination; *VDRL*, venereal disease research laboratory.

The two algorithms commonly used by laboratories are shown in Figs. 87.3 and 87.4.

Cerebrospinal fluid (CSF) analysis may be considered in certain cases of syphilis. CSF analysis should be done if there are signs and/or symptoms of neurosyphilis (including ocular symptoms without clinical evidence of cranial nerve dysfunction or ocular abnormalities on ophthalmologist examination). Other times to consider CSF analysis are when a patient does not improve serologically (i.e., at least a four-fold decline) despite appropriate treatment or when a patient is diagnosed with tertiary syphilis (CSF should be obtained prior to starting therapy). CSF analysis is not necessary in cases of isolated otosyphilis (without any other clinical concern for neurosyphilis). No single test can be used to diagnose neurosyphilis. CSF abnormalities are common in patients with early syphilis, and their significance is unknown in those without symptoms or signs of neurosyphilis. CSF abnormalities may include lymphocytic pleocytosis and elevated protein. CSF venereal disease research laboratory (VDRL) is very specific, and if it is reactive in a symptomatic patient (in the absence of CSF blood contamination), then a

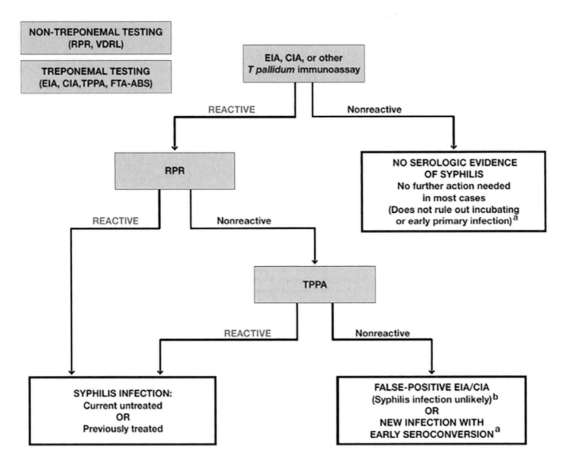

Figure 87.4 – Reverse algorithm. If suspected, then empiric treatment should be provided; if still suspicious, consider repeating RPR in several weeks

[a]if exposure in preceding 90 days or clear-cut manifestation of primary syphilis (i.e., chancre), then empiric treatmen should be considered.

[b]this could also represent early infection especially if history consistent so consider empiric treatment vs repeat serologic testing in 2-4 weeks

CIA, Chemiluminescence immunoassay; *EIA*, enzyme immunoassay; *FTA-ABS*, fluorescent treponemal antibody absorption; *RPR*, rapid plasma reagin; *TPPA*, Treponema pallidum particle agglutination; *VDRL*, venereal disease research laboratory.

diagnosis of neurosyphilis can be made. CSF VDRL is insensitive, so a negative test cannot rule out neurosyphilis. If there is ongoing suspicion in these cases, then CSF treponemal antibody testing should be considered. Compared with the CSF VDRL, CSF FTA-ABS is less specific but is more sensitive and may be helpful in ruling out neurosyphilis. In HIV-positive individuals, the use of a higher CSF pleocytosis cut-off (i.e., >20 cells/uL) may be more specific, because CSF abnormalities are fairly common in HIV patients (even those without syphilis).

Table 87.1 – Syphilis Serology

Nontreponemal Antibody Testing	Treponemal Antibody Testing
• Examples include rapid plasma reagin (RPR) and venereal disease research laboratory (VDRL)	• Examples include fluorescent treponemal antibody absorption, *Treponema pallidum* particle agglutination, syphilis IgG, etc.
• Antibody to cardiolipin antigens (provide qualitative and quantitative [titer] information)	• Antibody to treponemal antigens (provides qualitative information only)
• Titers correlate with disease activity and are followed for treatment response. The same nontreponemal antibody (NTA) test and laboratory should be used for serial testing/comparison (RPR titers tend to be higher than VDRL titers, so they cannot be compared)	• Levels do not correlate with disease activity and should not be followed
• A four-fold change (i.e., 1:4 to 1:16) in titer is considered significant	• Treponemal antibody (TA) tests are better than NTA tests for detecting early infection, because TA tests become positive 1–2 weeks after the development of the chancre
• Seroconversion or a four-fold increase in titer (in those with prior syphilis infection) is consistent with a new infection	
• Adequate treatment of syphilis is characterized by at least a four-fold decline in NTA titer over 12–24 months	• In general, in patients with prior syphilis exposure, TA remains positive for life. An exception occurs in those treated during the primary stage, because the TA can become nonreactive after 2–3 years in ~20% of cases
• Over time, the NTA will typically decline, regardless of whether or not treatment was given. In some individuals, the test will become nonreactive, but in others a new baseline will be established	
• False negatives may be seen with early infection, advanced/late-stage infections, and with very high antibody levels ("prozone reaction")	• These tests can also be positive with the endemic treponematoses
• False positives may be seen with some infections (malaria, brucellosis, mononucleosis, leprosy, HIV, hepatitis C), endemic treponematoses (yaws, pinta, bejel), autoimmune diseases (i.e., lupus, etc.), vaccinations, IV drug use, and pregnancy	

The diagnosis of syphilis can be very difficult to make at times. In most cases, erring on the side of caution and treating empirically is probably not a bad approach, especially because the treatment is not very difficult or risky in most cases. Treatment depends on the stage of disease, presence or absence of a penicillin allergy, or pregnancy status (Table 87.2). If the diagnosis is highly suspected, then empiric treatment should be given without waiting for testing to come back. A Jarisch–Herxheimer (JH) reaction may occur within 24 hours of treatment, and patients should be notified of this. In pregnancy, the JH reaction may induce early labor or fetal distress, but this should not preclude treatment. Sexual partners in the 90 days preceding the diagnosis of early syphilis (primary, secondary, or early latent) should be treated presumptively (i.e., not necessary to perform serologic testing). Sexual partners more than 90 days out should be tested and treated accordingly. If unable to do so or if concerned about unreliable follow-up, then presumptive treatment can be done for these partners as well. Sexual partners of patients diagnosed with later stages of syphilis should be evaluated with serology and treated accordingly.

Follow-up clinical evaluation and nontreponemal antibody (NTA) titers should be performed regularly (frequency and duration of follow-up depends on HIV status and pregnancy status).

Table 87-2 – Treatment of Syphilis

Situation	Preferred Treatment	Alternative Treatment if Penicillin-Allergic
Early syphilis—primary, secondary, and early latent	• Benzathine penicillin-G 2.4 million units IM once	• Doxycycline or tetracycline for 14 days
Late latent syphilis or latent syphilis of unknown duration[a]	• Benzathine penicillin-G 2.4 million units IM once weekly for three doses	• Doxycycline or tetracycline for 28 days
Tertiary syphilis + normal cerebrospinal fluid (CSF) exam and no clinical concern for neurosyphilis[a]	• Benzathine penicillin-G 2.4 million units IM once weekly for three doses • CSF examination is recommended before initiating therapy	• N/A
Neurosyphilis, ocular syphilis, and otosyphilis	• Penicillin-G 18–24 million units IV daily for 10–14 days	• Procaine penicillin-G 2.4 million units IM daily + probenecid 500 mg PO QID for 10–14 days • Ceftriaxone 2 g IV daily for 14 days
Pregnant patient with syphilis[a]	• Benzathine penicillin-G as for nonpregnant patients • A second dose of penicillin-G in early syphilis may be beneficial to prevent congenital syphilis	• Desensitize and treat with benzathine penicillin-G • Doxycycline should not be used in pregnancy

[a]The interval between doses should not exceed 9 days in most cases. If it does, then the series should be restarted.

Successful treatment is associated with at least a four-fold reduction in nontreponemal titer within 12 to 24 months. As previously stated, some patients become nonreactive, while others establish a new baseline titer level. If the appropriate titer decline does not occur, then considerations should include treatment nonadherence, reinfection, HIV infection, and neurosyphilis (if not previously considered). If there is no clinical concern for neurosyphilis, then retreatment with a regimen similar to that used for late latent syphilis/latent syphilis of unknown duration can be considered. Of note, 10% to 20% of patients with primary or secondary syphilis may not achieve a four-fold reduction in titer after 12 months. Repeat CSF analysis is unnecessary in most cases of appropriately treated neurosyphilis, especially if the patient clinically improves. Long-term, patients should receive annual NTA titer testing to assess for reinfection (i.e., at least a four-fold rise in titer from previous baseline).

Desensitize and administer benzathine penicillin-G once (**option A**) would be the treatment for early syphilis in pregnant patients. Desensitize and administer aqueous (intravenous) penicillin-G for 14 days (**option C**) would be the treatment for neurosyphilis in pregnancy. Ceftriaxone for 14 days (**option D**) is a regimen that is used as an alternative for the treatment of neurosyphilis, but it has not been validated in pregnancy. Doxycycline for 28 days (**option E**) is an alternative option for treating late stages of syphilis, but it should not be used in pregnant patients.

KEY LEARNING POINT

The treatment of choice for all stages of syphilis in pregnant patients is penicillin-G. If the patient is allergic to penicillin, then they should be desensitized and treated with penicillin-G.

REFERENCES AND FURTHER READING

- Carmine L. Genital ulcer disease—a review for primary care providers caring for adolescents. *Curr Probl Pediatr Adolesc Health Care*. 2020;50(7):100834. https://doi.org/10.1016/j.cppeds.2020.100834.
- Radolf JD, et al. Syphilis (*Treponema pallidum*). In: Bennet JE, Dolin R, Blaser MJ, eds. *Mandell, Douglas, and Bennett's Principles and Practice of Infectious Diseases*. 9th ed . Elsevier; 2020:2865–2892.
- Workowski K, Bachmann L, Chan P, et al. Sexually transmitted infections guideline, 2021. *MMWR Recomm Rep*. 2021;70(4):27–39. https://doi.org/10.15585/mmwr.rr7004a1.

A 55-year-old male presents to the emergency room with concern for an infection in his foot. He has had a nonhealing ulcer over the plantar side of his left foot for the past several months. His primary provider has tried to manage the ulcer with wound care, off-loading, and several courses of antibiotics. He has a history of poorly controlled type 2 diabetes mellitus complicated by retinopathy, peripheral neuropathy, and chronic kidney disease. Medications include metformin, insulin, atorvastatin, lisinopril, furosemide, and gabapentin. He has no medication allergies. Vital signs show temperature 99° F, heart rate 85 beats per minute, blood pressure 145/90 mmHg, and respiratory rate 16. Examination of the left is shown in figure. 88.1. He has no sensation in his feet up to the midshins bilaterally. Pulses are 1+ in both feet. The remainder of the examination is unremarkable.

Laboratory analysis reveals white blood cell (WBC) count 10,000 cells/µL, hemoglobin 10 g/dL, platelet count 450,000 cells/µL, creatinine 1.5 mg/dL (baseline creatinine range 1.3–1.6 mg/dL), and C-reactive protein (CRP) 6 mg/dL (normal <0.9 mg/dL).

What is the most appropriate next step in the management of this patient?

A. Start ceftriaxone and metronidazole.
B. Obtain blood cultures.
C. Obtain an MRI of the left foot with and without contrast.
D. Obtain an x-ray of the left foot.
E. Obtain a surgical consultation.

The most appropriate next test to obtain is an x-ray of the left foot (**option C**). The nonhealing ulcer in this patient plus the elevated C-reactive protein (CRP) should make you suspicious for chronic osteomyelitis (OM).

Diabetics are at an increased risk for skin and soft tissue infections (SSTIs; and consequently deeper infections) for several reasons. These include uncontrolled hyperglycemia and associated immune dysregulation, disruption of skin barriers, sensory and autonomic neuropathy, trauma/pressure, and vascular insufficiency. Infections are typically polymicrobial, especially if they are chronic, more severe, or deeper infections. The usual organisms are skin organisms such as *Staphylococcus aureus* (including methicillin-resistant *S. aureus* [MRSA] in certain cases), coagulase-negative staphylococci (CoNS), and streptococci. In patients with prior antibiotic exposure or more complicated infections (i.e., chronic, severe, or deeper), anaerobes, enterococci, and gram-negative organisms become more prevalent. In addition, anaerobic organisms should be suspected in patients with necrosis, gas, or malodorous discharge. *Pseudomonas* spp. are not as common as was once thought. *Pseudomonas* spp. should be considered in those with water exposure (i.e., soaking feet) or puncture wounds. Prior hospitalization and/or antibiotic exposure increases the risk for resistant organisms. An overview of the classification of diabetic foot infections (DFIs) is provided in Figure. 88.1.

As evident from Figure. 88.2, infections can be superficial (i.e., cellulitis, abscesses, etc.), deep (i.e., necrotizing fasciitis, myositis, tenosynovitis, septic arthritis, OM), mild, or more severe.

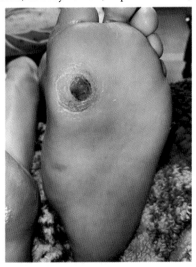

Figure 88.1 – Diabetic foot ulcer
Polk C, Sampson MM, Roshdy D, Davidson LE. Skin and soft tissue infections in patients with diabetes mellitus. *Infect Dis Clin North Am.* 2021;35(1):183–197. https://doi.org/10.1016/j.idc.2020.10.007.

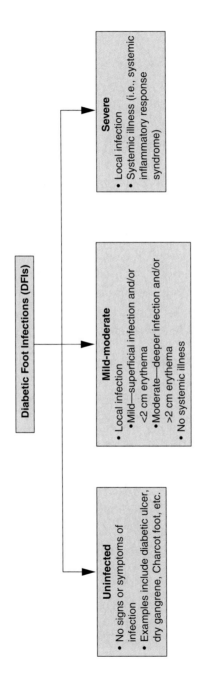

Figure 88.2 – Overview of diabetic foot infection

Infection in this diagram is defined as having at least two of the following manifestations: erythema, warmth, tenderness, swelling, purulence, or induration. This classification is important because it helps guide subsequent management decisions.

Chronic OM is classically seen in diabetics and most commonly develops as a consequence of contiguous spread from a neighboring focus (i.e., ulceration). Chronic OM should be suspected in patients with large and/or deep ulcers (>2 cm^2) or wounds that probe down to the bone, or if the infection fails to resolve or recurs despite appropriate therapy. It can be helpful to know how the wound or ulcer was previously managed (i.e., water exposure, antimicrobial use and response, etc.). In addition, patients should be asked about animal exposures (i.e., cat or dog messing with the wound) because this may modify the antibiotic choices. Examination should identify whether there is an acute infection present or not (i.e., the infectious signs discussed above). If an ulcer is present, then the size and depth should be assessed (i.e., Does it probe to bone?). Neurovascular assessment should be done as well.

The diagnosis of chronic OM should include synthesis of the presentation (history and physical exam), lab testing, microbiologic data, and imaging data. In chronic OM, white blood cell (WBC) count and inflammatory markers (erythrocyte sedimentation rate [ESR] and CRP) may be elevated, but they are nonspecific findings that can be seen in more superficial infections. An ESR greater than 70 mm/hr may be suggestive. Blood cultures (**option B**) should be obtained if the patient is systemically ill (i.e., fevers, chills, hemodynamic compromise, etc.). The best initial imaging test is actually an x-ray, because with prolonged infections (i.e., at least 2–3 weeks) x-ray will often identify OM, and an MRI may be avoided. X-ray may also show foreign bodies or gas. The most sensitive imaging test to diagnose OM is an MRI (**option C**). A negative MRI essentially excludes the diagnosis of OM. Contrast is actually not necessary for the diagnosis of OM, but it may be helpful to delineate associated abscesses. MRI is not very specific though. It may show reactive bone changes that may be confused with OM. In addition, Charcot arthropathy may be difficult to distinguish from OM on MRI. If an MRI is not feasible or possible, then alternative imaging tests include CT with contrast or bone scan combined with a leukocyte scan. A vascular assessment (i.e., ankle-brachial index, toe-brachial index, arterial ultrasound studies) may be necessary in some cases (i.e., if pursuing revascularization). The most accurate diagnostic test for identifying OM is a bone biopsy, but this is not commonly done. If an ulcer is present and appears infected (i.e., inflammatory signs or purulent drainage), then a deep tissue swab culture (after cleansing with iodine or chlorhexidine) may be helpful, mainly to exclude certain organisms (i.e., MRSA, resistant gram-negatives). Most of these ulcers/wounds are chronically colonized, so just because an organism is identified on a swab culture does not mean it is playing a significant role in the infection. This is also why uninfected ulcers should not be swabbed. Ideally, a surgical bedside debridement with deep tissue cultures (aerobic and anaerobic) should be obtained. Cultures should be obtained before antibiotics if possible or off of antibiotics for at least 2 weeks (in those previously on antibiotics). Unlike superficial swabs/culture, deep tissue cultures correlate well with bone infection. Lastly, noninfectious etiologies with similar presentations should be excluded, including crystalline arthropathy, Charcot arthropathy, fractures, venous stasis, and/or thrombosis.

The management of DFIs can be complex and may include medical (i.e., antimicrobials) and/or surgical (i.e., resection/amputation, debridement, etc.) interventions. All patients should receive good wound care, off-loading, and good diabetes control. If there is significant peripheral arterial disease, then revascularization may be necessary to ensure appropriate healing. Revascularization improves blood flow, which improves healing and antibiotic delivery and may reduce the incidence of amputation.

If the ulcer is not acutely infected and there is no concern for OM, then the mainstays of treatment are off-loading, good wound care, good diabetic control, and debridement of surrounding callus. Antibiotics are not helpful in these cases, mainly because of bacterial biofilm formation.

If there is an actual DFI, then antimicrobial therapy can get fairly complicated, and a complete discussion is beyond the scope of this book (and is probably unnecessary). The following are some useful generalizations:

- No single drug or drug combination has been shown to be superior to another.
- Antimicrobial therapy may actually be withheld (while obtaining culture data) in some cases of infection (i.e., OM) that have no surrounding SSTI and no systemic illness.
- If there is obvious infection (i.e., systemic illness, SSTI, etc.), therapeutic choice depends on the classification (i.e., the type/depth of infection and severity), prior and current organisms isolated, prior antimicrobial use and associated response, local microbial patterns, and certain historical features (i.e., foot soaking or dogs licking a wound).
- The antimicrobial therapy should almost always include coverage for beta-hemolytic streptococci and staphylococci. Empiric MRSA coverage should be considered in patients with prior MRSA isolation, purulent infections, or healthcare facility exposure.

- Broader empiric coverage (i.e., anaerobes and gram-negatives) may be considered for infections in the setting of considerable prior antibiotic exposure and infections that are more chronic, severe, and/or deeper.

- Anaerobic organisms can be difficult to isolate (even in cases where no prior antibiotics were given). Coverage for anaerobic organisms is probably useful in more severe/deeper infections or infections associated with necrosis, malodor, or gas/crepitus.

- Antimicrobials do not have to cover every single pathogen isolated on tissue culture. Certain pathogens (i.e., CoNS and enterococci) may be less important, especially when isolated in polymicrobial infections.

- In more severe cases, IV therapy is preferred over oral therapy (unless the oral agent has very high bioavailability, such as metronidazole, linezolid, or fluoroquinolones). Other agents with fairly high oral bioavailability that may be used as step-down oral agents include doxycycline, trimethoprim/sulfamethoxazole (TMP/SMX), clindamycin, amoxicillin/clavulanate, and first-generation cephalosporins.

- For OM, antibiotics with good bone penetration should be used. These include most IV antibiotics, fluoroquinolones, TMP/SMX, clindamycin, tetracyclines, and linezolid. Oral beta-lactams have poor bone penetration. It is unclear if the degree of bone penetration actually correlates with clinical outcomes.

- When the patient is not severely ill (i.e., severe sepsis or septic shock), it can be helpful to start narrower (i.e., avoid covering MRSA and resistant gram-negatives, including *Pseudomonas* spp.) and observe the clinical response. An example could be something like ampicillin/sulbactam (Unasyn) monotherapy or ceftriaxone/metronidazole (**option A**). If the patient improves clinically without covering these more resistant pathogens, then these pathogens are likely not involved in the infection.

- Prior response to antimicrobials should also be considered. If a patient failed to respond to a certain antibiotic in the recent past, then the offending organism(s) may not be covered by this antimicrobial, or the antimicrobial may not be effective enough for the infection (i.e., suboptimal oral absorption or tissue penetration).

- Once culture results are available and patient has improved, antimicrobial therapy should be de-escalated to cover the most relevant pathogens.

Surgical consultation (**option E**) may be necessary if there is an abscess that needs to be drained, callus/necrosis that needs debridement, revascularization is required, there is no improvement with antibiotics alone, or amputation/resection is warranted. More severe infections may benefit from concomitant surgical intervention. Typically, either an orthopedic surgeon or a podiatrist is consulted, but if revascularization is necessary, then a vascular surgeon should be involved.

Duration of therapy depends on the type/depth of infection and degree of source control. At least 1 week of therapy is necessary in most cases. Longer courses of therapy are needed for more complicated cases (i.e., deeper infections, poor source control, etc.). Chronic OM therapy is often coordinated with surgical management. For chronic OM with surrounding SSTI, the acute SSTI should be treated first before surgical intervention is performed. Often, patients will be kept on "suppressive" oral antibiotic therapy while awaiting definitive surgical therapy. If a surgery is performed and all of the infected/necrotic material is removed (i.e., based on discussion with the surgeon and pathologic margins), then antibiotics can be stopped within a day or two of surgery. If there is concern for residual infection in the bone, then a prolonged course of therapy (often 4–6 weeks) should be given. If there is concern for residual soft tissue infection (but not bone infection), then extending antibiotics for 1 to 2 weeks may be appropriate. If no surgical intervention is planned/done, then most providers will just treat SSTIs that may arise and avoid giving long-term antibiotics. The rationale for this is that antimicrobial therapy alone in cases of deep-seated chronic OM is often less successful in eradicating the infection (compared with combination surgery and antimicrobials), but the risk of developing antimicrobial side effects and resistance is significant. Some providers will try to provide long-term antibiotic therapy to achieve a cure. The success rate for this approach ranges from 50% to 75%, and 6 weeks of therapy is probably no worse than longer courses. Ultimately, the best approach involves an interdisciplinary discussion between the surgeon, the infectious disease specialist, and the patient. According to the Oral versus Intravenous Antibiotics for Bone and Joint Infection (OVIVA) trial, appropriately chosen oral therapy is noninferior to IV therapy for various bone and joint infections. During treatment, inflammatory markers should be monitored, as they should decline with treatment. Follow-up imaging is of no use in most cases.

THE OTHER CHOICES

Starting ceftriaxone and metronidazole (**option A**) is not necessary at this time, because the patient has no evidence of SSTI (i.e., overlying cellulitis) or systemic illness that would warrant urgently starting antibiotics. Obtaining blood cultures (**option B**) is likely going to be low-yield in this patient without systemic symptoms or signs of illness. Furthermore, this type of OM is most likely related to contiguous spread from the ulceration and not hematogenous dissemination. Obtaining an MRI of the left foot with and without contrast (**option C**) would be the most definitive test to evaluate for OM, but an x-ray should be done before an MRI. In most cases, contrast is not necessary to identify OM, but it can be helpful to identify associated soft tissue infections (i.e., abscesses). Obtaining a surgical consultation (**option E**) may become necessary at some point, but gathering more data is appropriate before consulting a surgeon.

KEY LEARNING POINT

The best initial test in the diagnosis of chronic contiguous osteomyelitis is an x-ray.

REFERENCES AND FURTHER READING

- Aicale R, Cipollaro L, Esposito S, Maffulli N. An evidence based narrative review on treatment of diabetic foot osteomyelitis. *Surgeon.*. 2020;18(5):311–320. https://doi.org/10.1016/j.surge.2020.01.007.
- Chastain CA, Klopfenstein N, Serezani CH, Aronoff DM. A clinical review of diabetic foot infections. *Clin Podiatr Med Surg*. 2019;36(3):381–395. https://doi.org/10.1016/j.cpm.2019.02.004.
- Polk C, Sampson MM, Roshdy D, Davidson LE. Skin and soft tissue infections in patients with diabetes mellitus. *Infect Dis Clin North Am*. 2021;35(1):183–197. https://doi.org/10.1016/j.idc.2020.10.007.
- Saeed K, Esposito S, Akram A, et al. Hot topics in diabetic foot infection. *Int J Antimicrob Agents*. 2020;55(6):105942. https://doi.org/10.1016/j.ijantimicag.2020.105942.

A 40-year-old male presents to the emergency room with a 1-week history of progressive, severe low back pain. He denies any recent injury. Acetaminophen and ibuprofen have not provided much relief. He has felt warm at times, but has not had any chills, night sweats, weight loss, weakness, sensory disturbances, or bowel or bladder incontinence. He does not have any major medical problems. He does not take any medications on a regular basis. He has no medication allergies. He admits to a remote history of IV drug use but denies any recent use. He denies any animal exposures. He does not consume unpasteurized dairy. Vital signs reveal temperature 99.5° F, heart rate 95 beats per minute, blood pressure 145/85 mmHg, and respiratory rate 16. On examination, he appears uncomfortable. Heart exam reveals a regular tachycardia. There is a grade 2 early systolic murmur heard over the apex. Lungs are clear. There is no abdominal distension or tenderness. There is percussion tenderness over his lower spine. Lower extremity motor and sensory examinations are normal. Rectal sphincter tone is normal. The remainder of the examination is unremarkable. Laboratory studies reveal white blood cell count 12,000 cells/μL, hemoglobin 13 g/dL, platelet count 500,000 cells/μL, creatinine 1.1 mg/dL, and C-reactive protein 10 mg/dL (normal <0.9 mg/dL). Two sets of blood cultures are obtained. MRI of the lower spine with and without contrast is shown in Fig. 89.1.

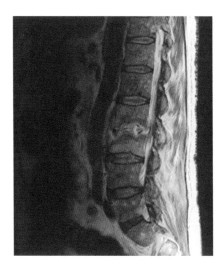

Figure 89.1 – MRI of lower spine
Tande AJ, et al. Osteomyelitis. In: Bennet JE, Dolin R, Blaser MJ, eds. *Mandell, Douglas, and Bennett's Principles and Practice of Infectious Diseases*. 9th ed. Elsevier; 2020.

What is the next best step in the management of this patient?

A. Start vancomycin.

B. Start vancomycin and cefepime.

C. Urgent neurosurgical consultation.

D. Await result of blood cultures before starting antibiotic therapy.

E. Obtain *Brucella* serology.

The next best step in this patient with vertebral discitis/osteomyelitis (D/OM) without associated systemic illness or neurologic compromise is to await the results of blood cultures before starting antibiotic therapy (**option D**).

In general, OM can be subdivided as shown in Fig. 89.2.

This figure is just meant to be an overview, and discussing all of these is beyond the scope of this book. I encourage you to familiarize yourself with these other conditions because they do occasionally show up in practice and on medical board exams. The discussion here will focus on vertebral D/OM.

Vertebral D/OM typically occurs as a consequence of hematogenous dissemination from a bacteremia. In fact, vertebral D/OM is the most common form of hematogenous OM in older adults. Rarely, vertebral D/OM may occur via direct/contiguous extension (i.e., postoperative). Risk factors include IV drug use, hemodialysis (especially with indwelling lines), immune compromise, and infections in other locations (i.e., skin and soft tissue, genitourinary, infective endocarditis, bloodstream infection, etc.). The most common cause of vertebral D/OM is *Staphylococcus aureus*. Other causes include coagulase-negative staphylococci (CoNS), streptococci, and various gram-negatives (especially the Enterobacteriaceae). Less common causes that may be seen in the appropriate epidemiologic context are *Mycobacterium tuberculosis* (Pott disease), *Mycobacterium bovis* (classically associated with intravesicular

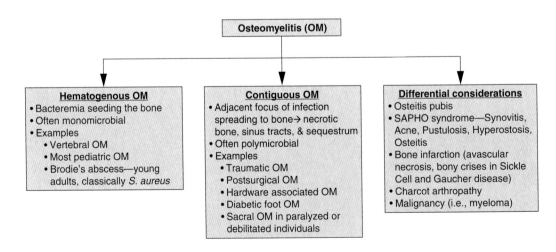

Figure 89.2 – Overview of osteomyelitis

Bacillus–Calmette–Guerin instillations for bladder cancer), nontuberculous mycobacteria (i.e., *Mycobacterium avium* complex in advanced HIV), fungal organisms, and *Brucella* spp. Most CoNS are associated with spinal hardware infections and are unlikely to cause native vertebral D/OM. One exception is the CoNS *Staphylococcus lugdunensis*, which often behaves very similar to *S. aureus* and should be treated as such.

The diagnosis can be very difficult to make, because the presentation is highly variable and the symptoms can mimic other more common disorders (i.e., musculoskeletal back pain). An overall approach to the diagnosis is shown in Fig. 89.3.

Fever is present in approximately 50% of patients. Most patients will have spinal pain and/or percussion tenderness. There may be associated muscle spasm and reduced spinal range of motion. More advanced cases or those associated with abscess (i.e., epidural, paraspinal, etc.) may present with neurologic dysfunction. Patients should be asked about IV drug use, certain exposures (i.e., unpasteurized dairy consumption), and recent infections at other sites. Less than 50% of patients will have leukocytosis. Elevated inflammatory markers (i.e., erythrocyte sedimentation rate and/or C-reactive protein [CRP]) may be seen, but this finding is not specific. HIV screening should always be considered, especially in those with risk factors for HIV. At least two sets of blood cultures (before antibiotics) should be obtained, and, if *Brucella* is suspected, then these blood cultures should be held for a longer period of time (up to 2 weeks), and serologic testing (**option E**) should be obtained. If the history is suggestive, then testing for mycobacterial and fungal infection may be pursued, as shown in Fig. 89.3. It is important to note that, anytime *Brucella* is suspected, the microbiology lab should be notified, as it represents a laboratory biohazard, and it may increase the chance that *Brucella* will be identified.

Spinal x-ray is very insensitive and typically takes several weeks to show abnormalities. The imaging test of choice is an MRI of the spine with and without contrast, because it is highly sensitive (Se) and specific (Sp). In addition, MRI can evaluate differentials (i.e., degeneration, malignancy, etc.) and detect associated complications such as spinal cord compression and abscesses (i.e., epidural, psoas, paraspinal). Alternative imaging modalities include gallium-67/Tc-99 bone scan (Se/Sp >90%) and PET/CT (highly sensitive and helpful to rule out the diagnosis). If no organism is identified on blood cultures or the additional testing discussed above, then image-guided aspiration biopsy should be considered. The biopsy yield (if done before antibiotics are given) is reported to range from 50% to 90% and is higher for open biopsy than for percutaneous aspiration. Repeat aspiration biopsy improves culture sensitivity, and PEDD is better (i.e., more accurate or high-yield) than aspiration biopsy.

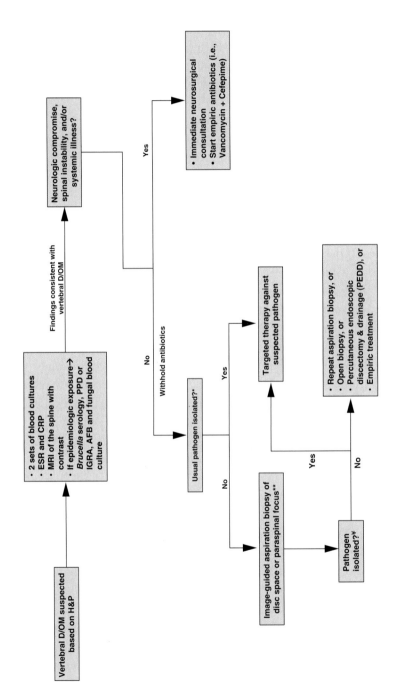

Figure 89.3 – Diagnosis of vertebral discitis/osteomyelitis. (D/OM). AFB, Acid-fast bacillus; **CRP,** C-reactive protein; **ESR,** erythrocyte sedimentation rate; **H&P,** history and physical; **IGRA,** interferon-gamma release assay; **PPD,** purified protein derivative.

*The usual pathogens are Staphylococcus aureus, Staphylococcus lugdunensis, streptococci, gram-negatives (especially Enterobacteriaceae), Candida spp., or Brucella spp. S. aureus bloodstream infection in the preceding 3 months and compatible MRI findings may preclude the need for disc space aspiration. If coagulase-negative staphylococci other than S. lugdunensis are isolated on culture, they are most commonly contaminants. If they are persistently positive or found in the setting of prosthetic devices, then they may be real pathogens, and clinical judgment needs to be used.**Typically, routine aerobic and anaerobic cultures are sent and, if tissue permits, pathology is performed to confirm infection and rule out other differentials. If history suggests mycobacterial, fungal, or Brucella infection, then appropriate cultures for these should be requested. In addition, if the routine cultures do not grow anything, then these same tests should be considered (regardless of history) along with nucleic acid amplification testing (i.e., broad-range PCR). *Certain pathogens, such as most coagulase-negative staphylococci, Cutibacterium acnes, and diphtheroids are often contaminants. They may cause true infections in the right host, but clinical judgment should be used when interpreting the significance of these organisms.

Management is relatively straightforward. Every effort should be made to identify the organism before initiating antimicrobial therapy. If the patient is not severely ill (i.e., sepsis, hemodynamic instability, and/or neurologic compromise), then antimicrobials may be withheld while working to identify the responsible pathogen. If any of these severe factors are present, then empiric therapy (**options A and B**) should be started with coverage for streptococci, staphylococci including methicillin-resistant *S. aureus* (i.e., vancomycin) and gram-negatives (either a third- or fourth-generation cephalosporin). In penicillin-allergic patients, gram-positives can be covered with daptomycin, and gram-negatives can be covered with aztreonam or a fluoroquinolone (FQ). If there is neurologic compromise, then an urgent neurosurgical consultation (**option C**) is warranted. If surgical intervention is performed, then appropriate samples should be sent for cultures and pathology as discussed above. If there are associated abscesses or fluid collections, then every effort should be made to aspirate or drain these in order to reduce the burden of infection, obtain culture data, and obtain the best possible source control. Once culture data are available, then antimicrobial therapy should be de-escalated to cover the pathogen(s) isolated. The definitive treatment is IV in most cases. Treatment duration is typically at least 6 weeks. Patients should be seen in follow-up toward the end of therapy. Sometimes, we will see patients halfway through the course and de-escalate to highly bioavailable oral therapy (i.e., metronidazole, linezolid, FQ, trimethoprim-sulfamethoxazole, etc.) if it is clinically feasible. Inflammatory markers (especially CRP) can be monitored during treatment, as appropriate therapy is associated with a decline in inflammatory markers. Follow-up imaging is not necessary in most cases, as a natural progression (apparent worsening on imaging) of the infection will be seen in most cases. Follow-up imaging is typically done if there is an undrained abscess to follow or if the patient does not clinically improve (i.e., persistent or worsening pain, recurrence of bloodstream infection or systemic symptoms, persistently elevated inflammatory markers without another reason, etc.). If patients fail to improve with antimicrobial therapy, then consider poor adherence, inadequate coverage, development of a new complication (i.e., fracture or abscess), or need for surgical debridement/stabilization. *Brucella* infection is treated with a 3-month course of either doxycycline and rifampin or doxycycline and streptomycin. Mycobacterial infections require significantly longer courses of therapy.

KEY LEARNING POINT

If patients with vertebral discitis/osteomyelitis are not severely ill (i.e., sepsis, hemodynamic instability, and/or neurologic compromise), then antimicrobials may be withheld while working to identify the responsible pathogen.

REFERENCES AND FURTHER READING

- Berbari EF, Kanj SS, Kowalski TJ, et al. 2015 Infectious Diseases Society of America (IDSA) clinical practice guidelines for the diagnosis and treatment of native vertebral osteomyelitis in adults. *Clin Infect Dis.* 2015;61(6):e26–e46. https://doi.org/10.1093/cid/civ482.
- Tande AJ, et al. Osteomyelitis. In: Bennet JE, Dolin R, Blaser MJ, eds. *Mandell, Douglas, and Bennett's Principles and Practice of Infectious Diseases*. 9th ed. Elsevier; 2020.

A 40-year-old male presents to the emergency room with a 1-week history of fevers, chills, cough, pleuritic chest pain, and shortness of breath. He has no known medical problems and does not take any medications routinely. He has no medication allergies. He drinks a six-pack of "tall-boys" daily. He smokes one pack of cigarettes daily. He denies any illicit drug use. Vital signs reveal temperature 102° F, heart rate 110 beats per minute, blood pressure 105/68 mmHg, respiratory rate 24, and oxygen saturation 88% to 90% on room air. He appears ill and malnourished. He has several missing teeth, and the remaining teeth have extensive caries. Heart exam reveals a regular tachycardia and no murmur. Lung exam reveals decreased breath sounds and dullness to percussion over the right lower lung fields posteriorly. The remainder of the examination is unremarkable. Laboratory analysis shows white blood cell count 15,000 cells/uL, hemoglobin 10 g/dL (mean corpuscular volume 105 fL), platelet count 500,000 cells/uL, creatinine 1.3 mg/dL, blood urea nitrogen 26 mg/dL, AST 120 U/L, ALT 55 U/L, total bilirubin 1.4 mg/dL, alkaline phosphatase 150 U/L, albumin 2.5 g/dL, total protein 5 g/dL, and lactate dehydrogenase (LDH) 200 IU/L. Blood cultures are obtained. Chest x-ray reveals a moderate-sized right-sided pleural effusion. Methicillin-resistant *Staphylococcus aureus* (MRSA) nasal swab (PCR) is negative. Thoracentesis is performed and reveals turbid-appearing fluid with 25,000 total nucleated cells (90% neutrophils), LDH 1200 IU/L, total protein 3.5 g/dL, pH 7.10, and glucose 20 mg/dL. Gram stain and culture are pending.

What is the most appropriate next step in management?

A. Start vancomycin and ampicillin/sulbactam.

B. Start ampicillin/sulbactam.

C. Start vancomycin and ampicillin/sulbactam and place a chest tube.

D. Start ampicillin/sulbactam and place a chest tube.

E. Video-assisted thoracoscopic surgery (VATS) with decortication.

This patient has a complicated parapneumonic effusion (PPE), likely related to aspiration in the setting of alcoholism and poor dentition. Therefore, the most appropriate next step is to start ampicillin/sulbactam and place a chest tube (**option D**). Vancomycin (**options A and C**) is unnecessary in light of the likely etiology, community onset, and negative MRSA swab.

Pleural effusions have various causes, which can be differentiated as shown in Fig. 90.1.

The focus of this discussion will be PPEs. Risk factors for PPE include alcoholism, poor dentition, immune suppression (including diabetes and malignancy), and illicit drug use. The infection commonly develops after aspiration of oropharyngeal microbes or following a community-acquired pneumonia. Less commonly, PPE can develop as a result of hematogenous dissemination, postoperative infection, or contiguous spread from a neighboring area (i.e., abdomen, mediastinum, or lungs). Uncomplicated PPE is characterized by a sterile exudative pleural effusion. Complicated PPE is characterized by bacterial invasion into the pleural space, which leads to the findings associated with complicated effusions (i.e., low glucose and pH, loculations, pus). With time, complicated PPE evolves to form an organized, pleural thickening called a "pleural peel." Empyema is a type of complicated PPE characterized by frank pus or positive Gram stain and/or culture.

Various organisms can cause pleural infections. The predominant pathogens depend on the exposure history, the type of host (immune-compromised vs. not), and the location of acquisition (i.e., community- vs. hospital-acquired). Community-acquired infections are somewhat similar to community-acquired pneumonias, including those caused by streptococci (especially *Streptococcus pneumoniae*, beta-hemolytic streptococci, and viridans-group streptococci like the *Streptococcus anginosus* group), staphylococci, anaerobes, gram-negatives, and occasionally viruses. Hospital-acquired infections are more commonly associated with *Staphylococcus aureus* (including MRSA) and resistant gram-negatives (including *Pseudomonas* spp.). Less common pathogens include *Actinomyces* spp., *Nocardia* spp., *Burkholderia* spp., mycobacteria (especially *Mycobacterium tuberculosis*), various zoonotic organisms, fungi, and even parasites (echinococcosis, amebiasis, paragonimiasis).

The presentation is very similar to most pneumonias, as demonstrated in this case. More chronic/indolent infections may present with additional constitutional symptoms (i.e., night sweats, weight loss, anorexia, etc.). PPE should be suspected if a patient with routine pneumonia fails to respond to antibiotics within a few days. Blood cultures should be obtained, even though the yield is low. The best initial test in most cases is a chest x-ray

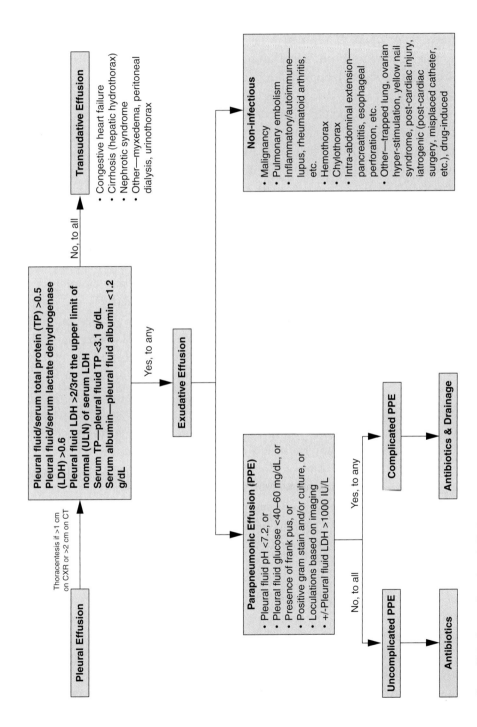

Transudative Effusion

- Congestive heart failure
- Cirrhosis (hepatic hydrothorax)
- Nephrotic syndrome
- Other—myxedema, peritoneal dialysis, urinothorax

Non-infectious

- Malignancy
- Pulmonary embolism
- Inflammatory/autoimmune—lupus, rheumatoid arthritis, etc.
- Hemothorax
- Chylothorax
- Intra-abdominal extension—pancreatitis, esophageal perforation, etc.
- Other—trapped lung, ovarian hyper-stimulation, yellow nail syndrome, post-cardiac injury, iatrogenic (post-cardiac surgery, misplaced catheter, etc.), drug-induced

No, to all

Yes, to any

Exudative Effusion

Pleural fluid/serum total protein (TP) >0.5
Pleural fluid/serum lactate dehydrogenase (LDH) >0.6
Pleural fluid LDH >2/3rd the upper limit of normal (ULN) of serum LDH
Serum TP—pleural fluid TP <3.1 g/dL
Serum albumin—pleural fluid albumin <1.2 g/dL

Thoracentesis if >1 cm on CXR or >2 cm on CT

Pleural Effusion

Parapneumonic Effusion (PPE)

- Pleural fluid pH <7.2, or
- Pleural fluid glucose <40–60 mg/dL, or
- Presence of frank pus, or
- Positive gram stain and/or culture, or
- Loculations based on imaging
- +/-Pleural fluid LDH >1000 IU/L

Yes, to any

Complicated PPE

Antibiotics & Drainage

No, to all

Uncomplicated PPE

Antibiotics

Figure 90.1 – Approach to pleural effusions

(ideally posteroanterior/lateral chest x-ray). X-ray may miss approximately 10% of effusions. If the chest x-ray is negative or inconclusive but suspicion is high, then chest CT or lung ultrasound should be considered. Imaging findings in complicated PPE may include loculations, necrosis/gas, or lung abscess. If the effusion is large enough to sample (typically >1 cm on chest x-ray or >2 cm on CT), then thoracentesis should be performed. If the effusion is significantly loculated, then it is usually best to proceed straight to chest tube drainage. The pleural fluid should be sent for cell count with differential, lactate dehydrogenase, and total protein (to be compared with the serum values for Light's criteria, as shown in Fig. 90.1), glucose, pH (tested with arterial blood gas machine and prone to error), and Gram stain and culture (typically aerobic and anaerobic culture, but acid-fast and fungal cultures may be considered if suspicion exists). Ideally, all cultures should be obtained before administering antibiotics. In addition, culturing the pleural fluid in blood culture bottles improves yield. If there is concern for malignancy, then cytology should be sent. The appearance of the fluid may be useful as well. For example, if the fluid comes out as "pus," then most of the additional testing (except for Gram stain/culture) is often unnecessary. Culture directly from a chest tube in patients who have had a chest tube in place for some time should be avoided, as organisms colonize the chest tube tubing, leading to misleading results. Additional testing may include HIV screening, tuberculosis rule-out (sputum acid-fast bacillus smear/culture and PCR testing), MRSA nasal swab (PCR), respiratory viral panel, sputum cultures, and *Legionella* urine antigen.

Management depends on the classification (complicated vs. uncomplicated). Uncomplicated PPE can often be managed with antibiotics alone (more on antibiotics later) and close clinical and radiographic follow-up. Uncomplicated PPE should typically get at least 2 weeks of therapy. Complicated PPE requires drainage for source control. The typical first-line approach is chest tube (tube thoracostomy) drainage, typically done with small-bore chest tubes nowadays. Based on the imaging appearance and clinical trajectory, more than one chest tube may be necessary. In addition, most patients (especially those with poor chest tube drainage) end up receiving concomitant therapy with intrapleural fibrinolytics and DNase. These additional therapies have been shown to reduce hospital length of stay and need for surgical decortication. Surgical decortication (i.e., VATS – **option E**) is done in select cases, especially in advanced cases and those that fail to respond to drainage and antibiotics. Decortication may reduce hospital length of stay, but no high-quality head-to-head trial has compared decortication with chest tube drainage plus fibrinolytic/DNase.

Antimicrobial therapy can get complicated and depends largely on the mechanism of infection, illness severity, local microbial resistance patterns, and location of acquisition.

Table 90.1 – Empiric Antimicrobial Therapy for Complicated Parapneumonic Effusion/Empyema

Situation	First-Line	Alternative	Comments
Community-acquired	• Ceftriaxone + metronidazole or • Ampicillin/sulbactam (Unasyn)	• Piperacillin/tazobactam • Ertapenem • Levofloxacin + metronidazole • Alternative to vancomycin —linezolid, daptomycin if there is no primary pneumonia associated	• Coverage may need to be broader in patients who are more severely ill (i.e., shock) • If there is a previous history of resistant organisms, then coverage for these pathogens may be necessary • If due to an upper gastrointestinal tract perforation, then coverage for *Candida* spp. may be warranted (i.e., echinocandin or fluconazole, depending on severity and prior azole exposure)
Hospital-acquired	• Vancomycin + cefepime + metronidazole	• Alternatives to cefepime + metronidazole → piperacillin/tazobactam or meropenem	

If the patient is hemodynamically stable, not in significant respiratory failure/distress, and not systemically ill, then antibiotics should be withheld until the necessary work-up is done to try to identify a pathogen. Otherwise, empiric therapy should be started. In most cases, empiric coverage for anaerobes is necessary because these are often involved but are difficult to isolate. Likewise, definitive management should also include anaerobic coverage in many cases. Atypical coverage is often not necessary unless there is strong suspicion for an atypical organism (i.e., *Legionella*, *Chlamydophila*, or *Mycoplasma*). In patients with a low pretest probability of *S. aureus* pneumonia (i.e., not a postviral pneumonia, no necrotizing features, etc.), a negative MRSA nasal PCR makes MRSA coverage unnecessary. Table 90.1 summarizes the empiric antimicrobial management.

Definitive therapy should be based on available Gram stain and culture data and clinical progress. As noted above, anaerobic coverage is often necessary. Treatment duration depends largely on the degree of source control. In most cases, the duration is 4 to 6 weeks. In cases with excellent clinical and radiographic improvement, then 2 weeks may be appropriate. Initially therapy is IV in most cases, except for if using certain drugs that have excellent oral bioavailability (i.e., linezolid, fluoroquinolone, metronidazole). If able to take oral medications and clinically improved with good source control, then de-escalation to highly bioavailable oral therapy may be considered (if susceptibility data allow). Patients are typically followed up by the involved surgical team (i.e., thoracic surgeons) and the infectious disease provider. Repeat imaging (often a CT) and clinical evaluation should be done at follow-up. These two factors help determine the endpoint of therapy.

An issue that arises commonly in patients with PPE who have drains in place is treatment failure. Treatment failure typically shows up as worsening sepsis (i.e., fevers, hemodynamics, leukocytosis, etc.). When this occurs, the following should be considered:

- **Source control, source control, and source control!** Drains may get dislodged, kinked, and/or clogged. This may manifest as decreased drain output. Repeat imaging, drain adjustment (repositioning, replacement, or placing more drains) and fibrinolytics/DNase (if not already done) may be helpful in these cases. If conservative management does not work, then surgical intervention needs to be considered.

- **Is there another source of "sepsis" or "sepsis-like" presentation?** This may include hospital-acquired infection (i.e., *Clostridiodes difficile*, line infection or phlebitis, surgical site infection, etc.), repeat aspiration event/pneumonitis, postoperative state, thrombosis, or drug-induced.

- **Is the coverage suboptimal?** If managed appropriately, this should not be an issue. If considering broadening therapy, then repeat cultures (i.e., sputum, blood and/or fresh pleural fluid sample) should obtained.

KEY LEARNING POINT

Complicated parapneumonic effusion (PPE) is managed with drainage and appropriate antibiotics. Uncomplicated PPE can be managed with antibiotics and close follow-up (i.e., drainage often unnecessary).

REFERENCES AND FURTHER READING

- Bibby AC, Maskell NA. *Pleural infections. Murray & Nadel's Textbook of Respiratory Medicine.* 7th ed. Elsevier; 2022.
- Broaddus CV, Light RW. *Pleural effusion. Murray & Nadel's Textbook of Respiratory Medicine.* 7th ed. Elsevier; 2022.
- Parta M. Pleural effusion and empyema. In: Bennet JE, Dolin R, Blaser MJ, eds. *Mandell, Douglas, and Bennett's Principles and Practice of Infectious Diseases.* 9th ed. Elsevier; 2020.
- Shen KR, Bribriesco A, Crabtree T, et al. The American Association for Thoracic Surgery consensus guidelines for the management of empyema. *J Thorac Cardiovasc Surg.* 2017;153(6):e129–e146. https://doi.org/10.1016/j.jtcvs.2017.01.030.

A 50-year-old male is hospitalized for severe alcohol-induced pancreatitis complicated by shock, respiratory failure with acute respiratory distress syndrome, and acute kidney injury with anuria. Consequently, he is now requiring mechanical ventilation, vasopressor support, and continuous renal replacement therapy (CRRT). Current medications include fentanyl, propofol, pantoprazole, norepinephrine, and piperacillin/tazobactam. On hospital day 7, he develops a new fever up to 102° F associated with an increased heart rate and a decline in mean arterial blood pressure requiring escalation of the norepinephrine dose. Ventilator settings are unchanged over the past several days. On examination, he is sedated and unable to cooperate with the exam. When his sedation is weaned, he gets very agitated. Scleral icterus is present. He has a nasogastric tube in place. An endotracheal tube is in place, and suctioning the tube reveals thin, clear secretions. Lung exam reveals diffuse crackles. Heart exam shows a regular tachycardia and no murmur. Abdomen is mildly distended. A Foley catheter is in place with cloudy-appearing, amber-colored urine. There is a hemodialysis line inserted at the right neck that is functioning normally. There is a peripherally-inserted central catheter in the right brachial region. He has a peripheral IV catheter in the left antecubital region. There is no erythema, induration, or drainage associated with any of these lines. Serum laboratory analysis reveals white blood cell (WBC) count 16,000 cells/μL (12,000 cells/μL the day prior), creatinine 1 mg/dL (while on CRRT), AST 250 μ/L, ALT 110 μ/L, total bilirubin 20 mg/dL, alkaline phosphatase 200 μ/L, and lactic acid 4.5 mmol/L. Urinalysis reveals positive nitrite and leukocyte esterase on dipstick. Urine microscopy shows greater than 100 WBCs per high-power field (hpf). Chest x-ray shows diffuse bilateral opacities that appear stable compared with chest x-rays done the past few days. Cultures are obtained, and empiric vancomycin is added. Endotracheal aspirate culture eventually grows *Stenotrophomonas maltophilia*. Peripheral blood cultures grow methicillin-resistant *Staphylococcus aureus* (MRSA) in one out of four bottles. Blood cultures were not obtained from any of the intravascular catheters. Urine culture grows greater than 100,000 CFU/mL of *Enterobacter aerogenes*.

Which of the following organisms should be treated?

A. MRSA, *S. maltophilia*, and *E. aerogenes*.
B. MRSA and *S. maltophilia*.
C. MRSA and *E. aerogenes*.
D. MRSA only.
E. None of these organisms need to be treated.

The best answer to this question is MRSA only (**option D**). Isolation of *S. aureus* in a blood culture (even if it is only in one bottle) should never be regarded as a contaminant because of the high mortality of *S. aureus* bacteremia. This patient has no clinical evidence of a ventilator-associated pneumonia at this time; therefore, *S. maltophilia* (**options A** and **B**) does not need to be covered. In fact, this organism is often a nosocomial colonizer seen in critically ill patients with prior antibiotic exposure and/or foreign materials (i.e., endotracheal tube, catheters, etc.). Catheter-associated urinary tract infections (UTIs) are actually very uncommon causes of fever in the intensive care unit. Most urine specimens from catheterized patients will appear "infected," as evidenced by positive leukocyte esterase, positive nitrites, pyuria (>10 whie blood cells per highpower field [WBC/hpf]), and even bacteriuria (like the *E. aerogenes* in this patient). However, unless the patient has unequivocal symptoms of a UTI, meets criteria for treatment of asymptomatic bacteriuria (i.e., pregnancy or impending urologic procedure), or has no other explanation for sepsis, then treatment is not necessary (**options A** and **C**).

Fever in hospitalized patients is very common, and having a good approach to this entity is very important. Many of the principles that will be discussed here can be applied to acute leukocytosis (without fever) in a hospitalized patient. The following are some useful generalizations about fevers that develop in patients during their hospitalization:

- Ruling out an infectious etiology is the most important initial goal. If there is no clinical evidence of infection, then consider the noninfectious etiologies of fever (Table 91.1).
- If an infection is present, then it is typically nosocomial (hospital-acquired). Very rarely will you see a community-onset infection manifesting for the first time well into a hospitalization. Community-acquired infections typically manifest prior to hospitalization or very soon after hospitalization (i.e., within 48 hours of admission).
- As shown in Table 91.1, a systematic head-to-toe approach should be taken when evaluating for infection in these patients. In addition, it can be helpful to talk with the primary physician or team and the patient's nurse when evaluating these patients.
- Any abnormality should be correlated clinically. For example, if the patient has an opacity on chest x-ray, then correlate for clinical signs and symptoms of pneumonia.
- Table 91.1 outlines the various infectious and noninfectious causes of fever and/or leukocytosis.

Table 91.1 – Etiologies of Fever and/or Leukocytosis in the Hospital

Category	Clinical Considerations	Work-Up to Consider
Central nervous system (CNS) infection	• Headaches, confusion, nuchal rigidity, etc. • Often postsurgical (head, neck, spine)	• CNS imaging—head CT, brain and/or spine MRI • Lumbar puncture (cerebrospinal fluid analysis)
Ears, nose, and throat (ENT) infection	• Symptoms/signs of otitis, sinusitis, upper respiratory infection, parotitis, or odontogenic infection	• Dedicated ENT imaging (typically head CT) • Respiratory viral panel (film-array)
Cardiovascular infection	• Bacteremia, line-associated infection, septic thrombophlebitis, or very rarely, endocarditis • Presentation is often nonspecific (i.e., fevers, rigors) • Perform heart examination and examine all lines for inflammatory signs (i.e., erythema, warmth, tenderness)	• At least two sets of blood cultures should be obtained for every febrile patient in the hospital (include a line culture as well if suspicious) • Vascular ultrasound or echocardiogram
Pulmonary infection	• New or worsening cough, chest pain, shortness of breath, or respiratory failure • Aspiration events/pneumonitis	• Respiratory cultures, *Legionella* urine antigen, respiratory viral panel, and/or chest imaging • Thoracentesis to evaluate effusions • Swallow evaluation
Abdominal infection	• New or worsening abdominal pain, vomiting, diarrhea, etc. • Common considerations include *Clostridioides difficile*, intra-abdominal abscess, and acalculous cholecystitis	• Liver function testing, lipase, abdominal imaging, and/or *C. difficile* testing (if ≥3 watery stools/day without another explanation) • Other stool studies (i.e., stool culture, ova and parasites, etc.) if high suspicion or symptoms started before admission or within 3 days of admission • If ascites is present, then paracentesis to rule out peritonitis
Genitourinary infection	• Vomiting, flank pain, hematuria, dysuria, suprapubic pain, etc. • Digital rectal exam to evaluate for prostatitis	• Urinalysis (UA) with microscopy ± urine culture (depending on UA result) • Imaging (i.e., ultrasound or CT) should be considered to rule out obstruction and/or stones • May need to exchange indwelling urinary catheter or, ideally, remove an unnecessary catheter
Skin and soft tissue infection (SSTI)	• Look for skin breakdown or decubitus ulcers, rashes, cellulitis, and abscesses	• May need incision and drainage of abscess for culture • May need imaging to rule out deeper infections
Bone and/or joint infection	• Arthralgia and/or arthritis • Examine all large joints for inflammation and percuss the spine • Closely examine all areas with hardware	• Arthrocentesis—cell count with differential, crystal analysis, Gram stain, and culture

(Continued)

Table 91.1 – Etiologies of Fever and/or Leukocytosis in the Hospital *(Cont'd)*

Category	Clinical Considerations	Work-Up to Consider
Surgical site infection	• Assess all surgical sites/wounds closely	• May need to obtain deep tissue samples for culture
Poor source control	• Examples include decreased drain output (i.e., clogged, dislodged, etc.), retained infected/inflamed tissue, or incomplete debridement	• Work to obtain the best possible source control
Noninfectious causes of fevers (and leukocytosis)	• Hyperthermia syndromes (i.e., malignant hyperthermia, serotonin syndrome, neuroleptic malignant syndrome, heat stroke, endocrine disorders, etc.) • Drug- or substance-related—excess or withdrawal • Inflammation—gout/pseudogout, pancreatitis, etc. • Transfusion reaction • Intracranial pathology—stroke, hemorrhage, or seizures • Thrombosis or phlebitis • Hematoma • Malignancy-related (esp. leukemias and lymphoma)	
Leukocytosis	• The etiologies will depend on the white blood cell differential • General causes of leukocytosis include inflammatory states, hypovolemia, stress (postop state), steroids (neutrophilia, eosinopenia, and lymphopenia), malignancy (esp. leukemia), postsplenectomy, drug-related (often eosinophilia), and many of the other noninfectious fever causes	

KEY LEARNING POINT

It is very important to have a systematic approach to fever in hospitalized individuals. Any abnormal findings need to be clinically correlated (i.e., do not just treat everything you find).

A 50-year-old male is admitted to the hospital with a 3-day history of fevers, chills, and shortness of breath. Medical history is notable for a bicuspid aortic valve with mild aortic valve stenosis and previously treated hepatitis C virus infection with documentation of sustained virologic response. He does not take any medications. He has no drug allergies. He drinks two to three beers daily. He smokes a pack of cigarettes daily. He previously used IV drugs but denies any recent use. He denies any animal exposures. Vital signs reveal temperature 101.5° F, heart rate 110 beats per minute, blood pressure 95/70 mmHg, respiratory rate 24, and oxygen saturation 90% on room air. On examination, he appears ill and is breathing heavily. There is no icterus or conjunctival abnormality. Oral mucosa is dry. Heart exam reveals a regular tachycardia and a grade 3 early diastolic decrescendo murmur heard best over the left lower sternal border. Lung exam reveals bibasilar crackles. Skin and nail examinations are normal. The remainder of the examination is unremarkable. Labs reveal white blood cell (WBC) count 13,500 cells/uL, hemoglobin 12 g/dL, platelet count 500,000 cells/uL, creatinine 1.1 mg/dL, rheumatoid factor 80 IU/mL (normal <24 IU/mL), and C-reactive protein 8 mg/dL (normal <0.9 mg/dL). Blood cultures are obtained, and empiric vancomycin and ceftriaxone are started. Chest x-ray shows cardiomegaly and bilateral interstitial opacities in the lower lung lobes. Transthoracic echocardiogram (TTE) reveals a bicuspid aortic valve with severe aortic valve regurgitation and no valvular vegetation. Transesophageal echocardiogram (TEE) shows similar findings.

What is the next best step in management?

A. Repeat TEE in 3 to 5 days.
B. Obtain PET/CT.
C. Obtain tagged WBC scan.
D. Await blood culture results prior to pursuing further testing.
E. Obtain *Coxiella burnetii* serology.

The best next step is to await blood culture results prior to pursuing further testing (**option D**). Based on the Duke criteria (see below), this patient's presentation is consistent with infective endocarditis (IE). Therefore, additional testing to diagnose IE is not necessary at this time, unless the blood cultures fail to identify an organism. An overview of IE is shown in Fig. 92.1.

There are various classifications of IE:
- **Native-valve endocarditis versus prosthetic-valve endocarditis (PVE)**
  - The predominant organisms that cause IE differ between these two groups, as shown in Fig. 92.1.

- **Culture-positive versus culture-negative**
  - Culture-negative IE may occur in up to 20% of cases and is often due to administration of antibiotics before obtaining blood cultures
  - Other etiologies of culture-negative IE include infection with organisms that are difficult to isolate (i.e., fastidious organisms like the nutritionally variant streptococci), infection with atypical pathogens (i.e., *C. burnetii, Bartonella* spp., etc.), or noninfectious etiologies (see Fig. 92.1)

- **Acute versus subacute/chronic**
  - Acute IE is typically due to virulent organisms (i.e., *Staphylococcus aureus*, group A streptococci, *Streptococcus pneumoniae*, etc.); patients are typically acutely ill; the classic stigmata of IE (i.e., Osler nodes, Roth spots, etc.) are unlikely to be present, as these take time to develop
  - Subacute/chronic IE is typically due to less virulent organisms (i.e., viridans-group streptococci, *Enterococcus* spp., etc.); patients are less ill and often have constitutional symptoms; the classic stigmata of IE are more likely to be seen

- **Left-sided (aortic and/or mitral) versus right-sided (pulmonic and/or tricuspid)**
  - Left-sided (especially mitral valve) is far more common than right-sided
  - Right-sided is mainly seen in IV drug users and those with indwelling lines. Right-sided IE may be associated with septic pulmonary emboli. The typical organisms in IV drug abusers are *S. aureus, Pseudomonas* spp., *Candida* spp., *Corynebacterium jeikeium,* and *Serratia marcescens*

Risk factors for IE include intravenous penetration (i.e., IV drug abuse, hemodialysis, indwelling lines, etc.), structural heart disease (i.e., congenital heart disease, prosthetic devices,

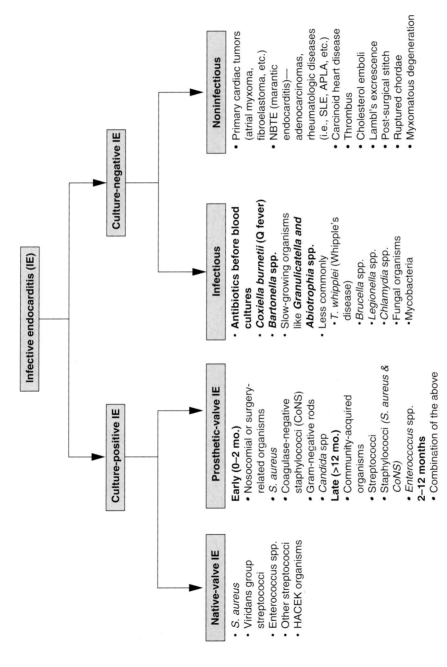

Figure 92.1 – Overview of infective endocarditis

APLA, Antiphospholipid antibody syndrome; *HACEK, Haemophilus* spp., *Aggregatibacter* spp., *Cardiobacterium hominis, Eikenella corrodens, and Kingella* spp; *NBTE*, nonbacterial thrombotic endocarditis; *SLE*, systemic lupus erythematosus.

abnormal valves, etc.), prior IE, prolonged bacteremia, gastrointestinal tract disruption (i.e., dental manipulation, colon cancer, etc.), and immune compromise.

The pathophysiology of IE involves two major components: an abnormal heart valve and the right type of organism (i.e., an organism that is "sticky" or poorly immunogenic, which allows the organism to persist in the blood). In the setting of an abnormal valve, there can be platelet-fibrin deposition that forms a sterile vegetation (i.e., nonbacterial thrombotic endocarditis [NBTE]). NBTE may also occur with hypercoagulability and/or endothelial damage (i.e., antiphospholipid antibody syndrome, malignancy, etc.). This sterile vegetation may get colonized by the right type of organism that promotes more platelet-fibrin deposition to form a mature vegetation. The classic vegetation is typically located along the line of closure of a valve leaflet on the atrial surface of the atrioventricular valves or on the ventricular surface of the semilunar valves. The immune response is characterized by humoral and cellular components including complement, cryoglobulin, immune complexes, rheumatoid factor (RF), and antinuclear antibody formation.

The clinical presentation is highly variable and depends on the factors discussed in the classification section above. In addition, the infection can be localized or metastatic (i.e., local extension or emboli to any organ). The various potential manifestations of IE are shown in Table 92.1.

Some of the more classic manifestations of IE are shown in Fig. 92.2.

If IE is suspected, then at least three sets of blood cultures should be obtained from different sites (at least 1 hour between the first and third set) and before administration of antibiotics. This protocol is used because the bacteremia in IE is often continuous but low-grade. Blood culture clearance should be documented as well. Basic laboratory evaluation typically includes complete blood count with differential, complete metabolic profile (i.e., renal function, hepatic function, electrolytes), urinalysis with microscopy, and inflammatory markers. HIV screening should always be considered. In IV drug users, testing for hepatitis B and hepatitis C may be warranted as well. Additional supportive testing may include RF and serum complement levels. If suspicious, then testing for culture-negative IE pathogens may be considered. ECG is often done and may show cardiac conduction disturbances. If warranted, then dedicated imaging of any potentially involved area should be pursued. This may include imaging of the central nervous system, chest, and abdomen/pelvis. A cardiothoracic surgeon should be involved, as they may help guide some of the necessary imaging, especially if

Table 92.1 – Manifestations of Infective Endocarditis

Category	Manifestations
Nonspecific symptoms	• Constitutional and cardiopulmonary symptoms—fevers, chills, anorexia, weight loss, night sweats, myalgias, arthralgias, chest pain, palpitations, shortness of breath
Cardiac	• New or worsening heart murmur, new or worsening valvular insufficiency, heart failure, local pyogenic complications (i.e., abscesses, fistula formation, prosthetic valve dehiscence, etc.), local conduction disturbances, myopericarditis, mycotic aneurysms (most commonly in the central nervous system, but can form anywhere)
Pulmonary	• May see evidence of heart failure (i.e., pulmonary edema). • In right-sided IE, may see "cannonball lesions" of septic pulmonary emboli
Renal	• Renal abscess, infarction, or glomerulonephritis (acute kidney injury, hematuria, proteinuria, etc.)
Central nervous system	• Cerebral emboli → encephalopathy, strokes, or abscesses • Cerebral mycotic aneurysms → intracranial hemorrhage • Roth spots (retinal hemorrhage surrounding pale central area)—not pathognomonic
Abdominal	• Splenomegaly, splenic infarction, or abscess
Skin	• Petechiae (conjunctival, palatal, skin) • Osler nodes (immunologic)—painful lesions on pads of fingers and/or toes • Janeway lesions (vascular/septic)—painless lesions on palms and/or soles • Subungual (splinter) hemorrhages
Laboratory	• Anemia of chronic disease • Elevated inflammatory markers—erythrocyte sedimentation rate, C-reactive protein, thrombocytosis • May see elevated rheumatoid factor, hypocomplementemia, hypergammaglobulinemia, cryoglobulinemia

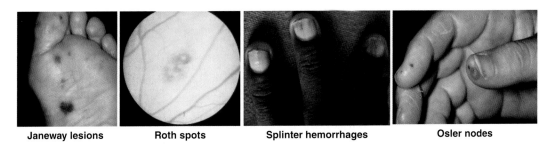

Janeway lesions   Roth spots   Splinter hemorrhages   Osler nodes

Figure 92.2 – Classic stigmata of infective endocarditis

Holland TL, et al. Endocarditis and intravascular infections. In: *Mandell, Douglas, and Bennett's Principles and Practice of Infectious Diseases*. 9th ed. Elsevier Inc; 2020;1068–1108. Accessed 9/14/21 from: https://www.clinicalkey.com/service/content/pdf/watermarked/3-s2.0-B9780323482554000801.pdf?locale=en_US&searchIndex=
Yang E, Frazee BW. Infective endocarditis. *Emerg Med Clin North Am*. 2018 Nov;36(4):645–663. https://doi.org/10.1016/j.emc.2018.06.002. PMID: 30296997. From Sande MA, Strausbaugh LJ. Infective endocarditis. In: Hook EW, Mandell GL, Gwaltney JM Jr, et al, eds. Current Concepts of Infectious Diseases. New York: Wiley Press; 1977.

pursuing surgical intervention. In addition, infectious disease and cardiology should be involved in these cases. One of the most important tests to obtain is the echocardiogram. The approach to echocardiography is shown in Fig. 92.3.

All patients should initially receive a transthoracic echocardiogram (TTE). TTE is less sensitive than transesophageal echocardiogram (TEE) and cannot rule out endocarditis. Interestingly, the performance of TTE may be similar to that of TEE for tricuspid valve endocarditis. If the suspicion/pretest probability of IE is high (i.e., PVE, IV drug use, etc.), then a TEE should be done. TEE is more sensitive in cases with prosthetic valve endocarditis and smaller vegetations. If the initial TEE is negative, but suspicion is sufficiently high, then a repeat TEE should be performed 3 to 5 days later, or sooner if there is a clinical change concerning for a new IE complication. It is important to remember that an echo may be falsely negative with early IE, small vegetations, or embolized vegetations. Lastly, an echocardiogram is also recommended at the completion of therapy to establish a new baseline for valvular function/morphology and ventricular function.

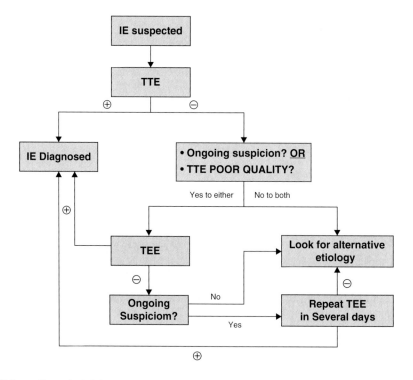

Figure 92.3 – Echocardiography in infective endocarditis
IE, Infective endocarditis; *TEE*, transesophageal echocardiogram; *TTE*, transthoracic echocardiogram.

Based on the information discussed so far, one should be able to utilize the modified Duke criteria to establish the likelihood of IE. The modified Duke criteria are shown in Table 92.2.

The Duke criteria should only be used as a guide and should not supersede clinical judgment. The sensitivity of these criteria is reduced in the setting of PVE. Based on these criteria, the patient in this case has definite IE.

Repeating TEE in 3 to 5 days (**option A**) can be considered if the patient develops a new complication (i.e., heart block, etc.) or the diagnosis of IE is still up in the air (not the case here). Obtaining a PET/CT (**option B**) or a tagged WBC scan (**option C**) is probably the most beneficial in prosthetic valve endocarditis. PET/CT may be falsely positive in the first 3 months post–cardiac surgery. PET/CT may be able to reclassify patients labeled as having "possible IE" via the Duke criteria as either "rejected IE" or "definite IE." Obtaining *C. burnetii* serology (**option E**) is unlikely to be helpful in this patient with no exposure history consistent with Q fever infection.

Table 92.2 – Modified Duke Criteria

Pathologic Criteria

- Microorganisms demonstrated on culture or histopathology of a vegetation or intracardiac abscess
- Active endocarditis demonstrated by histopathology of a vegetation or intracardiac abscess

Major Clinical Criteria	**Minor Clinical Criteria**

1. **Positive blood cultures**
  • Typical microorganisms consistent with infective endocarditis (IE) from two separate blood cultures or
  • Microorganisms consistent with IE from persistently positive blood cultures or
  • Single positive blood culture for *Coxiella burnetii* or antiphase I IgG antibody titer ≥1:800
2. **Positive echocardiogram**
  • Valvular vegetation or oscillating cardiac mass
  • Intracardiac abscess
  • New valvular regurgitation
  • New prosthetic valve dehiscence
	1. **Predisposing condition**—heart disease, IV drug use, etc.
	2. **Fever 38° C or higher**
	3. **Vascular phenomena**—arterial emboli, septic pulmonary emboli/infarcts, mycotic aneurysm, intracranial hemorrhage, conjunctival hemorrhage, Janeway lesions
	4. **Immune phenomena**—Osler nodes, Roth spots, elevated rheumatoid factor, glomerulonephritis
	5. **Microbiologic evidence**—positive blood culture but does not meet a major criterion (excludes single positive cultures for coagulase-negative staphylococci and organisms that do not cause endocarditis) or serological evidence of active infection with organism consistent with IE

- **Definite IE** = presence of pathologic criteria; or two major criteria; or one major and three minor criteria; or five minor criteria
- **Possible IE** = presence of one major and one minor criteria; or three minor criteria
- **Rejected IE** = firm alternative diagnosis explaining evidence of IE; or resolution of IE syndrome with antibiotic therapy for ≤4 days; or no pathological evidence of IE at surgery or autopsy with antibiotic therapy for ≤4 days; or does not meet criteria for possible IE as above

KEY LEARNING POINT

The modified Duke criteria should be used to diagnose infective endocarditis but should not supersede clinical judgment.

REFERENCES AND FURTHER READING

- Baddour LM, Wilson WR, Bayer AS, et al. Infective endocarditis in adults: diagnosis, antimicrobial therapy, and management of complications: a scientific statement for healthcare professionals from the American Heart Association. *Circulation.* 2015;132(15):1435–1486. https://doi.org/10.1161/CIR.0000000000000296. Erratum in: *Circulation.* 2015;132(17):e215. Erratum in: *Circulation.* 2016;134(8):e113. Erratum in: *Circulation.* 2018;138(5):e78-e79.
- Holland TL, et al. Endocarditis and intravascular infections. In: Bennet JE, Dolin R, Blaser MJ, eds. *Mandell, Douglas, and Bennett's Principles and Practice of Infectious Diseases.* 9th ed. Elsevier; 2020:1068–1108.
- Hubers SA, DeSimone DC, Gersh BJ, Anavekar NS. Infective endocarditis: a contemporary review. *Mayo Clin Proc.* 2020;95(5):982–997. https://doi.org/10.1016/j.mayocp.2019.12.008.
- Palraj R, et al. Prosthetic valve endocarditis. In: Bennet JE, Dolin R, Blaser MJ, eds. *Mandell, Douglas, and Bennett's Principles and Practice of Infectious Diseases.* 9th ed. Elsevier; 2020.
- Yang E, Frazee BW. Infective endocarditis. *Emerg Med Clin North Am.* 2018;36(4):645–663. https://doi.org/10.1016/j.emc.2018.06.002.

A 60-year-old male is admitted to the hospital with a 1-day history of fevers and chills. Due to prior issues with poor vascular access, he has a peripherally inserted central catheter (PICC) in place. Medical history is notable for type 2 diabetes mellitus, hypertension, and coronary artery disease requiring cardiac stenting 2 years ago. Medications include aspirin, atorvastatin, lisinopril, metformin, and metoprolol. Vital signs reveal temperature 102° F, heart rate 120 beats per minute, blood pressure 92/55 mmHg, and respiratory rate 18. On examination, he appears ill with visible rigors. Heart exam reveals a regular tachycardia with no heart murmur. There is a PICC line in the right brachial region that appears slightly red at the site of insertion. There is no purulence, tenderness, or swelling in the right upper extremity. The remainder of the examination is unremarkable. Laboratory studies reveal white blood cell count 16,000 cells/uL, creatinine 1.2 mg/dL (creatinine clearance 55 mL/min), and glucose 200 mg/dL. Blood cultures are simultaneously drawn from the PICC line and peripheral circulation. Vancomycin and cefepime are initiated. Eventually, the PICC line blood culture grows methicillin-resistant *Staphylococcus aureus* (MRSA) in 8 hours and 30 minutes. The peripheral blood culture grows MRSA in 11 hours. Cefepime is discontinued, and blood cultures are repeated.

What is the most appropriate next step in management for this patient?

A. Ultrasound of the right upper extremity.

B. Transthoracic echocardiogram.

C. Retain the PICC line and utilize concurrent antibiotic-lock therapy.

D. Exchange the PICC line over a guidewire.

E. Remove the PICC line.

The most appropriate next step is to remove the PICC line (**option E**). This patient has a catheter-associated bloodstream infection (CRBSI) due to *S. aureus*. In light of this and his hemodynamic instability, line removal is recommended.

As shown in Fig. 93.1, catheter infections may originate in multiple ways.

Short-term catheters (i.e., those in place <14 days) are typically contaminated by skin organisms at device insertion (extraluminal). Contamination of the catheter hub-lumen (intraluminal) is the most common cause of bacteremia associated with long-term catheters. Several types of infections are possible, as shown in Table 93.1.

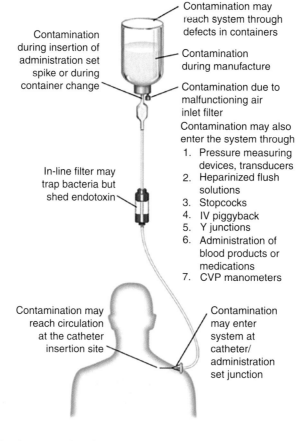

Contamination may reach system through defects in containers

Contamination during insertion of administration set spike or during container change

Contamination during manufacture

Contamination due to malfunctioning air inlet filter

Contamination may also enter the system through
1. Pressure measuring devices, transducers
2. Heparinized flush solutions
3. Stopcocks
4. IV piggyback
5. Y junctions
6. Administration of blood products or medications
7. CVP manometers

In-line filter may trap bacteria but shed endotoxin

Contamination may reach circulation at the catheter insertion site

Contamination may enter system at catheter/administration set junction

Figure 93.1 – Etiologies of catheter-associated infections
CVP, Central venous pressure.
Beekman SE, Henderson DK. Infections caused by percutaneous intravascular devices. In: Bennet JE, Dolin R, Blaser MJ, eds. *Mandell, Douglas, and Bennett's Principles and Practice of Infectious Diseases*. 3560–3575.

Table 93.1 – Catheter-Related Infections

Infection	Definition and Considerations
Catheter colonization	• Significant growth of at least one organism in a quantitative or semiquantitative culture of the catheter tip, subcutaneous catheter segment, or catheter hub. By definition, peripheral blood culture is negative. • Management is typically individualized depending on clinical status, organism, and necessity of the line.
Phlebitis	• Induration, erythema, warmth, pain, or tenderness along the tract of a catheterized or recently catheterized vein. • Suppurative (septic) thrombophlebitis is the term used when there is an associated bloodstream infection. This entity requires line removal and at least 2–3 weeks of antimicrobial therapy. Anticoagulation is a controversial topic.
Exit-site infection	• Induration, erythema, warmth, pain, or tenderness within 2 cm of the catheter exit site or purulent discharge from the exit site. • If discharge is present, then it can be swabbed for Gram stain/culture.
Tunnel infection	• Induration, erythema, warmth, pain, or tenderness >2 cm from the catheter exit site, along the subcutaneous tract of a tunneled catheter.
Pocket infection	• Infected fluid in the subcutaneous pocket of a totally implanted intravascular device often associated with tenderness, erythema, and/or induration over the pocket, spontaneous rupture and drainage, or necrosis of the overlying skin.

Catheter-related bloodstream infection	• Bacteremia or fungemia (attributable to the catheter as defined below) in a patient with an intravascular device, sepsis (i.e., fevers, chills, etc.), and no other source of bloodstream infection.
	• Bloodstream infection attributable to a catheter:
	  • Same organism grows from peripheral culture and catheter tip culture
	  • Differential time-to-positivity—growth from line blood culture at least 2 hours quicker than growth from peripheral blood culture
	  • Quantitative blood culture positivity—colony count from the line blood culture is at least three-fold greater than the colony count from the peripheral blood culture

The approach to the diagnosis and management of CRBSI is summarized in Fig. 93.2.

Empiric therapy in most cases should include gram-positive coverage (including MRSA). The typical choice for gram-positive coverage is vancomycin, but if there is a history of prior infection or colonization with more resistant gram-positives (i.e., vancomycin-resistant enterococci), then daptomycin or linezolid may be more appropriate. Empiric gram-negative coverage (including resistant pathogens such as *Pseudomonas* spp.) should be provided in patients who are severely ill, neutropenic, have prior colonization or infection with resistant gram-negatives, or have a femoral line. Typical options include piperacillin/tazobactam, cefepime, or a carbapenem. Empiric *Candida* coverage should be considered in patients who are severely ill, have a femoral line, have prior colonization with *Candida* spp., or have risk

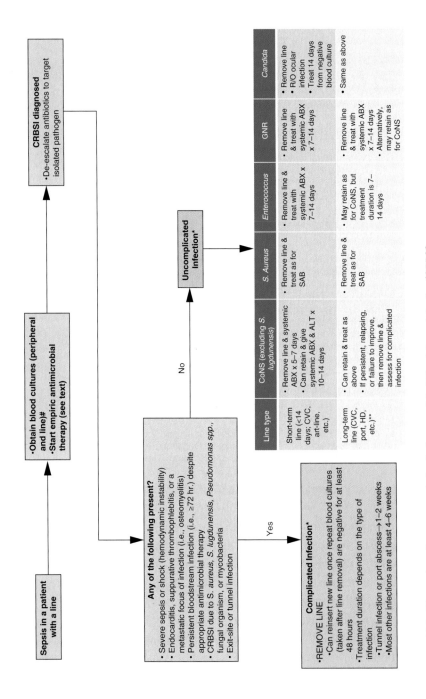

Figure 93.2 – Diagnosis and management of catheter-associated bloodstream infection (CRBSI)

ABX, Antibiotics; *ALT*, antibiotic-lock therapy; *CoNS*, coagulase-negative Staphylococcus; *CVC*, central venous catheter; *GNR*, gram-negative rod; *HD*, hemodialysis; *SAB*, Staphylococcus aureus bacteremia.

#If a blood sample cannot be drawn from a peripheral vein, it is recommended that two blood samples should be drawn through different catheter lumens. If the colony count from one lumen is at least three-fold greater than the colony count from the other lumen, then CRBSI is possible.

*Treatment start day is the day of blood culture clearance. If the line is retained, then should consider obtaining a surveillance set of blood cultures ~1 week after completion of therapy.

**For HD patients, can consider line-exchange via guidewire if unable to remove (i.e., line holiday).

factors for invasive candidiasis such as total parenteral nutrition, prolonged use of broad-spectrum antibiotics, hematologic malignancy, or bone marrow transplantation. The best initial antifungal is an echinocandin, but in patients who are not severely ill and have no risk factors for resistant *Candida* spp. infections (i.e., recent azole exposure), fluconazole may be used. Once the causative organism is identified, then therapy should be de-escalated to target the offending organism. Indications for line removal and definitive management are shown in Fig. 93.2. If the catheter cannot be removed but removal is indicated, then exchanging the catheter over a guidewire may be considered. If a catheter is retained (i.e., catheter salvage), then antibiotic lock therapy (ALT) should be considered. If ALT is not feasible, then systemic antimicrobial therapy should be administered through the colonized catheter.

Ultrasound of the right upper extremity (**option A**) can be considered if there is concern for thrombophlebitis or catheter-associated venous thrombosis, but this patient has no signs of either of these. Transthoracic echocardiogram (**option B**) should be done in almost every case of *S. aureus* bacteremia, but removal of the line takes precedence. Retaining the PICC line and utilizing concurrent ALT (**option C**) is not recommended for patients with *S. aureus* CRBSI. Exchanging the PICC line over a guidewire (**option D**) should only be done if removal of the line is not feasible (often arises in HD patients). In this case, removal of the line is possible and should be done.

KEY LEARNING POINT

In patients with catheter-associated bloodstream infection (CRBSI; suspected or proven), the catheter should be removed if any of the following are present:

- *Severe sepsis or shock (hemodynamic instability)*
- *Endocarditis, suppurative thrombophlebitis, or a metastatic focus of infection (i.e., osteomyelitis)*
- *Persistent bloodstream infection (i.e., ≥72 hours) despite appropriate antimicrobial therapy*
- *CRBSI due to* **Staphylococcus aureus, Staphylococcus lugdunensis, Pseudomonas** *spp., fungal organism, or mycobacteria*
- *Exit-site or tunnel infection*

REFERENCES AND FURTHER READING

- Beekman SE, Henderson DK. Infections caused by percutaneous intravascular devices. In: Bennet JE, Dolin R, Blaser MJ, eds. *Mandell, Douglas, and Bennett's Principles and Practice of Infectious Diseases.* 3560–3575.
- Mermel LA, Allon M, Bouza E, et al. Clinical practice guidelines for the diagnosis and management of intravascular catheter-related infection: 2009 update by the Infectious Diseases Society of America. *Clin Infect Dis.* 2009;49(1): 1–45. https://doi.org/10.1086/599376.

A 70-year-old male is admitted to the hospital with a 1-week history of fevers, chills, and malaise. His medical history is significant for diabetes mellitus, chronic kidney disease with baseline creatinine ranging from 1.5 to 2 mg/dL (creatinine clearance 30–45 mL/min), and previously treated colon cancer. Approximately 2 weeks ago he underwent a surveillance colonoscopy. Medications include metformin, atorvastatin, lisinopril, and furosemide. He has no medication allergies. Vital signs reveal temperature 101° F, heart rate 95 beats per minute, blood pressure 110/70 mmHg, respiratory rate 16, and oxygen saturation 98% on room air. On examination, he appears ill. There is no icterus or conjunctival abnormalities. Heart is regular rate and rhythm. There is a grade 2 holosystolic murmur heard best over the apex. Lungs are clear. Abdomen is soft and nontender. There is a surgical scar in the midabdomen. The remainder of the examination is unremarkable. Labs reveal white blood cell count 13,000 cells/uL, creatinine 1.6 mg/dL, normal liver function testing, and C-reactive protein 10 mg/dL (normal <0.9 mg/dL). Blood cultures are obtained, and vancomycin and piperacillin/tazobactam are started. Eventually, the blood cultures grow *Enterococcus faecalis* sensitive to penicillin, ampicillin, vancomycin, and gentamicin. An echocardiogram shows an oscillating echodensity on the mitral valve. Repeat blood cultures are clear.

What is the most appropriate management of this patient?

A. Penicillin-G and gentamicin for 6 weeks.
B. Ampicillin and gentamicin for 4 weeks.
C. Ampicillin and ceftriaxone for 6 weeks.
D. Vancomycin for 6 weeks.
E. Vancomycin and gentamicin for 6 weeks.

The most appropriate management in this case is ampicillin and ceftriaxone for 6 weeks (**option C**). This patient has native mitral valve endocarditis due to *E. faecalis*. In light of his age and renal dysfunction, Vancomycin and Gentamicin based regimens (**options A, B, D, and E**) should be avoided. The dual beta-lactam combination of ampicillin and ceftriaxone is the preferred regimen in these cases. The management of infective endocarditis (IE) should involve a multidisciplinary approach that includes infectious disease specialists, cardiologists, and cardiothoracic surgeons. Antimicrobial therapy is summarized in Table 94.1.

Table 94.1 – Antimicrobial Management of Infective Endocarditis

Organism	Native-Valve Endocarditis (NVE)	Prosthetic-Valve Endocarditis (PVE)
Empiric therapy	• If the patient is hemodynamically stable, then antimicrobial therapy can be withheld until an organism is identified • If starting therapy, then reasonable initial choice is vancomycin + (CFTX 2 g IV once daily or gentamicin 1 mg/kg IV every 8 hours) • Some advocate for rifampin in PVE, but this is not typically given upfront, due to the risk of rapid development of resistance, especially with *Staphylococcus aureus*	

Viridans-group streptococci or *Streptococcus gallolyticus*	• PCN MIC ≤0.12
	  • PCN-G or CFTX for 4 weeks (can do 2 weeks if uncomplicated IE and give with gentamicin 3 mg/kg IV once daily)
	  • Alternative—vancomycin for 4 weeks
	• PCN MIC 0.12–0.5
	  • CFTX for 4 weeks
	  • Alternative—PCN-G for 4 weeks + gentamicin 3 mg/kg IV once daily for 2 weeks
	    • Alternative—vancomycin for 4 weeks
	• PCN MIC ≥0.5 or *Abiotrophia defectiva* or *Granulicatella* spp.
	  • (Ampicillin or PCN-G) + gentamicin (similar to enterococcal IE)
	  • Alternative—vancomycin alone
		• PCN MIC ≤0.12
		  • (PCN-G or CFTX) for 6 weeks +/- gentamicin 3 mg/kg IV daily for 2 weeks
		  • Alternative—vancomycin for 6 weeks
		• PCN MIC >0.12
		  • (PCN-G or CFTX) + gentamicin 3 mg/kg IV daily for 6 weeks
		  • Alternative—vancomycin for 6 weeks

Methicillin-susceptible staphylococci	• Nafcillin or oxacillin 12 g/day or • Cefazolin 6 g/day (only use if no concern for CNS infection, because cefazolin does not penetrate well into the CNS) • Alternative—vancomycin or daptomycin (≥8 mg/kg daily) • Duration = at least 6 weeks, but if uncomplicated right-sided IE, then can do 2 weeks	• (Nafcillin or oxacillin or cefazolin) for 6 weeks + rifampin 900 mg daily (divided TID) for 6 weeks + gentamicin 3 mg/kg IV daily (divided BID-TID) for 2 weeks • Verify isolate is sensitive to gentamicin if using gentamicin. If not sensitive, then use a different aminoglycoside to which the isolate is susceptible or a fluoroquinolone (FQ; if susceptible)

(Continued)

Answer and Explanation

Table 94.1 – Antimicrobial Management of Infective Endocarditis *(Cont'd)*

Organism	Native-Valve Endocarditis (NVE)	Prosthetic-Valve Endocarditis (PVE)
Methicillin-resistant staphylococci	• Vancomycin or Daptomycin (≥8 mg/kg daily; if no concern for primary pneumonia) × 6 weeks	• Vancomycin for 6 weeks + rifampin 900 mg daily (divided TID) for 6 weeks + gentamicin 3 mg/kg IV daily (divided BID-TID) for 2 weeks • Verify isolate is sensitive to gentamicin if using gentamicin. If not sensitive, then use a different aminoglycoside to which the isolate is susceptible or a FQ (if susceptible)

Enterococcus spp.	• **If sensitive to PCN and gentamicin**
	  • (PCN-G or ampicillin) + gentamicin 3 mg/kg IV daily (divided BID-TID) for 4–6 weeks (only use 4 weeks if NVE and symptom duration <3 months) or
	  • CFTX (higher dose—2 g IV q12h) + ampicillin for 6 weeks
	• **If sensitive to PCN, resistant to gentamicin, but sensitive to streptomycin**
	  • CFTX (higher dose—2 g IV q12h) + ampicillin for 6 weeks
	  • (PCN-G or ampicillin) + streptomycin 15 mg/kg IV daily (divided BID) for 4–6 weeks (only use 4 weeks if NVE and symptom duration <3 months)
	• **If resistant to PCN but sensitive to vancomycin and aminoglycosides**
	  • Vancomycin + gentamicin (3 mg/kg IV daily divided TID) for 6 weeks
	• **If resistant to PCN, aminoglycoside, and vancomycin**
	  • Linezolid or daptomycin (10–12 mg/kg IV daily) for at least 6 weeks	

HACEK group	• CFTX or ampicillin • Alternative—ciprofloxacin • Duration = 4 weeks (NVE); 6 weeks (PVE)	
Other GNR	• Beta-lactam + (aminoglycoside or FQ) for 6 weeks	
Fungi	• Surgery is highly recommended • Treatment of choice is amphotericin-B for 6 weeks. After that, lifelong oral azole suppression is reasonable due to considerable risk of relapse	

CFTX, Ceftriaxone; *CNS*, central nervous system; *GNR*, gram-negative rods; *HACEK*, *Haemophilus* spp., *Aggregatibacter* spp., *Cardiobacterium hominis, Eikenella corrodens*, and *Kingella* spp.; *IE*, infective endocarditis; *MIC*, minimum inhibitory concentration; *PCN*, penicillin.

The first day of therapy is the day of blood culture clearance in most cases. If a patient undergoes valve surgery, and the valve culture grows the organism and/or an abscess is found, then the first day of therapy is the day of the surgery. Of note, a positive gram stain of the valve tissue (without actual growth) represents dead organisms; thus, the first day of therapy in these cases should still be the day of blood culture clearance. In native-valve IE, the duration ranges from 2 to 6 weeks or more, but in most cases of prosthetic-valve IE, the duration is typically at least 6 weeks. The therapy is typically given intravenously for the entire duration, but a recent trial has challenged this concept. The Partial Oral Treatment of Endocarditis trial was a multicenter, randomized, unblinded, noninferiority trial that enrolled patients ($n = 400$) with left-sided native and prosthetic valve IE due to streptococci, S. *aureus* (0% MRSA), coagulase-negative staphylococci, and enterococci. Patients were randomized to either standard IV therapy or an oral therapy group that received 10 days of IV therapy followed by de-escalation to highly bioavailable oral therapy thereafter (various agents, including amoxicillin, linezolid, rifampin, and moxifloxacin). The oral therapy was noninferior to the IV therapy for the primary outcomes (all-cause mortality, unplanned cardiac surgery, clinically evident embolic events, or relapse of bacteremia at 6 months). Despite these data, most practitioners still use IV therapy to treat IE, but may fall back to this trial if long-term IV therapy is not an option (i.e., an IV drug user who cannot be sent home with a long-term IV line).

Indications for early surgical intervention (i.e., during the initial hospitalization and before completion of the antibiotic course) in left-sided endocarditis include:

- Valve dysfunction resulting in heart failure
- Infection due to fungal organisms or drug-resistant organisms (i.e., vancomycin-resistant enterococci, multi-drug resistant gram-negative organisms, etc.)
- Complicated infections—heart block, annular or aortic abscess, penetrating lesions, etc.
- Persistent bloodstream infection (>1 week) despite optimal treatment
- Recurrent emboli while on appropriate treatment
- Persistent or enlarging vegetation while on appropriate treatment
- Mobile vegetation with size >1 cm
- Relapsing prosthetic valve endocarditis

Valve surgery should be delayed by at least 4 weeks if there is evidence of a central nervous system (CNS) bleed or a major ischemic stroke. In addition, in the setting of a CNS bleed, anticoagulation should be withheld for at least 2 weeks. Additional management considerations include drug rehabilitation referral for IV drug users, education on signs and symptoms of IE and the need for antibiotic prophylaxis for certain procedures, and thorough dental evaluation and treatment. Echocardiogram is recommended at completion of therapy to establish new baseline for valve function and morphology, and ventricular size/function.

IE prophylaxis guidelines have evolved over the twenty-first century. The most recent guidance can be summarized as follows:

- **Patient population to consider IE prophylaxis in**:
  - Prosthetic heart valve or prosthetic material used for valve repair (i.e., annuloplasty ring)
  - Previous IE
  - Unrepaired cyanotic congenital heart defect or repaired congenital heart defect, with residual shunts or valvular regurgitation at the site adjacent to the site of a prosthetic patch or prosthetic device
  - Cardiac transplant with valve regurgitation due to a structurally abnormal valve

- **Procedures to consider IE prophylaxis**:
  - Dental procedures with manipulation of gingiva/periapical region, or perforation of oral mucosa

- **IE prophylaxis regimens**:
  - No antibiotic allergies
    - **Can tolerate PO**—Amoxicillin 2 grams PO
    - **Cannot take PO**—Ampicillin 2 grams IV/IM
  - Penicillin allergy (severity of reaction will affect choice)
    - **Can tolerate PO**—Cephalexin 2 grams PO, or clindamycin 600 mg PO
    - **Cannot take PO**—Cefazolin 1 gram IV, or clindamycin 600 mg IV/IM, or vancomycin (not to exceed 2 g)
  - Typically, the antibiotic is given 30 to 60 minutes prior to the procedure

KEY LEARNING POINT

Enterococcal endocarditis in patients with renal dysfunction or high-level aminoglycoside resistance, or in whom the adverse effects of aminoglycosides are unacceptable, can be managed with the combination ampicillin and ceftriaxone.

REFERENCES AND FURTHER READING

- Baddour LM, Wilson WR, Bayer AS, et al. Infective endocarditis in adults: diagnosis, antimicrobial therapy, and management of complications: a scientific statement for healthcare professionals from the American Heart Association. *Circulation.* 2015;132(15):1435–1486. https://doi.org/10.1161/CIR.0000000000000296. Erratum in: Circulation. 2015;132(17):e215. Erratum in: Circulation. 2016;134(8):e113. Erratum in: Circulation. 2018;138(5):e78e79.
- Hubers SA, DeSimone DC, Gersh BJ, Anavekar NS. Infective endocarditis: a contemporary review. *Mayo Clin Proc.* 2020;95(5):982–997. https://doi.org/10.1016/j.mayocp.2019.12.008.
- Yang E, Frazee BW. Infective endocarditis. *Emerg Med Clin North Am.* 2018;36(4):645–663. https://doi.org/10.1016/j.emc.2018.06.002.

A 60-year-old Filipino male presents to the emergency room with a 2-week history of fevers, night sweats, weight loss, anorexia, arthralgias, malaise, cough, and shortness of breath. Medical history is notable for type 2 diabetes mellitus. Medications include metformin, insulin, lisinopril, and atorvastatin. He has no medication allergies. He smokes one pack of cigarettes daily. He drinks three to four beers daily. He denies illicit drug use. He denies any animal exposures. He moved to New Mexico 6 weeks ago. He enjoys dirt-biking. Vital signs reveal temperature 101° F, heart rate 95 beats per minute, blood pressure 125/75 mmHg, respiratory rate 24, and oxygen saturation 92% on room air. On examination, he appears tired. Lung exam reveals increased work of breathing and diffuse crackles. Heart exam reveals a regular tachycardia with no murmur. There are tender erythematous plaques over his shins bilaterally. Examination of the left knee shows a small effusion, tenderness, and reduced range of motion. The remainder of the examination is unremarkable. Laboratory studies reveal white blood cell count 14,000 cells/μL (70% neutrophils, 20% lymphocytes, 10% eosinophils), glucose 220 mg/dL, creatinine 1.2 mg/dL, and normal liver function testing. HIV p24 antigen/antibody testing is negative. *Legionella* urine antigen is negative. Respiratory pathogen panel (multiplex polymerase chain reaction) is negative. Tuberculosis interferon-gamma release assay (TB-IGRA) 1 year prior was negative. Chest x-ray shows bilateral airspace opacities with consolidation and mediastinal lymphadenopathy. Blood and sputum cultures are sent.

What is the most appropriate initial therapy for this patient?

A. Ceftriaxone and azithromycin.
B. Rifampin, isoniazid, pyrazinamide, ethambutol.
C. Amphotericin-B.
D. Fluconazole.
E. No treatment is necessary.

The most appropriate initial therapy is fluconazole (**option D**). This patient's presentation is highly concerning for coccidioidomycosis (also known as San Joaquin Valley fever). Coccidioidomycosis is an endemic mycosis caused by a soil dwelling dimorphic fungus (*Coccidiodes immitis* or *Coccidiodes posadasii*). This fungus is endemic to the southwest United States, including central and southern California, Arizona, New Mexico, Utah, Nevada, and West Texas. It can also be found in Washington State, Central America, and South America. The infection is acquired by inhalation of arthroconidia, but direct cutaneous inoculation and reactivation of an existing dormant (latent) infection may occur as well. Once inhaled, the arthroconidia change into spherules (which contain endospores). As these spherules mature, they rupture to release the endospores which can spread via the blood or lymphatic system to infect essentially any organ.

Most patients (~60%) actually present with an asymptomatic or mild, self-limited illness. Symptomatic patients typically present within 1 month of exposure. The differences in the presentation reflect the variable host immune response to infection. Risk factors for severe and/or disseminated infection include age over 65 years, male sex, high inoculum exposure, pregnancy (especially the third trimester), diabetes mellitus, smoking, nonwhite ethnicity (especially African Americans, Filipinos, and Pacific Islanders), complement-fixation (CF) titer greater than 1:16, and cell-mediated immune deficiencies. Many of the manifestations can take weeks to months to resolve (especially the fatigue). The various potential manifestations are summarized in Table 95.1.

The diagnosis of coccidioidomycosis is somewhat complicated. The whole presentation needs to be considered when interpreting diagnostic testing. A history of exposure to an endemic region is very important. Patients may occasionally have peripheral eosinophilia. Always consider if there is an underlying immune suppression (especially if severe/disseminated infection) and check HIV status. The various available tests for the diagnosis of *Coccidioides* are shown in Table 95.2.

Central nervous system (CNS) infection can be challenging to diagnose. Cerebrospinal fluid (CSF) analysis should be done only if the presentation is concerning for CNS infection (i.e., compatible signs and/or symptoms). The diagnosis *Coccidioides* CNS infection is made based on a compatible presentation, CSF profile, and positive testing based on tests discussed above. CSF fungal culture is positive in only approximately 25%. Antibodies by immunodiffusion (ID)/CF are more sensitive than culture, but approximately 10% of patients with *Coccidioides* meningitis will not have antibody in the CSF. CSF beta-D-glucan

Table 95.1 – Presentation of Coccidioidomycosis

Presentation	Description
Constitutional	• Fevers, night sweats, weight loss, malaise, etc.
Pulmonary disease	• Community-acquired pneumonia (CAP)—25% of CAP in endemic regions is attributable to coccidioidomycosis, may be associated with erythema nodosum or erythema multiforme; a more severe diffuse pneumonia may be associated with acute respiratory distress syndrome • Chronic pneumonia—fibrocavitary and fibronodular • Asymptomatic cavitary lesion or solitary lung nodule (may resemble malignancy and may require biopsy to distinguish) • Pleural effusion—often exudative with lymphocytic or eosinophilic cell count
Disseminated disease	• Dissemination can occur to any organ, but common sites include the skin, bone/joints, central nervous system, lymph nodes, and genitourinary organs • Patients with disseminated disease may have no evidence of pulmonary disease
Cutaneous disease	• Can occur at site of inoculation or as a consequence of disseminated disease • Many of these manifestations are actually immunologic phenomena • Erythema nodosum, erythema multiforme, maculopapular rash, chronic skin ulceration, and/or abscesses
Bone/joint disease	• Most commonly involves the spine and can be associated with abscesses • Peripheral joint arthralgia and arthritis ("desert rheumatism")—often a symmetric process involving the lower extremities (most commonly the knee)
Central nervous system	• Lymphohematogenous spread to the leptomeninges may occur weeks to months after the initial infection and is nearly always fatal if untreated • Meningitis (can be basilar)—pleocytosis can be lymphocytic, neutrophilic, or eosinophilic, elevated protein, low or normal glucose • Patients can develop hydrocephalus, cranial neuropathies, stroke, vasculitis, arachnoiditis, mass lesions or abscesses, or myelopathy with syrinx

and CSF *Coccidioides* antigen can be helpful/supportive, and CNS imaging (MRI, etc.) can be useful to evaluate for complications.

Treatment of coccidioidomycosis depends on the location of the infection, the severity of the infection, and the host immune status. Treatment is summarized in Table 95.3.

Ceftriaxone and azithromycin (**option A**) would be appropriate coverage for typical community-acquired pneumonia, but this case is more consistent with *Coccidioides* pneumonia. Rifampin, isoniazid, pyrazinamide, and ethambutol (**option B**) would be the treatment for pulmonary tuberculosis (TB). TB can present in a very similar way, but the recent negative TB-IGRA suggests that TB is less likely in this case. Amphotericin-B (**option C**) is

Table 95.2 – Diagnosis of Coccidioidomycosis

Platform	Description
Serology	• Most common method for diagnosis
	• In general, a positive antibody test suggests either recent or active *Coccidioides* infection, because most of these tests revert to normal after infection resolves
	• Immunoglobulin (Ig)M usually detectable within 1–3 weeks of infection (may linger for a while but often [not always] disappears after 6 months); whereas IgG usually detectable within 2–3 weeks of infection (and can persist for months to years)
	• A negative serologic test cannot rule out *Coccidioides* infection
	• Always consider repeating serologic testing after several weeks, because serology can easily miss early infections (antibodies take time to develop). A four-fold rise in titer is considered positive
	• Immune suppression may also cause false-negative serologic results.
	• Infection with other dimorphic fungi (esp. *Histoplasma* and *Blastomyces*) can cross-react to cause false-positives
	• **Enzyme immunoassay (EIA) for IgM and/or IgG (qualitative)**
	• Typically used as initial (screening) test as more sensitive for early infection but negative test does NOT rule out infection. Positive EIA should be confirmed by immunodiffusion (ID)/complement-fixation (CF) testing
	• Positive IgM EIA (by itself) is often a false positive (the least compelling diagnostic evidence)
	• **Standard ID for IgM and IgG (qualitative ± quantitative)**
	• Less sensitive but more specific than EIA
	• Can be done on serum and cerebrospinal fluid(CSF)
	• IgM ID (serum) — "IDTP (tube precipitins)"
	• IgG ID (serum) — "IDCF (complement-fixation)" — can also ask for titer (see CF below)
	• Presence of CSF ID suggests *Coccidioides* meningitis
	• **CF for IgG (quantitative)**
	• Can be done on serum or CSF
	• Most useful in immune-competent patients and for monitoring disease activity during therapy (esp. the IgG test)
	• Successful treatment leads to decreasing titer, whereas rising titer is associated with persistent or relapsing infection
	• Typically wait at least 1 month prior to repeating during treatment monitoring
Antigenic testing	• Can be done on CSF, urine, or serum. Antigen is most useful in extensive or disseminated infection, in immune-compromised patients, or in CNS infection
Polymerase chain reaction	• Can be done on various tissues, but not commonly available. Sensitivity similar to culture but considered highly specific and can even be done on formalin-fixed tissue
Culture and/or histopathology	• Identification by staining for spherules (potassium hydroxide, periodic acid-Schiff, calcofluor, hematoxylin and eosin, Grocott-Gomori's methenamine silver) or growing in culture is always considered abnormal/pathologic. See Figure. 95.1
	• *Coccidioides* can grow on virtually any lab media
	• Further identification can be done via probing
	• Always notify micro lab that you are concerned about *Coccidioides* infection (lab biohazard)

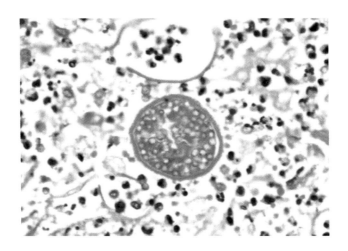

Figure 95.1 – *Coccidioides* spherules in tissue
Galgiani JN. Coccidioidomycosis (*Coccidioides species*). In: Bennet JE, Dolin R, Blaser MJ, eds. *Mandell, Douglas, and Bennett's Principles and Practice of Infectious Diseases*. 9th ed. Elsevier; 2020:3190–3200. Courtesy Richard Sobonya, MD, University of Arizona.

Table 95.3 – Treatment of Coccidioidomycosis

Manifestation	Treatment[a]
Acute pneumonia (uncomplicated)	• Treat if debilitating illness, extensive pulmonary disease, or high risk for severe/disseminated disease • Drug of choice (expert opinion) = fluconazole ≥400 mg PO daily (no studies available regarding optimal dose or duration), alternative is itraconazole 200 mg PO BID • Variable duration but typically at least 3–6 months and until signs/symptoms and inflammatory markers have normalized and serology and radiographic studies have stabilized
Asymptomatic pulmonary nodule	• Close observation if immune-competent • Consider risk factors for malignancy (age, smoking history, PET/CT avidity, etc.) and clinical history (recent illness c/w *Coccidioides*) to decide whether to monitor with imaging (goal is to show stability for 2 years) or purse biopsy to rule out malignancy
Asymptomatic cavitary lesion	• Recommendation is close observation if immune-competent • These can progress, rupture → empyema, hemoptysis, etc., or get superinfected
Symptomatic chronic (>3 month) pneumonia	• Recommendation is to treat with fluconazole or itraconazole • Duration is at least 1 year, but one-third may recur after treatment is stopped • Consider surgical removal (video-assisted thoracoscopic surgery preferred) if fail to respond to medical treatment, rupture, and cavity present >2 years
Soft tissue infection	• Recommendation is to treat with fluconazole (≥400 mg PO daily) or itraconazole 200 mg PO BID • IV amphotericin-B if azole failure or synovitis • Alternative options are posaconazole and voriconazole • Duration should be at least 6–12 months

Table 95.3 – Treatment of Coccidioidomycosis *(Cont'd)*

Bone/joint infection	• Milder disease—azole therapy recommended (fluconazole ≥800 mg PO daily or itraconazole 200 mg PO BID; itraconazole may be superior)
	• Severe/life-threatening disease (i.e., vertebral disease causing cord compromise)—amphotericin-B (once daily initially and then thrice weekly for up to 3 months) followed by azole therapy; surgical consultation recommended
	• Alternative options include posaconazole and voriconazole
	• Duration is variable—3 years to lifetime depending on severity and host immune status
Central nervous system infection	• First-line treatment is fluconazole 400–1200 mg PO daily (normal renal function)
	• Alternative is itraconazole 200 mg BID to QID. There are also some data (less than for the azoles above) for voriconazole and posaconazole
	• Intrathecal amphotericin-B used as rescue therapy in cases of azole failure
	• Amphotericin-B is used in refractory cases—deoxycholate has not been shown to be efficacious in central nervous system infection, and liposomal formulation has been shown to be efficacious in animal models and case reports
	• Management of intracranial pressure—serial lumbar punctures (similar protocol to cryptococcal meningitis) and, if refractory, then shunting
	• Corticosteroids (anecdotal evidence) may be used for vasculitis/stroke, cranial neuropathy, or arachnoiditis
	• Treatment success is judged by clinical improvement and cerebrospinal fluid parameters—goal is to get to near-normal status
	• Treatment duration is typically lifelong, as relapse rate is fairly high when treatment is stopped

[a]Immune-compromised hosts with pulmonary disease typically require treatment. In pregnant patients, Amphotericin-B is preferred in the first trimester and azole antifungals are preferred in the 2nd/3rd trimesters.

BID, twice daily; *CT*, computed tomography; *IV*, intravenous; *PET*, positron emission tomography; *PO*, per os (oral route); *QID*, four times daily.

often considered second-line or salvage therapy in most cases of *Coccidioides* infection. No treatment (**option E**) may be appropriate for patients with acute uncomplicated *Coccidioides* pneumonia or an asymptomatic pulmonary nodule or cavity due to *Coccidioides*.

KEY LEARNING POINT

Treatment (typically with fluconazole) is recommended for patients with acute Coccidioides *pneumonia with risk factors for severe and/or disseminated infection.*

REFERENCES AND FURTHER READING

• Bays DJ, Thompson GR 3rd. Coccidioidomycosis. *Infect Dis Clin North Am.* 2021;35(2):453–469. https://doi.org/10.1016/j.idc.2021.03.010.
• Galgiani JN. Coccidioidomycosis *(Coccidioides species)*. In: Bennet JE, Dolin R, Blaser MJ, eds. *Mandell, Douglas, and Bennett's Principles and Practice of Infectious Diseases.* 9th ed. Elsevier; 2020:3190–3200.
• Galgiani JN, Ampel NM, Blair JE, et al. 2016 Infectious Diseases Society of America (IDSA) clinical practice guideline for the treatment of coccidioidomycosis. *Clin Infect Dis.* 2016;63(6):e112–e146. https://doi.org/10.1093/cid/ciw360.

A 24-year-old male is referred to the infectious disease clinic for evaluation of hepatitis C virus (HCV) infection. He does not have any fevers, weight loss, night sweats, fatigue, anorexia, pruritus, jaundice, rashes, or abdominal distension. He has no medication allergies. He does not take any medications routinely, as he does not have any known medical problems. There is no family history of liver disease or hepatocellular carcinoma. He does not drink alcohol. He is an active IV drug user. He is not sexually active. Vital signs are normal. Body mass index is 19 kg/m². Physical examination is within normal limits. Laboratory analysis reveals:

- White blood cell count 8,000 cells/uL (normal differential)
- Hemoglobin 14 g/dL
- Platelet count 200,000 cells/uL
- Creatinine 0.8 mg/dL
- AST 55 U/L
- ALT 60 U/L
- Total bilirubin 1.0 mg/dL
- Alkaline phosphatase 70 U/L
- Serum albumin 3.8 g/dL
- International normalized ratio 1.0

- HIV p24 antigen/antibody negative
- Hepatitis C serum antibody positive
- Hepatitis C serum RNA 1.5 million copies/mL
- Hepatitis C genotype 2
- Hepatitis B surface antigen negative
- Hepatitis B surface antibody positive
- Hepatitis B total core antibody negative
- Hepatitis A antibodies (IgM and IgG) negative
- Alpha fetoprotein normal

Liver ultrasound is normal. Elastography (Fibroscan) shows no evidence of fibrosis or cirrhosis.

What is the best next step in management?

A. Sofosbuvir + ledipasvir (Harvoni) for 8 weeks.

B. Sofosbuvir + ledipasvir (Harvoni) for 12 weeks.

C. Sofosbuvir + velpatasvir (Epclusa) for 12 weeks.

D. Glecaprevir + pibrentasvir (Mavyret) for 8 weeks.

E. Hold off on treatment until no longer using IV drugs.

The best next step in this patient with chronic HCV infection (genotype 2) without cirrhosis is glecaprevir plus pibrentasvir (Mayvret) for 8 weeks (**option D**). Sofosbuvir plus velpatasvir (Epclusa) for 12 weeks (**option C**) would also be reasonable, but the shorter duration of Mavyret makes it a more attractive option. Sofosbuvir plus ledipasvir (Harvoni) for 8 to 12 weeks (**options A and B**) can be used for genotypes 1, 4, 5, and 6 only.

HCV is a flavivirus that affects people with certain risk factors that reflect its bloodborne transmission. These risk factors include birth between 1945 and 1965, receipt of a blood transfusion prior to 1992, IV drug abuse, hemodialysis, HIV, men who have sex with men, unregulated tattooing, and healthcare work. Upon acquisition, a few patients develop acute hepatitis and may even clear the infection on their own. Unfortunately, most patients (~80%) actually develop chronic infection, which is defined as viremia for more than 6 months. Patients are often asymptomatic or may have mild, nonspecific symptoms (i.e., fatigue, pruritus, etc.), which is why undetected (and thus untreated) HCV may result in cirrhosis and hepatocellular carcinoma. Certain extrahepatic manifestations should prompt consideration of HCV, including porphyria cutanea tarda, nephrotic syndrome, lichen planus, or cryoglobulinemia.

The best initial screening and/or diagnostic test is the HCV antibody test. This highly sensitive test may be falsely negative in the first 2 months postexposure and in HIV patients. A positive HCV antibody test may reflect prior infection with spontaneous clearance or ongoing, active infection. The way to differentiate these possibilities is to obtain the HCV viral load (serum RNA level). The viral load is positive in active/ongoing chronic infection and negative in previously cleared infection. HCV genotype is often unnecessary, especially if using pangenotypic treatments.

The evaluation and management of chronic HCV is summarized in Fig. 96.1.

Essentially every patient with HCV infection and a significant life expectancy should be treated. Active substance abuse (**option E**) is not a contraindication to HCV treatment. The goals of therapy are:

1. Achieve a cure (sustained virologic response)—undetectable viral load at 12 weeks posttreatment completion
2. Slow disease progression to cirrhosis or hepatocellular carcinoma
3. Reduce disease transmission

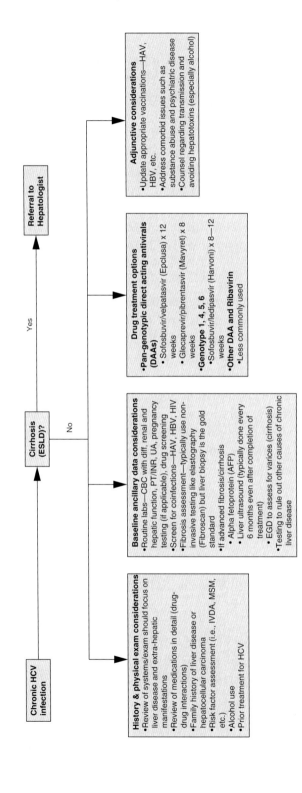

Figure 96.1 – Evaluation and treatment of hepatitis C virus (HCV) infection

CBC, Complete blood count; *DAA*, direct acting antivirals; *EGD*, esophagogastroduodenoscopy (upper endoscopy); *ESLD*, end-stage liver disease; *HAV*, hepatitis A virus; *HBV*, hepatitis B virus; *IVDA*, intravenous drug abuse; *MSM*, men who have sex with men; *PT/INR*, prothrombin time/international normalized ratio; *UA*, urinalysis.

The following text appears within the figure:

Chronic HCV infection

Cirrhosis (ESLD)?

Yes → **Referral to Hepatologist**

No

History & physical exam considerations
- Review of systems/exam should focus on liver disease and extra-hepatic manifestations
- Review of medications in detail (drug-drug interactions)
- Family history of liver disease or hepatocellular carcinoma
- Risk factor assessment (i.e., IVDA, MSM, etc.)
- Alcohol use
- Prior treatment for HCV

Baseline ancillary data considerations
- Routine labs—CBC with diff, renal and hepatic function, PT/INR, UA, pregnancy testing (if applicable), drug screening
- Screen for coinfections—HAV, HBV, HIV
- Fibrosis assessment—typically use non-invasive testing like elastography (Fibroscan) but liver biopsy is the gold standard
- If advanced fibrosis/cirrhosis
  - Alpha fetoprotein (AFP)
  - Liver ultrasound (typically done every 6 months even after completion of treatment)
  - EGD to assess for varices (cirrhosis)
- Testing to rule out other causes of chronic liver disease

Drug treatment options
- Pan-genotypic direct acting antivirals (DAAs)
  - Sofosbuvir/velpatasvir (Epclusa) x 12 weeks
  - Glecaprevir/pibrentasvir (Mavyret) x 8 weeks
- Genotype 1, 4, 5, 6
  - Sofosbuvir/ledipasvir (Harvoni) x 8—12 weeks
- Other DAA and Ribavirin
  - Less commonly used

Adjunctive considerations
- Update appropriate vaccinations—HAV, HBV, etc.
- Address comorbid issues such as substance abuse and psychiatric disease
- Counsel regarding transmission and avoiding hepatotoxins (especially alcohol)

The treatment regimens typically involve direct acting antivirals (DAAs) with or without ribavirin. The choice of agent may depend on the genotype and if (and to what degree) fibrosis/cirrhosis is present. The DAAs all carry a black box warning for hepatitis B virus (HBV) reactivation when being used to treat patients with HBV/HCV coinfection. Therefore, coinfected patients may need intensive monitoring for HBV during treatment, or concurrent treatment for HBV while treating HCV. Drug-drug interactions always need to be considered when using DAAs as well. Ribavirin is occasionally given. It is teratogenic and may cause a dose-dependent, reversible hemolytic anemia. Lastly, after starting treatment, liver function testing is typically repeated in 8 weeks, and HCV viral load is repeated in 12 weeks.

KEY LEARNING POINT

If accepted by the patient's insurance, the two easiest hepatitis C virus treatment regimens are sofosbuvir plus velpatasvir (Epclusa) for 12 weeks and glecaprevir plus pibrentasvir (Mavyret) for 8 weeks.

REFERENCE AND FURTHER READING

- AASLD-IDSA. Recommendations for testing, managing, and treating hepatitis C. http://www.hcvguidelines.org. Accessed on October 31, 2021.

A 65-year-old female is admitted to the hospital in July with a 3-day history of fevers, confusion, headache, and right lower extremity weakness. She has a history of type 2 diabetes mellitus. Medications include atorvastatin, lisinopril, metformin, and insulin. She has not traveled abroad recently. Vital signs reveal temperature 101.5° F, heart rate 110 beats per minute, blood pressure 110/80 mmHg, and respiratory rate 16. On physical examination, she is confused, and she has a hard time following basic commands. Cranial nerves are intact. Right patellar reflex is absent. Left patellar reflex is 2+. Right lower extremity strength is 2+. Left lower extremity strength is 5+. Babinski sign is negative. Lower extremity sensation is intact. There are no skin rashes or mucosal lesions. The remainder of the examination is unremarkable. Cerebrospinal fluid (CSF) analysis reveals glucose 80 mg/dL (serum glucose 120 mg/dL), protein 150 mg/dL, red blood cells (RBCs) 0/mm^3, and white blood cells 50/mm^3 (50% lymphocytes). CSF multiplex PCR panel is done, and the results are as follows:

Cytomegalovirus (CMV) PCR: negative
Herpes simplex virus (HSV)-1 and HSV-2 PCR: negative
Human herpes virus (HHV)-6 PCR: positive
Varicella-zoster virus (VZV) PCR: negative
Human parechovirus PCR: negative
Enterovirus PCR: negative

Contrast MRI of the brain is normal.

What is the most likely cause of this presentation?

A. Poliovirus.
B. West Nile virus (WNV).
C. VZV.
D. HHV-6.
E. HSV.

The most likely cause of this presentation is WNV (**option B**). WNV is a flavivirus transmitted by the *Culex* mosquito, which is most active in the late summer/early fall. Rarely, transmission can occur via blood transfusion (blood supply is screened in the United States), organ donation, accidental lab exposure, or obstetric-related (i.e., vertically or breastfeeding). Most infections are asymptomatic (~80%). The other 20% of patients will develop an influenza-like illness that may or may not be associated with a maculopapular rash. Less than 1% develop neuroinvasive disease (typically elderly and/or immune-compromised), which can include aseptic meningitis (typically with the CSF profile shown in the case), encephalitis (classically associated with extrapyramidal signs), or acute flaccid paralysis (myelitis resembling poliomyelitis pathologically and clinically).

Diagnosis is typically established with serologic testing. Typically, this is done via IgM antibody testing in the serum and/or the CSF. The IgM assay can cross-react with other flaviviruses, so specialized confirmatory testing is often necessary. The IgM assay may also persist for a very long time, which can confound the results. A four-fold rise in titer between acute and convalescent sera can be very useful, but obviously is unlikely to change the course of management. A PCR test (serum or CSF) can be done but is only helpful if done during the initial week after infection (i.e., when the patient is likely to be viremic). Other conditions with similar presentations should be ruled out as well. Management is largely supportive. Long-term neurologic sequelae are common in those with neuroinvasive disease.

Poliovirus (**option A**) is an enterovirus that is spread by the fecal-oral route. Poliovirus can present similar to WNV, especially when it comes to the acute flaccid paralysis that both of these infections can cause. Polio is incredibly rare nowadays and is only seen in the Middle East.

VZV (**option C**) causes chickenpox (varicella), shingles (zoster), and in rare cases, central nervous system (CNS) disease (encephalitis, meningitis, myelitis, or vasculopathy). VZV CNS infection can occur during primary infection or with reactivation. VZV vasculopathy is particularly interesting, because it represents a granulomatous arteritis, which can result in strokes. MRI will show multifocal hyperintense lesions (typically in the white matter or at gray–white matter junction) on T2-weighted fluid-attenuated inversion recovery (FLAIR) images. Diagnosis is made by demonstration of intrathecal synthesis of VZV-specific antibody or by detection of VZV DNA in CSF with PCR. Treatment of CNS disease is with IV acyclovir for 14 days with or without steroids.

HHV-6 (**option D**) often comes up positive on meningitis/encephalitis (CSF multiplex PCR) panels. This is because HHV-6 integrates into the DNA in lymphocytes, and PCR assays pick up on this. In most cases, it is nothing to worry about, as this virus is almost exclusively a disease of children, and low-grade, subclinical reactivations in the setting of other illnesses are common. In severely immune-compromised individuals (i.e., stem-cell transplant patients), HHV-6 can cause limbic encephalitis characterized by amnesia, insomnia, and seizures. MRI characteristically shows increased hyperintense T2 signal in the medial temporal lobe. Treatment is similar to CMV and includes ganciclovir.

HSV (**option E**) causes a characteristic-appearing encephalitis that is commonly tested on board exams. Most often, the encephalitis is caused by HSV-1. The diagnostic test of choice is the CSF PCR for HSV DNA, as it is highly sensitive and specific. This test can be falsely negative in early infections (typically within the first 48–72 hours after symptom onset), so repeat testing may be necessary. Elevated CSF RBC count may be a tip-off. MRI is the most sensitive imaging test and may show T2 and FLAIR hyperintensity involving the medial temporal lobe and the inferior frontal lobes, with relative sparing of the adjacent white matter (Fig. 97.1).

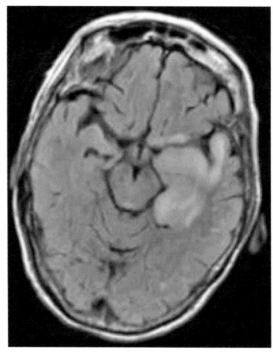

Figure 97.1 – Herpes simplex virus encephalitis
McKnight C, Kelly AM, Petrou M, et al. A simplified approach to encephalitis and its mimics: key clinical condition points in the setting of specific imaging abnormalities. *Academ Radiol.* 2017;24(6):667–676. https://doi.org/10.1016/j.acra.2016.04.013.

The treatment of HSV encephalitis is IV acyclovir for 14 to 21 days. IV acyclovir should be given as soon as the diagnosis is suspected (i.e., do not wait to get work-up prior to starting).

KEY LEARNING POINT

Most viral encephalitis cases have a similar presentation. Knowing the distinguishing features of these can be very helpful clinically and on board exams.

Etiology	Distinguishing Features
Herpes simplex virus	• Most common viral cause; temporal/frontal lobe involvement; red blood cells in cerebrospinal fluid
Varicella-zoster virus	• Vasculopathy → stroke; may or may not have zoster rash
Human herpes virus-6	• Severely immune-compromised; medial temporal lobe
Cytomegalovirus	• Severely immune-compromised; periventricular involvement
West Nile virus	• Extrapyramidal symptoms; flaccid paralysis; summer/fall (mosquitos)
Poliovirus	• Travel to Middle East (especially Afghanistan or Pakistan); flaccid paralysis
Lymphocytic choriomeningitis virus	• Rodent exposure • Cell count disturbances (cytopenia)
JC virus	• Progressive multifocal leukoencephalopathy seen in advanced AIDS or with certain drugs (i.e., natalizumab)
Japanese encephalitis	• Travel to southeast Asia and not vaccinated • Extrapyramidal symptoms; flaccid paralysis
Rabies	• High-risk animal exposure—homeless, traveler, veterinarian, etc. • Hydrophobia, aerophobia, dysphagia
Herpes B virus	• Exposure to macaque monkeys

REFERENCES AND FURTHER READING

- Beckham D, et al. Encephalitis. In: Bennet JE, Dolin R, Blaser MJ, eds. *Mandell, Douglas, and Bennett's Principles and Practice of Infectious Disease*. 9th ed. Elsevier; 2020. 1226-1247.e4.
- McKnight C, Kelly AM, Petrou M, et al. A simplified approach to encephalitis and its mimics: key clinical condition points in the setting of specific imaging abnormalities. *Academ Radiol*. 2017;24(6):667–676. https://doi.org/10.1016/j.acra.2016.04.013.

98

CASE

A 30-year-old male is admitted to the hospital with a 1-week history of fevers, nausea, anorexia, dark urine, and jaundice. 98He is otherwise healthy and does not take any medications. There is no family history of liver disease. He denies any alcohol use. He is an active IV drug user. Vital signs reveal temperature 100.6° F, heart rate 95 beats per minute, blood pressure 115/75 mmHg, and respiratory rate 16. On examination, he appears well. Scleral icterus is present. Heart and lung exams are normal. Abdominal exam reveals tenderness in the right upper quadrant. There is minimal distension but no fluid wave. Skin is jaundiced. The remainder of the exam is unremarkable. Laboratory studies reveal white blood cell count 11,000 cells/μL, hemoglobin 12 g/dL, platelet count 110,000 cells/μL, creatinine 1.0 mg/dL, AST 1500 μ/L, ALT 1770 μ/L, alkaline phosphatase 150 Iμ/L, total bilirubin 5.0 mg/dL (direct bilirubin 4.0 mg/dL), albumin 3.2 g/dL, and international normalized ratio (INR) 1.2. Additional studies include:

Hepatitis A virus IgM—negative	Hepatitis B DNA—30,000 IU/mL
Hepatitis A virus IgG—positive	Hepatitis C antibody—negative
Hepatitis B surface antigen—positive	Hepatitis D antibody—negative
Hepatitis B surface antibody—negative	HIV p24 antigen/antibody—negative
Hepatitis B total core antibody—positive	Acetaminophen drug level—undetectable
Hepatitis B e antigen—positive	Ethanol level—undetectable
Hepatitis B e antibody—negative	

Abdominal ultrasound is unremarkable.

What is the next best step in the management of this patient?

A. Supportive care.
B. Entecavir.
C. Tenofovir.
D. Pegylated interferon.
E. Lamivudine.

482

The next best step is supportive care (**option A**). This patient's presentation is most consistent with acute hepatitis B virus (HBV) infection. HBV infection is acquired by exposure to infected bodily fluids (i.e., sexual, bloodborne, vertical, etc.). Infection can be acute or chronic in nature. Acute HBV is often subclinical (anicteric), but approximately 25% of patients will present with acute hepatitis, as in this case. In rare cases, fulminant hepatitis may occur. The likelihood of developing chronic HBV infection is inversely proportional to the age at which the infection is acquired (i.e., >90% of perinatally-acquired HBV infections become chronic infection, whereas <5% of adult-acquired infections go on to chronic infection). Chronic HBV is often asymptomatic or minimally symptomatic (i.e., fatigue, pruritus, etc.). The major consequences of untreated HBV infection may include cirrhosis and hepatocellular carcinoma (HCC) (which can occur even without cirrhosis). Extrahepatic manifestations may include serum sickness-like syndrome, polyarteritis nodosa, cryoglobulinemia, or glomerulopathy (membranous nephropathy and membranoproliferative glomerulonephritis).

The natural history (and phases) of chronic HBV infection is summarized in Fig. 98.1.

Diagnosis of HBV infection can sometimes be confusing. The main tests/markers and their significance are shown in Table 98.1 and Fig. 98.2.

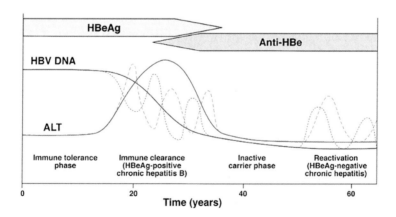

Figure 98.1 – Natural history of hepatitis B virus *(HBV)* infection. The natural course of chronic HBV infection consists of four phases. The immune tolerance phase is characterized by the presence of HBV e antigen *(HBeAg)*, high HBV DNA levels, and persistently normal ALT levels, but no evidence of active liver disease. The immune clearance phase is characterized by the presence of HBeAg and high/fluctuating HBV DNA and ALT levels. An outcome of the immune clearance phase is HBeAg seroconversion. Most patients then enter the inactive HBV carrier phase, which is characterized by the absence of HBeAg and the presence of anti-HBe, low or undetectable HBV DNA levels (<2000 IU/mL), normal ALT levels, and no/minimal inflammation on liver biopsy. The reactivation phase is characterized by the absence of HBeAg, intermittent/persistently increased ALT and HBV DNA levels, and inflammation on liver biopsy.

Table 98.1 – Hepatitis B Virus (HBV) Infection Markers/Tests

Marker	Significance
HBV surface antigen (HBsAg)	• A marker of activation infection • If present for >6 months, then defines chronic HBV infection
HBV DNA	• Presence in the serum correlates with active viral replication in the liver
HBV e antigen (HBeAg)	• A marker of active viral replication and increased infectivity (often associated with high HBV DNA levels) • The HBV precore mutant is an exception, because this mutant does not produce HBeAg but typically follows a more aggressive course
HBV core antibody (anti-HBc)	• IgM appears first and indicates either acute infection or flare (relapse) of chronic infection • IgG persists for life in those with prior HBV infection (resolved or ongoing)
HBV surface antibody (anti-HBs)	• Indicates resolution of acute disease and immunity • This is the only marker that is positive in individuals vaccinated against HBV
HBV e antibody (anti-HBe)	• Indicates reduced viral replication and infectivity

Some commonly encountered patterns in real-life practice and on the boards are shown in Table 98.2.

Treatment of HBV is a bit nuanced, but the overall approach is outlined in Fig. 98.3.

Most cases of acute HBV infection do not require treatment, because the overwhelming majority of these patients recover on their own. Treatment is only needed in those with acute liver failure or a protracted course (elevated INR and/or jaundice >4 weeks).

Chronic HBV infection is a bit more complicated. Baseline evaluation to consider prior to treatment includes:

- Appropriate history including risk factors for HBV, family history of HCC, liver disease, or hepatitis, signs/symptoms of chronic liver disease, and alcohol use
- Baseline HBV testing may include HBsAg, HBsAb, HBcAb, HBeAg, HBeAb, and HBV DNA
- Additional lab testing may include complete blood count with differential, complete metabolic panel, prothrombin time/INR, urinalysis, HIV screening, screening for other hepatitis viruses (hepatitis A virus, hepatitis C virus, hepatitis D virus), alpha-fetoprotein (AFP), pregnancy testing (if applicable), and testing to rule out other causes of liver disease

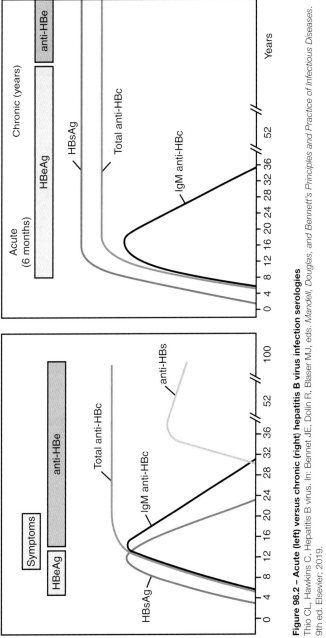

Figure 98.2 – Acute (left) versus chronic (right) hepatitis B virus infection serologies
Thio CL, Hawkins C, Hepatitis B virus. In: Bennet JE, Dolin R, Blaser MJ, eds. *Mandell, Douglas, and Bennett's Principles and Practice of Infectious Diseases.* 9th ed. Elsevier; 2019.

Table 98.2 – Hepatitis B Virus (HBV) Scenarios

HBsAg	Anti-HBc	Anti-HBs	ALT	Interpretation(s)
+	+ (IgM)	-	↑↑↑	• Acute HBV infection
-	+	+	-	• Immunity due to natural infection
-	-	+	-	• Immunity due to immunization
+ (>6 months)	+ (IgG)	-	Variable	• Chronic infection

-	+	-	-	• Isolated positive core antibody → five possibilities:
				  • Prior HBV infection with undetectable anti-HBs
				  • Recovery from acute infection (window period; would be IgM core antibody in this case)
				  • False-positive anti-HBc
				  • Mutations in HBsAg leading to false-negative HBsAg
				  • Chronic infection with undetectable HBsAg

Approach to Treatment of HBV

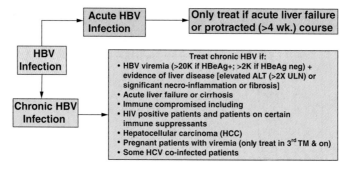

Figure 98.3 – Hepatitis B virus *(HBV)* treatment approach
HCV, Hepatitis C virus; *TM*, trimester; *ULN*, Upper limit of normal.

- Additional considerations may include:
  - Fibrosis evaluation (i.e., FibroScan)
  - If cirrhosis or advanced fibrosis, HCC screening with liver ultrasound plus or minus AFP every 6 months
  - If cirrhosis, upper endoscopy for varices surveillance
  - Liver biopsy to rule out other causes of liver dysfunction
  - Counseling regarding transmission and testing relevant family members
  - Counseling regarding avoiding hepatotoxins (i.e., alcohol, acetaminophen, etc.)

- HBV resistance testing typically only if treatment-experienced or failed prior treatment
- HBV genotype if planning to use interferon for treatment

Some useful treatment generalizations to remember:

- Treatment is associated with reduced liver disease progression (cirrhosis and HCC) and transmission
- Goals of therapy include HBsAg clearance (very rare to actually occur), HBeAg conversion, HBV DNA suppression (if HBeAg neg), and reduction of disease progression
- In most cases, single-drug therapy is sufficient, but in HIV-positive patients, the patient should be on antiretroviral therapy (ART) and have at least two HBV active agents. Entecavir used as monotherapy for HBV in a patient with HBV/HIV coinfection can lead to HIV cross-resistance to lamivudine and emtricitabine (development of M184V resistance mutation). This is why HIV coinfected patients need to be on appropriate ART when treating the HBV infection. Fortunately, many of the ART regimens used nowadays satisfy this requirement (i.e., contain tenofovir, emtricitabine, lamivudine)
- In many cases, drug treatment is continued lifelong, and patients should be aware of this and agreeable to it
- The drug regimens considered to be first-line are:
- Tenofovir (DF or AF formulation, **option C**)
- Entecavir (**option B**)
- Pegylated interferon (**option D**)
  - Once-weekly subcutaneous injection for 48 weeks
  - Associated with many side effects and requires monitoring
  - This is the drug of choice for HDV infection
  - This drug should be avoided in decompensated cirrhosis

The second-line regimens are:

- Lamivudine (concurrent HIV coverage; **option E**)
- Emtricitabine (concurrent HIV coverage)
- Telbivudine
- Adefovir

KEY LEARNING POINT

Most patients with acute hepatitis B virus infection recover on their own without treatment. Treatment may be considered in those with acute liver failure or a protracted course (>4 weeks of elevated international normalized ratio and/or jaundice).

REFERENCES AND FURTHER READING

- Thio CL, Hawkins C, Hepatitis B virus. In: Bennet JE, Dolin R, Blaser MJ, eds. *Mandell, Douglas, and Bennett's Principles and Practice of Infectious Diseases*. 9th ed. Elsevier; 2019.
- Yapali S, Talaat N, Lok AS. Management of hepatitis B: our practice and how it relates to the guidelines. *Clin Gastroenterol Hepatol*. 2014;12(1):16–26. https://doi.org/10.1016/j.cgh.2013.04.036.
- Zamor PJ, Lane AM. Interpretation of HBV serologies. *Clin Liver Dis*. 2021;25(4):689–709. https://doi.org/10.1016/j.cld.2021.06.012.

A 35-year-old male with a history of IV drug abuse is hospitalized for methicillin-resistant *Staphylococcus aureus* bacteremia. He has to stay in the hospital for his treatment because he cannot be discharged with a long-term IV line in light of his drug use history. Approximately 3 weeks into his vancomycin treatment course, he develops the rash shown in Fig. 99.1. He has not started any new medications during the hospitalization. Vital signs reveal temperature 102° F, heart rate 110 beats per minute, blood pressure 115/70 mmHg, respiratory rate 18, and oxygen saturation 98% on room air. On exam, he appears ill. He has periorbital edema. There is no conjunctivitis or oral mucosal lesions. He has anterior cervical lymphadenopathy. Skin exam is shown in Fig. 99.1. The remainder of the exam is unremarkable. Laboratory analysis reveals white blood cell count 14,000 (neutrophils 70%, lymphocytes 20% with atypical lymphocytes, eosinophils 10%), creatinine 1.7 mg/dL (creatinine clearance 40 mL/min), and ALT 95 IU/L. What is the best next step in management?

A. Topical steroids.

B. Systemic steroids.

C. Stop vancomycin.

D. Consult dermatology.

E. Obtain skin biopsy.

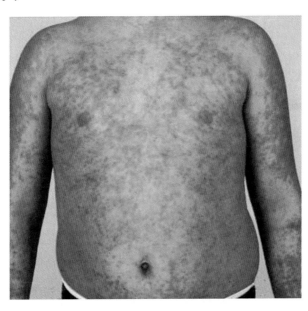

Figure 99.1 – Skin rash
Heelan K, Shear NH. Cutaneous drug eruptions. In: *Dermatological Signs of Systemic Disease*. 5th ed. Elsevier; 2017:425–436.

The best next step is to stop vancomycin (**option C**). This patient most likely has a drug reaction with eosinophilia and systemic symptoms (DRESS) syndrome, also known as drug-induced hypersensitivity syndrome (DIHS). Infectious disease specialists encounter plenty of drug eruptions, so having some familiarity with these is important.

Table 99.1 – Drug Eruptions

Drug Reaction	Distinguishing Features	Management
Allergic	• Timing—minutes to hours • Urticaria—pruritic wheals (hives) • Angioedema/anaphylaxis	• Stop offending agent • Antihistamines • Epinephrine • Steroids
Exanthematous (morbilliform)	• Timing—1 to 2 weeks (quicker if repeat exposure) • Measles-like rash (maculopapular erythematous eruption) similar to Fig. 99.1 • Resolves without sequelae, but some may have desquamation	• Stop offending agent • May be able to treat through in some cases (esp. if unable to stop or switch offending agent)
Fixed drug eruption	• Timing—1 to 2 weeks (quicker if repeat exposure) • Often a solitary lesion (dusky plaque or bulla) that recurs at the same site with repeat exposure (Fig. 99.2) • Lips, hands, and genitalia are common sites	• Stop offending agent • Topical steroids • If erosion, then antimicrobial ointment and dressing
DIHS (DRESS)	• Timing—at least a couple weeks after exposure and up to 6 weeks (quicker if repeat exposure) • Cutaneous eruption (various morphologies) • Facial edema and/or lymphadenopathy • Systemic features—fevers, etc. • Leukocytosis (± eosinophilia or atypical lymphocytosis) • Organ injury—hepatitis, nephritis, carditis, pneumonitis, thyroiditis, etc.	• Stop offending agent and any unnecessary medications • Dermatology consultation • Topical steroids if mild/limited • Systemic steroids with prolonged taper with more severe cases • May develop delayed cardiac and/or thyroid abnormalities
AGEP	• Timing—within 1 week (quicker if repeat exposure) • High fever • Sterile pustules within edematous erythema, especially on face or intertriginous regions (Fig. 99.3)	• Discontinue the offending agent • Supportive/symptomatic care
SJS/TEN	• Skin pain and sloughing • Mucous membrane involvement • Targetoid lesions with dusky appearance • Systemic toxicity	• Stop offending agent and any unnecessary medications • Dermatology consultation • Burn unit care • Intensive support—fluid, electrolytes, etc.

AGEP, Acute generalized exanthematous pustulosis; *DIHS*, drug-induced hypersensitivity syndrome; *DRESS*, drug reaction with eosinophilia and systemic symptoms; *SJS*, Stevens–Johnson syndrome; *TEN*, toxic epidermal necrolysis.

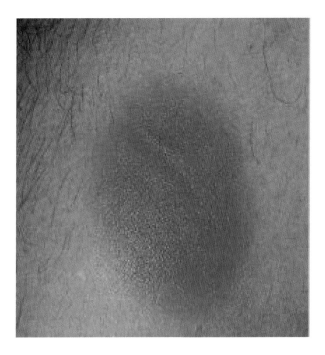

Figure 99.2 – Fixed drug eruption
Valeyrie-Allanore. Drug reactions. In: *Dermatology*. 4th ed. Elsevier; 2018:348–375.

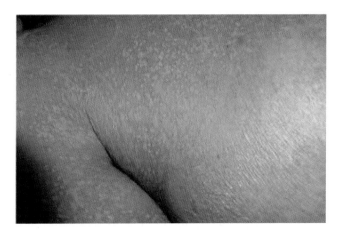

Figure 99.3 – Acute generalized exanthematous pustulosis
Valeyrie-Allanore. Drug reactions. In: *Dermatology*. 4th ed. Elsevier; 2018:348–375.

When a patient develops a rash while on an antibiotic, the first step is to take an appropriate history. This includes identifying when a medication was started or changed (i.e., dose increased) and when the rash started. Physical examination should involve a thorough examination of the entire skin (including mucous membranes, hair, and nails) and lymph nodes. Red flag findings include:

- Systemic symptoms—fevers, tachycardia, hypotension, wheezing/stridor, and so on.
- Mucous membrane involvement—genitalia, eyes, oral ulceration
- Facial swelling (edema)
- Lymphadenopathy
- Skin pain, burning, or sloughing
- Dusky-appearing lesions
- Visceral involvement—kidney injury, liver injury, etc.

Some common drug eruptions are compared in Table 99.1.

Topical steroids (**option A**) can be used in milder cases of DIHS/DRESS but would not be enough for this patient. Systemic steroids (**option B**) should be given, but stopping the offending agent is the best next step. Consulting dermatology (**option D**) is recommended but should not take precedence over stopping the offending agent. Obtaining a skin biopsy (**option E**) could be considered, but a clinical diagnosis is often sufficient in many of these cases.

KEY LEARNING POINT

In most drug eruptions, stopping the offending agent is the most important initial step in management.

REFERENCES AND FURTHER READING

- Heelan K, Shear NH. Cutaneous drug eruptions. In: *Dermatological Signs of Systemic Disease*. 5th ed. : Elsevier; 2017:425–436.
- Valeyrie-Allanore. Drug reactions. In: *Dermatology*. 4th ed. : Elsevier; 2018:348–375.

A 50-year-old man is admitted to the hospital with a 2-day history of right lower extremity swelling, redness, and pain. He notes associated low-grade fevers. He is allergic to penicillin. He thinks he had a rash when he received penicillin as a child. He thinks he has taken cephalexin without any issue. Medical history is notable for diabetes mellitus and bilateral lower extremity lymphedema. Medications include metformin, insulin, lisinopril, furosemide, and atorvastatin. Vital signs reveal temperature 100.8° F, heart rate 90 beats per minute, blood pressure 110/70 mmHg, and respiratory rate 16. Body mass index is 35 kg/m². On examination, his right leg is swollen, tender, and erythematous with a well-defined border of erythema. There is no purulence or skin breakdown. There is no inguinal or popliteal lymphadenopathy. The left leg is edematous but not tender or erythematous. The remainder of the examination is unremarkable. Laboratory studies reveal white blood cell count 14,000 cells/uL and creatinine 1.0 mg/dL. Ultrasound of the right leg shows no evidence of thrombosis. Blood cultures are obtained.

What is the next best step in management?

A. Intravenous penicillin-G.

B. Cefazolin.

C. Ceftriaxone.

D. Vancomycin.

E. Trimethoprim-sulfamethoxazole.

The best next step is to start cefazolin (**option B**).

Penicillin allergies are commonly reported, so having an approach to penicillin allergy is very useful for the infectious disease specialist (and any other medical provider). Most patients with reported penicillin allergies can actually tolerate penicillin, because many penicillin allergies wane over time. Penicillin allergy evaluation and management improves healthcare quality and reduces exposure to unnecessarily broad antibiotic therapy (which is associated with more adverse effects and development of drug resistance).

The questions to ask the patient with a reported penicillin allergy include:

1. **What was the reaction and its timing relative to drug administration?**

   IgE-mediated (immediate) may include hives, angioedema, or anaphylaxis.

   Delayed reactions (T-cell–mediated) include maculopapular (morbilliform or exanthematous) drug eruption, Stevens–Johnson syndrome/toxic epidermal necrolysis, acute interstitial nephritis, drug-induced hypersensitivity syndrome/drug reaction with eosinophilia and systemic symptoms (DRESS), etc.

   Reactions may also be an adverse effect of the antimicrobial or a nonspecific reaction.

2. **When did it occur?**

   In addition, it can be helpful to inquire as to why the antibiotic was prescribed, how the reaction was treated, and whether any other drugs were given at around the time of the reaction.

3. **Has the patient tolerated similar antibiotics (i.e., amoxicillin, cephalexin, etc.) in the past (based on history or chart review)?**

   If the patient tolerated amoxicillin, then a real penicillin allergy is extremely unlikely.

MANAGEMENT CONSIDERATIONS

1. **Penicillin skin testing and management based on type of reaction**

   Penicillin skin testing is the most reliable method for evaluation of penicillin allergy. With regard to serious immediate-type (IgE-mediated) reactions, the negative predictive value of penicillin skin testing is 97% to 99%. There is no predictive value of penicillin skin testing for non–IgE-mediated reactions.

   If the history is clearly consistent with IgE-mediated reaction, then penicillin skin testing is the most appropriate test, if feasible. Skin testing should not be done in unstable patients. If skin testing is positive or not feasible, then options include using a different antibiotic (later-generation cephalosporins [third- or fourth-generation], carbapenems, or aztreonam using a graded challenge procedure; or non–beta-lactam antibiotic) or desensitization (if penicillin is the best therapy).

If the history is consistent with a severe non–IgE-mediated reaction (i.e., DRESS), then most beta-lactams should be avoided. Aztreonam is the exception.

If the reaction is nonspecific or unknown or a mild, non–IgE-mediated reaction (i.e., morbilliform drug eruption), then the approach depends on the stability of the patient. In unstable patients, alternative therapy or aztreonam may be the best strategy. In stable patients, the approach is similar to the approach for IgE-mediated reactions.

2. **Cross-reactivity**

Studies involving patients with a history of penicillin allergy (and positive skin testing) who subsequently received cephalosporins found an overall reaction rate of approximately 2%. This rate is probably even lower for cefazolin, because it does not share any common side chains with other antimicrobials. In addition, the cross-reactivity is less with later-generation cephalosporins (i.e., third- and fourth-generation). The cross-reactivity between penicillins and carbapenems is less than 1%. Lastly, the monobactam aztreonam is the drug of choice for gram-negative coverage in patients with penicillin or cephalosporin allergies. The main exception to this rule is allergy to ceftazidime or ceftolozane (as they have the same side chain as aztreonam).

Intravenous penicillin-G **(option A)** is the drug of choice for beta-hemolytic streptococcal infections, but given this patient's reported penicillin allergy, cefazolin is a better option, as the coverage is still narrow, and the patient tolerated cephalexin, which makes it likely that he would tolerate cefazolin. Ceftriaxone **(option C)** would be unnecessarily broad for this patient's infection. Vancomycin **(option D)** and trimethoprim-sulfamethoxazole **(option E)** would be more appropriate for a purulent skin and soft tissue infection, which is more likely to be caused by *Staphylococcus aureus*. This patient's infection is most likely caused by beta-hemolytic streptococci.

KEY LEARNING POINT

The cross-reactivity between penicillin and cephalosporins is fairly low (~2%). It is probably even lower for cefazolin and late-generation cephalosporins.

REFERENCE AND FURTHER READING

• Pongdee T, Li JT. Evaluation and management of penicillin allergy. *Mayo Clin Proc.* 2018;93(1):101–107. https://doi.org/10.1016/j.mayocp.2017.09.020.

Index